BOYS IN WHITE

HOWARD S. BECKER

BLANCHE GEER

EVERETT C. HUGHES

ANSELM L. STRAUSS

BOYS IN WHITE

STUDENT CULTURE IN MEDICAL SCHOOL

Transaction Publishers
New Brunswick (U.S.A.) and London (U.K.)

Tenth printing 2007
First Paperback Edition, 1977 by Transaction Publishers.
Copyright © 1961 by The University of Chicago Press.

This book is printed on acid-free paper that meets the American National
Standard for Permanence of Paper for Printed Library Materials.

Library of Congress Catalog Number: 76-26951
ISBN: 978-0-87855-622-9
Printed in the United States of America

Library of Congress Cataloging-in-Publication Data

Becker, Howard Saul, 1928-
   Boys in White.

   Reprint of the 1961 ed. published by University of Chicago Press, Chicago.
   1. Medical students—United States.   2. Medical education—Social
aspects—United States.   3. Kansas University. School of Medicine.
   I. Title.

[R745.B38   1976]   610'.739   76-26951
ISBN: 0-87855-622-2

"The reflective experience, the world, and the things within it exist in the form of situations. . . ."

"The perspective is the world in its relationship to the individual and the individual in his relationship to the world."

"In experience the individual perspectives arise out of a common perspective. The common perspective is not built up out of individual perspectives."

GEORGE HERBERT MEAD, *The Philosophy of the Act*

Acknowledgments

Many people and organizations helped make this study possible. We are grateful to them. The students, faculty, and administration of the University of Kansas Medical School allowed us the intimate access to their activities without which we could not have proceeded. Interested members of the faculty participated in seminars during which we discussed preliminary drafts of portions of this volume. They took the time to read these drafts and give us their thoughts on them. Dean W. Clarke Wescoe (now chancellor of the university), Dr. Mahlon Delp, Dr. C. Arden Miller (now dean of the medical school), and Dr. Robert Hudson read a version of the manuscript and assisted us with their comments. Dr. Vernon Wilson, now dean of the medical school of the University of Missouri, helped us during the study as did Mrs. Frances Hiatt, the registrar.

Our work has been carried on under the auspices of Community Studies, Inc., of Kansas City, Missouri, a non-profit research organization of whose staff two of us (Becker and Geer) are full-time members. We wish to thank Dr. W. D. Bryant, executive director of Community Studies, for making the study possible and for his continuing aid and encouragement. The University of Chicago also assisted in various ways.

Miss Audrey Forrest prepared the analyses of the student interviews used in the text. Dr. Bahjat Khleif assisted us in preparing for analysis the interviews with students. Mrs. Dorothy Seelinger, project secretary, typed most of the field notes and interviews as well as innumerable memos and drafts of the present manuscript; we are much indebted to her for her loyalty, devotion, and skill. Mrs. Joy Hadden and Mrs. Kathryn James also typed portions of the final manuscript. Mr. Robert Hines drew the charts and illustrations.

We wish to thank the following organizations for providing funds: the Kansas City Association of Trusts and Foundations and its executive director, Mr. Homer C. Wadsworth; the National Institutes of Health; and the Carnegie Corporation of New York.

Sociological colleagues have read sizable portions of this manuscript for us, and their comments have been of great value in solving problems of substance, method, and style. David Riesman has been close to our work from its beginnings, and his comments, questions, and enthusiasm have aided us immensely. Eliot Freidson and Sheldon Messinger similarly helped us in our problems of analysis and presentation.

We wish to thank the following for permission to quote from our articles first published by them: *Administrative Science Quarterly*, *American Sociological Review*, *Harvard Educational Review*, The Society for Applied Anthropology, and the Dorsey Press.

Contents

Illustrations

Tables

Part One:
BACKGROUND AND METHODS

Chapter 1

Boys in White

In the fall of the year several thousand college seniors get out of their casual college clothing, put on the uniform of the young executive — dark suit with a line of white handkerchief at the decreed distance parallel above the breast pocket — and present themselves to be interviewed by the admissions committees of medical schools. They are a picked lot. They have done well in college, and they have given good account of themselves in the standard tests taken by all students who apply to enter medical schools in this country.

The interview is a serious affair. At stake is one's opportunity to enter one of the most honored and — at present in America — most lucrative of the professions. They comport themselves on this solemn occasion not as boys but as men. The teachers of medicine who interview them look at them seriously and anxiously. They ask themselves and one another, "Will this bright boy really make a medical man?" For medicine is man's work. It is also woman's work, and there is no theme of human history more interesting than the changes in the respective roles of man and woman in looking after those who are sick or in labor. But in this country, although an increasing proportion of the people who have a part in the medical system are women, the medical profession itself remains overwhelmingly male. In this book, we shall talk mainly of boys becoming medical men.

These boys, if examinations and interview go well, will enter the charmed circle of medicine next autumn, after their graduation from college. It is a crucial moment, the entry to medical school. Hints of future colleagueship may be heard in the words with which their teachers usher them in. They put on white, the color symbolic of modern medicine. For the rest of their lives they will spend a good many hours of every day among people who wear uniforms, more often white than not, which tell the place of each in the complicated division of work and the ranking system of the medical world, at whose top the medical student is destined to be. But the road is long. Although he has been accepted as a potential physician, he soon learns that for the present he is near the bottom of the heap. During the first two years he wears only a white laboratory coat. In the third and fourth years he puts on the white trousers, jacket, and shirt worn by interns and residents, but he is still not a physician, as they are. In fact, although he is at the end of one four-year undergraduate course, the new medical student is about to begin another one in which day-to-day discipline and routine are much more strict than in the first. In becoming medical students, the boys enter upon one of the longest rites of passage in our part of the world. A rite of passage is that series of instructions, ceremonies, and ordeals by which those already in a special status initiate neophytes into their charmed circle, by which men turn boys into fellow men, fit to be their own companions and successors.

In our society, among the most desired and admired statuses is to be a member of a profession. Such status is attained not by going into the woods for intense, but brief, ordeals of initiation into adult mysteries, but by a long course of professional instruction and supervised practice. In training for medicine, great emphasis is laid upon the learning of basic sciences and their application in the diagnosis and treatment of the sick. But science and skill do not make a physician; one must also be initiated into the status of physician; to be accepted, one must have learned to play the part of a physician in the drama of medicine.

As in other dramas, learning the lines is not enough. One must learn what others expect of him and how they will react to his words and actions. But in medical school, the student never, in his first day, or even in his first year, meets the situation in which physicians must play their part. There is no magic moment in which the student, as an understudy to a great actor who falls ill, is thrust on to the stage. Modern medicine is too well organized for that. The transition, from young layman aspiring to be a physician to the young physician skilled in technique and sure of his part in dealing with patients in the complex setting of modern clinics and hospitals, is slow and halting. The young man finds out quite soon that he must learn first to be a medical student; how he will act in the future, when he is a doctor, is not his immediate problem. A good deal of what follows in this book has to do precisely with the way in which students, at various points in their progress through medical school, see and solve the immediate problems of dealing with their teachers and the tasks they assign. The students of medicine, it turns out, see their world in a moving perspective. How to climb the distant mountain may be a question in the backs of their heads; how to make their way across the swamp they are floundering in now and over the steep hill just ahead engages their immediate attention.

In the above paragraphs we have indicated the emphasis of our study of the students of a medical school. We do not consider curriculum or subject-matter, in which we have no competence, except as they become objects of attention, interpretation and action on the students' part. But if our point of view is now clear, we still have said nothing about why we think it of importance to look at a medical school in this way.

A prolonged professional training is part of the experience of a large and increasing number of young people in our society, young people who are — physically and in most social respects — fully adult. They may be married and have children; they may have served in the armed services; and they may have worked at various jobs in which they have taken the full responsibilities of an adult. Yet in their chosen professions, they still have ahead of them a long period of a sort of adolescence during which they are asked to show adult competence and learning, without being given full adult responsibility.

Our social and technical order requires more and more services which depend upon esoteric knowledge and skills; so esoteric, in fact, that each of us — no matter how skilled and full of knowledge in his own specialty — must accept them on trust. When some people apply such knowledge and skill in performing services for other men, for organizations, or for society at large, and when these services are accepted on trust (at least in the short run), they are practicing a profession. Of professions so-defined, we have more than ever before and will have more in the future as scientific knowledge is increasingly applied and as social organization becomes more complex. As new occupations develop to apply technology and science — the tenders of rapid-calculating machines — or to fill new organizational niches — the hospital administrator — those who practice them are very likely to ask to have a license, a monopoly, in effect, over their line of work and control over admission to it. The license will be claimed on the ground that only those in the occupation are competent to do the work, or, what is more crucial, to judge when the work is well done.[1]

Such occupations, new or old, have in recent decades sought to increase the length of time required for educating and training those young people who aspire to them. Medicine took the lead in this; other professions have sought to follow with varying success. At the same time, most professions have set up lists of prerequisite courses without which a candidate may not enter the professional school itself. Thus the point in school and the age at which a youngster must commit himself to a profession by declaration and action are pushed back. The time between the point of crucial decision to enter the profession and actual admission to full and free colleagueship in it is thus increased. The aspirant must decide earlier; he will reach his goal later. As the time between increases, the aspirant must make his original commitment with an ever less full and accurate picture of what his professional work will really be. This may, in turn, lead to more and more use of tests of various kinds to predict whether the aspirant will successfully finish his training and practice the profession; these will probably be tests of personality, motivation, and ability rather than of substantive knowledge and interest, since the aspirants will be tested and chosen before they have had access to substantive knowledge and professional experiences. This might conceivably be carried to such a point that, instead of choosing his profession, the young person will be chosen, and will perhaps be told it is his duty to do what the tests say is best for him. For is it not his manifest duty to do what he is best at?

[1] For more general discussion of the professions, what they are and their place in modern society, see the following sources:

W. J. Goode, "Community Within a Community: The Professions," *American Sociological Review*, XXII (April, 1957), 194–200.

Everett C. Hughes, "Licence and Mandate," in *Men and Their Work* (Glencoe, Ill.: Free Press, 1958), pp. 78–87; and "The Professions in Society," *Canadian Journal of Economics and Political Science*, XXVI (February, 1960), 54–61.

T. H. Marshall, "The Recent History of Professionalism in Relation to Social Structure and Social Policy," *ibid.*, V (August, 1939), 325–40.

Robert K. Merton, "Some Preliminaries to a Sociology of Medical Education," in Robert K. Merton, George Reader and Patricia Kendall (eds.), *The Student-Physician* (Cambridge, Mass.: Harvard University Press, 1957), pp. 3–79.

Talcott Parsons, "The Professions and Social Structure," in revised edition of *Essays in Sociological Theory* (Glencoe, Ill.: Free Press, 1954), pp. 34–49; and "Social Structure and Dynamic Process: The Case of Modern Medical Practice," in *The Social System* (Glencoe, Ill.: Free Press, 1951), pp. 428–79.

Perhaps things will never come to such a pass. The picture is drawn simply to suggest that choice of professional occupation has to be made longer and longer in advance. There is a long period of pre-professional school, professional school, and of supervised practice. The chooser of a professional occupation makes his first steps toward it on the basis of second-hand images, not of immediate experience; before him is a long blind flight. What happens to him between commitment and final acceptance into professional colleagueship is an important part of his life and a process which a society dependent on professions should understand. Medicine is, in many respects, the crucial case. It should be added that the signs of some reaction against an over-long professional adolescence are also turning up first in medicine; medicine may lead the reaction, as it did the trend.[2]

We have mentioned two aspects of the professional trend — the increase in the number of professions and the increase in length of training for each. A third, of equal importance, is a trend toward the practice of the professions in organizations more complex than the old-fashioned doctor's or lawyer's office. Some of the newer professions — again, note the tender of electronic computers — are bound to machines which in turn can be run only by an organization; others — again, note the hospital administrator — are themselves by-products of new trends in organization. Medicine and law themselves, the two occupations most often taken as models of the very concept of profession, are not exempt from the trend. Indeed, the more renowned members of these professions are less likely to be found practicing alone or outside larger organizations than are the less renowned. There is some evidence that a man who wishes to choose his style of practice must either found an organization (group, clinic, hospital, firm, etc.) or attach himself to one. Furthermore, the trend toward practice in larger and more complicated organizations seems to occur quite independently of the degree of governmental control of the professions. It is rather a function of technology and of social organization itself.

A corollary of this trend is that the people in the professions have to work with a number of auxiliary occupations of which some also have or seek professional standing. Physicians find themselves work-

[2] The Johns Hopkins University has already adopted a plan to allow students to enter medical school a year earlier. Other schools are said to be considering similar steps. While such a change will, in the absence of further lengthening of specialty residencies, get young men into practice earlier, it also requires of them a still earlier decision to enter the profession.

ing with registered nurses, practical nurses, aides and maids, and
with several kinds of technicians and therapists not to mention ac-
countants, personnel men, and administrators.[3] In earlier times the
physician, midwife, surgeon, and apothecary were somewhat independent of each other. They might quarrel, as did the midwife and
doctor who were called in at the birth of Tristram Shandy. Now all
of these, and many more, are organized into one system in which the
physician is thought the most powerful figure. So he is, in some respects, but he who gains power by organization always finds that he
loses a good share of it. The physician, a great power in a small way
in his own private office, now works in a complex division of labor
in which he shares power not only with his numerous colleagues but
with the many people of other categories who are part of the modern
medical system.

This complexity affects professional educational institutions as
well, and none more than schools of medicine. A modern medical
school, associated generally with a university and always with one or
several large hospitals, with clinics and laboratories, is a far cry from
clerkship in its original sense. The student is not an apprentice working with a master; he has many masters. Some are physicians; some
are not. In a sense, the expensive plant, with its millions of dollars'
worth of precious equipment, is his master. The technicians, the
nurses, and the patients are all his masters insofar as their presence
affects his own behavior and his own fate. Finally, those who are most
clearly and avowedly his masters, the teachers of clinical medicine,
are usually removed in some measure from the nonacademic practice
of medicine. Even if they are in private practice, they are likely to
have had careers that are largely academic and to work under conditions somewhat different from those of nonacademic physicians. The
separation of academic from nonacademic careers appears in increasing measure in professions generally. It is accompanied by some
strain between professional schools and the practicing professions
out in the world.

All these trends are clearly marked in medicine, which is at once
a very old and a very new profession. Its clear place at the center of
the whole system of institutions concerned with health is a product
of the nineteenth century, when the present associations and licensing

[3] A recent report states that for every physician in practice in 1900 there was one
other health practitioner, while today there are four such persons for every physician
(U. S. Dept. of Health, Education, and Welfare, *Physicians for a Growing America*
[October, 1959], p. 65).

systems were developed. Science and medicine were married in that period; the union appears permanent, but is not always a peaceful one. At that time the union of medical education with universities, an old phenomenon, to be sure, was renewed in the English-speaking world; indeed, the reunion is not yet quite complete.

The young person who considers entering medicine may think he knows what he is getting into. Everyone knows about doctors. But he is also entering that profession which, in its more specialized branches, requires the longest training of all. Between the time he makes his commitment and takes his first premedical or even medical course and his final admission to practice, some of what he learns may have become obsolete, some new specialty may have been developed and may have sought separation from its parent, and new ways of organizing medical practice may have been invented. All of the professional trends of modern life are manifest in the medical profession and the medical school.

Levels and Directions of Effort

Among the problems common to educators and the professions nowadays is concern over the quality and the performance of those who apply and are admitted to colleges and the professional schools. It was the frequent expression of this concern by teachers of medicine and administrators of medical institutions that got us into the study which we here report. One of us had been approached on more than one occasion about possible studies of the problem. Eventually, on an opportune occasion, we talked of it to members of the staff of the School of Medicine of the University of Kansas.[4] They expressed the usual concern earnestly, but neither noticeably more nor less strongly than the faculties of other schools of equally vigorous and progressive leadership.

We do not mean to imply that there is a general belief that the present aspirants to professions are of poorer quality or are less devoted to their work than those of the past. Some teachers do, indeed, say that it is the case; others say that they are better. Some say that the school and college training of present medical (and other) students is poorer nowadays. Others point out the very greatly increased amount of knowledge required of the medical student. It is

---

[4] At that point Hughes wrote and circulated a memorandum of ideas on medical education, later published as "The Making of a Physician" in *Human Organization*, XIV (Winter, 1956), 21–25.

also noted that there are more professions, and the total number of professionally trained people required to operate our social and economic establishment is increasing rapidly; each profession, including medicine, has to compete for its share of capable people. Perhaps there are not enough talented people to go around — or enough devoted people.

In the medical profession, concern of this kind is complicated by the competing claims of general and specialized practice; of practice and teaching as against research; by competition among the specialties themselves for the limited supply of young physicians; and by a certain strain within the profession over the different ways in which medical practice may be organized.

That there should be this anxiety is in some respects an anomaly, for it is still not easy to get into medical schools. Undergraduate students work hard for the privilege. Of those who, after much informal screening, apply to be admitted, only about half are accepted. Nearly all who are accepted actually go to some medical school. The examinations required of aspirants are not taken idly and applications are not often submitted without serious intent. Those who entered North American medical colleges in 1956 had a median I.Q. of 127, three points higher than the median of graduate students generally; all but a few had attained an average of B or higher in their college work.[5] The medical students are not only ambitious but also individualistic in the sense of not wanting to work for a salary and of liking to be their own bosses.[6] In short, they have characteristics which would lead one to believe that they all would do their level best without paying much attention to what others do unless to keep ahead of them.

The concept of the individual's level best has, however, come to be suspect to students of human effort. There are many kinds of level best; the heroic and brilliant best of those superior in dedication as well as in ability; the desperate, but not very good, best of those beset by fear of failure; the consistent and collective best of a group working together under admired leadership. But, although students

[5] Dael Wolfle, "Medicine's Share in America's Student Resources" (Part A in Chapter 2), *Journal of Medical Education*, XXXII, 121 (October, 1957), 10–16.
[6] D. Cahalan, P. Collette, and N. A. Hilmar, "Career Interests and Expectations of U. S. Medical Students", *Journal of Medical Education*, XXXII (August, 1957) 557–563. Seven-eighths of a national sample of medical students say they prefer non-salaried practice. About one-fourth prefer an individual practice without any arrangements or pooling of facilities with other physicians. Of those who want to practice absolutely alone, 79 per cent say it is because "I want to be my own boss."

of human work have come to think it natural that the level of effort is likely to be arrived at in some collective fashion, they have tacitly assumed that higher levels are individual and that, where the level of effort is collectively determined, it is likely to be low. Studies of this problem have been confined largely to industry and to cases where the workers have set quotas of production lower than their supervisors think they should achieve. Likewise, it has been assumed that people who enter into implicit or explicit understandings about how much work to do have given up all thought of climbing to higher positions.

In short, while students of industrial behavior and even the managers of industry have accepted the fact that levels of effort are determined by social interaction and are, in some measure, collective phenomena, both the social scientists and those who teach candidates for professions have tended to see the problem of effort and achievement in the professional school as a matter of individual quality and motivation. We have been reluctant to apply to professional education the insights, concepts, and methods developed in study of lowlier kinds of work. This is but another instance of the highbrow fallacy in the study of human behavior; what we discover among people of less prestige, we hesitate to apply to those of higher.

Nevertheless, we did bring to our study of medical students the idea that their conduct, whatever it might be, would be a product of their interaction with each other when faced with the day-to-day problems of medical school.

We were also aware that physicians engaged in various kinds of practice have some influence on the students' ideas of what kinds of things they should learn in medical schools and what kinds of careers they might aspire to, and that these ideas might not coincide with those of their teachers. But we had no specific ideas about the results of the various experiences of the students and of the various influences upon them. We were convinced that it would be worthwhile, and a distinct innovation, to study medical students by the same methods of close day-to-day observation as have been applied in industry.

As said above, it has been generally assumed that when levels of effort are set collectively they are apt to be low. But we did not undertake this study with any such assumption. Levels of effort may be high or low; they may also be individual or collective. They may be, to be a bit tiresome about it, individual, high or low; they may also be collective, high or low. One of us, in lectures, emphasized the possibility that high levels of effort are as likely to be collectively determined as are low ones,[7] and that it would be an unusually disorganized group in which there would arise no common understanding about how much work to do. But what we had not foreseen, although it now seems obvious, is that in a group of professional students the collective understandings should have as much to do with the direction as with the level of their efforts. Automobile workers may determine the speed of the assembly line, but they make no attempt to alter the model of the cars they turn out. Medical students — and probably any group of people who are themselves to be the product of the organization in which they are at work under authority — have an interest in the nature of the work done as well as in the amount. About a year after we had started the field work of our study, we wrote, for our own discussion, a memorandum entitled "Levels and Directions of Effort." It dealt with a theme common to all educational and industrial institutions, for in each there is a chronic struggle of wills over both the nature and the amount of their product.

When we say that modern industry has destroyed craftsmanship we mean that the skills and judgments concerning direction of effort formerly built into the man are now built into the materials, the design, the machines, and the plan of assembly. Mass production is so called not merely to indicate that the product in toto and per manhour is colossal, but also that the items produced are so nearly identical that together they are a mass. They are, in turn, identical because power over the nature of the product is more completely concentrated in the hands of management than ever in the past. Even so, there is a residual struggle over direction of effort, for workers will invent small short cuts in performing the most standardized and fragmented tasks and will push hard against the limits of tolerance enforced by the most meticulous "quality control" inspectors.

Direction of effort has several aspects. One is the determination of the nature of one's work (what a worker will put his hand to); another is the control of the way of doing the work. It may be assumed that those in authority will always try to control direction of effort, but in varying degree. Some are content to define the end

[7] This idea was stated explicitly by Max Weber, German economist and sociologist, in a monograph entitled "Zur Psychophysik der industriellen Arbeit (1908–9)," published in *Gesammelte Aufsätze zur Soziologie und Sozialpolitik* (Tübingen, 1924), pp. 61–255. He was the first, so far as we know, who looked upon "restriction of production" as a natural and almost universal phenomenon rather than as a plot of agitators and trade union leaders.

product while allowing freedom as to ways of attaining it. Others, as management of an automated industry, work out in great detail control over ways of working as well.

In professional educational institutions the product is, as we have said, a person — the very person who is assigned work to do. It is assumed that the teacher is "management" and will himself put forth full effort as well as define how much and what work the student should do. The latter presumably works to change himself in ways which his teachers consider desirable. But he is only an intermediate product. The end product is the professional service which he will render to clients. Furthermore, a profession does not let the client decide exactly what service he wants, for only the profession can define his needs. While the profession may agree that only professionals may define medical (or other) needs, consensus may be rather less than complete as to what the needs are and how to treat them in any particular case. Those who, as teachers, "produce" physicians are not all agreed on what to teach or how to teach it. They are not completely at one concerning the directions of their own efforts, nor could they be without destroying a right of individual professional judgment very precious to them.

In short, the joints of the medical system have a great deal of play in them. The people who work in the system have — and use — a good deal of freedom in choosing both what to do and how to do it. Their students — the people who are told what to do and how to do it — are quick to discover that they, too, can and indeed must, in some measure, decide not merely how much work to do but in what directions to exert their energies. In showing how and why these well-intentioned and strongly motivated students do not and probably could not exactly follow the wishes of their teachers, we shall be contributing to an understanding of the essential nature and workings of all institutions in which some people teach others or in which some have manifest authority to control the efforts of others.

The Organization

A medical school is an organized enterprise with unusual singleness of purpose. In order to fulfil that purpose, the replenishment of the supply of physicians, it must perform other functions. Foremost among them is looking after a large number of people who need medical care; second, in our day, is medical research. Medical practice and research can be done in the absence of teaching; teaching cannot, however, be done without them. The whole requires a good deal of administration. Each member of the staff combines, in his work, some or all of these four activities — teaching, the practice of medicine, research, and administration — in varying proportions. Practically all of them teach, but not all practice medicine, do research, or engage in administration. They differ from each other in their opinions about the best combinations of these activities in the medical school, in medical curricula, and in their own careers. But all are strongly devoted to the purpose of training physicians. A majority of them are members of the medical profession. Practically all of the physicians are also members of some specialty. Others are members of scientific associations. The medical school is thus a very complex organization, composed of men who, in spite of devotion to one main goal, are involved in the school in quite different ways.

Because of its several functions, the school and its related hospitals, clinics, and laboratories have relations with many organizations and publics outside. Although we have not ignored these many facets of the medical school, and have taken account of them from time to time, our main emphasis remains fixed on the students in their interaction with each other and those who teach them. The following chapter will tell of our method. The fourth chapter of this section will say something about medical schools in general and the University of Kansas Medical School in particular.

Any organization — no matter what its purposes — consists of the interaction of men — of their ideas, their wills, their energies, their minds, and their purposes. The men who thus interact are involved in the organization in varying degree, for varying periods of time, and at different stages of their careers. Some of the staff are bound to the school we studied in many ways — as patriotic sons of Kansas, as alumni of the college and medical school of the university, as practitioners of medicine, and as long-time members of the staff. They are attached not merely to medicine and medical schools but to this school above all others. Other members are attached to medicine, science, and medical education but not to this school more than to some other where they might pursue their work. Some undoubtedly regard this school as a steppingstone in their careers.

But to all, regardless of the place of the school in their careers, a study made by outsiders may appear a risky thing. Although many members of the staff of this or any large organization may be critical of it, their criticism may be particular to their own view of how the organization should be run and what its product should be. The outside investigator may bring to it his own canons of criticism; or he may, by his very objectivity, appear to make light of the purposes, attachments, and the deeper sentiments of the people to whom the organization is dear.

We who study organizations do bring to our work, if we are worth our salt, a certain objectivity and neutrality. We assume that organizations can be compared with one another no matter how different their avowed purposes may be. We do not take it for granted that the sole purpose of an organization is what those concerned say it is. We do not expect any organization to be the perfect instrument for attaining its purposes, whatever they may be. This attitude, necessary as it is to increase of knowledge of social organizations, contains what may appear a criticism to those deeply involved in an organization.

But our purpose is not criticism, but observation and analysis. When we report what we have learned, it is important that we do so faithfully. We have a double duty — to our own profession of social observation and analysis and to those who have allowed us to observe their conduct. We do not report everything we observe, for to do so would violate confidences and otherwise do harm. On the other hand, we must take care not to bias our analyses and conclusions. Finding a proper balance between our obligations to our informants and the organization, on the one hand, and our scientific duty, on the other, is not easy. We have been at some pains to find such a balance.

Yet it will appear that there is a certain bias in our account, for we look at the medical school very largely through the eyes of the students.[8] The administrators and the teachers of our chosen school and of other medical schools may not find full expression given their own hopes and plans for the students. Instead, they may find what appears to them overemphasis on the points where their work has not been fully successful, where — in spite of their best efforts — things have gone awry. We remind those teachers that throughout the book we are saying, "This is how things look and feel down under. This is how, whether anyone intends it or not, it is for the students."

There is no organization in which things look the same from all positions. There is none in which aspirations and realities are identi-

---

[8] We interviewed at some length over fifty members of the full-time staff. While what was learned from them has been used in many ways, it seemed best to reserve systematic analysis of that material for another kind of report.

cal. To point out the disparities in any particular institution may
appear to those most concerned both an exaggeration and a criticism.
But the microscope — which exaggerates things — is an honored instrument. It makes hidden things clear to the eye. But it does not
criticize. Rather, it enables us to compare one thing with another.
Our aim is so to bring to view and so to analyze the experience and
actions of medical students in interaction with their teachers and
their tasks that the reader may compare them with other situations of
the same order.

Chapter 2   Design of the Study

I<small>N</small> one sense, our study had no design. That is, we had no well-worked-out set of hypotheses to be tested, no data-gathering instruments purposely designed to secure information relevant to these hypotheses, no set of analytic procedures specified in advance. Insofar as the term "design" implies these features of elaborate prior planning, our study had none.

If we take the idea of design in a larger and looser sense, using it to identify those elements of order, system, and consistency our procedures did exhibit, our study had a design. We can say what this was by describing our original view of our problem, our theoretical and methodological commitments, and the way these affected our research and were affected by it as we proceeded. We will, then, turn in the next chapter to a description of the point of view we finally adopted, from which this book is written, and the analytic procedures we adopted to implement it.

Our research problem, as we originally saw it, had nothing to do with problems of the level and direction of effort, for this concept was developed in the course of the research and became our central focus only when we were engaged in the final analysis of our materials. Instead, the problem we began with was to discover what medical school did to medical students other than giving them a technical education. It seemed reasonable to assume that students left medical school with a set of ideas about medicine and medical practice that differed from the ideas they entered with, ideas they could not have had in advance of the concrete foretaste of practice that school gave them. Such changes would presumably influence the career choices

17

students made once they became practicing physicians: whether to go into general practice or a specialty and, if the latter, which specialty to enter; where to practice; whether to practice alone, with a partner, or in some institution; and so on. Our original focus, then, was on the medical school as an organization in which the student acquired some basic perspectives on his later activity as a doctor.

It is important to note here some of the things we did not assume. For instance, we did not assume that we knew what perspectives the doctor would need in order to function effectively in practice, for we believed that only a study of doctors in practice could furnish that information and such studies were not available. We did not, furthermore, assume that we knew what ideas and perspectives a student acquired while in school. This meant that we concentrated on *what* students learned as well as on *how* they learned it. Both of those assumptions committed us to working with an open theoretical scheme in which variables were to be discovered rather than with a scheme in which variables decided on in advance would be located and their consequences isolated and measured.

This commitment raises both theoretical questions and questions of method. To start with the latter, we necessarily had to use methods that would allow us to discover phenomena whose existence we were unaware of at the beginning of the research; our methods had to allow for the discovery of the variables themselves as well as relationships between variables. We were committed, therefore, to the use of unstructured techniques, particularly at the beginning. "Unstructured techniques" refers here, obviously, to techniques in which the data-gathering operations are not designed, for instance, to see which of two or more alternative answers to a question someone will pick, but rather which questions he himself will ask. We will discuss later our choice of particular kinds of unstructured techniques. The important point is that our initial conceptions dictated techniques of this kind.

The assumptions discussed so far, being negative in nature, did not say much about what kinds of concepts and theories we would make use of in our study, nor, to put it another way, did they say much about which facets of the school's social structure or the experience of individual students we would focus on. These questions were decided in part by major a priori theoretical commitments, which we can explain briefly here. The first of these is to a sociological mode of analysis. By this we mean simply that we were interested in problems of a collective character, in what was true of medical students by virtue of the fact that they participated in a structured set of social relationships, both those of the school and of other organizations whose activities impinged on school activities. This theoretical premise suggested that we look at the medical school as an organization of collective forms of social action.

Since we were interested, at this time, in analyzing not only the collective forms of social action that made up the medical school as an institution, but also in the effects on the medical student of living and working in this institution, we needed also to make some decisions in the area of social psychological theory. Here we had more to choose from than in the area of sociological theory; although sociological theory contains basic assumptions and perspectives which are fairly well agreed upon by most workers in the field, social psychology contains many competing theories whose comparative worth has never been definitively tested. Thus, choice of a point of view must necessarily be somewhat arbitrary. (One is tempted to justify the choice of a theoretical viewpoint by saying that it is most suitable for the problems under investigation. But the problems are in part defined by the theory one chooses, so that such a justification is tautological.)

We decided to work with a theory based on the concept of symbolic interaction, the theory first enunciated by Charles Horton Cooley, John Dewey, and George Herbert Mead [1] and since used and expanded by many others.[2] This theory stresses the more conscious aspects of human behavior and relates them to the individual's participation in group life. It assumes that human behavior is to be understood as a process in which the person shapes and controls his conduct by taking into account (through the mechanism of "role-taking") the expectations of others with whom he interacts. Such a

[1] Charles Horton Cooley, *Human Nature and the Social Order* (Glencoe, Ill.: Free Press, 1956); John Dewey, *Human Nature and Conduct* (New York: Modern Library, 1930); George Herbert Mead, *Mind, Self and Society* (Chicago: University of Chicago Press, 1934), and *The Philosophy of the Act* (Chicago: University of Chicago Press, 1938).

[2] See, for example, Herbert Blumer, "Psychological Import of the Human Group," in M. Sherif and M. Wilson (eds.), *Group Relations at the Crossroads* (New York: Harper, 1953), pp. 185–202; Nelson N. Foote, "Concept and Method in the Study of Human Development," in M. Sherif and M. Wilson (eds.), *Emerging Problems in Social Psychology* (Norman, Okla.: Institute of Group Relations, 1957), pp. 29–53; Alfred R. Lindesmith and Anselm L. Strauss, *Social Psychology* (New York: Dryden Press, 1956); Robert E. Park, *Race and Culture* (Glencoe, Ill.: Free Press, 1950), pp. 345–92; and Anselm L. Strauss, *Mirrors and Masks: The Search for Identity* (Glencoe, Ill.: Free Press, 1959).

theory meshes well with most sociological theories, in which such concepts as "interaction" and "expectations" also play a central part, and so in this way is well adapted to use in a study working at the margins where collective behavior and individual conduct overlap.

Although the decision to work with sociological theory and social-psychological theory of the symbolic interactionist variety limited the area of things we might study and the concepts we might use to study them, it did not dictate specific concepts or objects of study. Even with these commitments, we still faced the problem of deciding which of the many phenomena that could be studied in the medical school and in the lives of the medical students to study. Symbolic interactionist theory lacks a body of substantive propositions that would have directed our attention to particular phenomena in the way that, for instance, a psychoanalytically based theory might do.

In explaining our further theoretical specification of the problem, we are tempted to make our decisions seem more purposeful and conscious than in fact they were. We did not have a well-worked-out rationale for these choices. Rather, we went into the field and found ourselves concentrating on certain kinds of phenomena; as we proceeded, we began to make explicit to ourselves the rationale for this concentration of our interest. The areas we found ourselves concentrating on were consistent with our general theoretical assumptions but did not flow logically and inevitably from them. We studied those matters which seemed to be of importance to the people we studied, those matters about which they themselves seemed interested or concerned. Second, we studied those matters which seemed to be the occasion of conflict or tension between the students and the other social categories of persons with whom they came into contact in the school.

We studied what was of interest to the people we were investigating because we felt that in this way we would uncover the basic dimensions of the school as a social organization and of the students' progress through it as a social-psychological phenomenon. We made the assumption that, on analysis, the major concerns of the people we studied would reveal such basic dimensions and that we could learn most by concentrating on these concerns. This meant that we began our study by looking for and inquiring about what concerned medical students and faculty and following up the connections of these matters with each other and with still other phenomena.

We studied phenomena that seemed to produce group tension and conflict because it seemed to us that the study of tensions was most likely to reveal basic elements of the relationships in which the medical student was involved.[3] If it is true that conflict and tension arise when the expectations governing social relationships are violated or frustrated, then it is clear that study of such instances will reveal just what those expectations are; and the discovery of such expectations is an important part of the sociological analysis of any organization. Operationally, this meant that we were eager to uncover "sore spots," to hear "gripes" and complaints. It might seem that in doing this we were deliberately looking for dirty linen and skeletons in the family closet, but this is not the case. The point of concentrating on instances where things do not work well is that it helps one discover how things work when they do work well, and these are discoveries that are more difficult to make in situations of harmony because people are more likely to take them for granted and less likely to discuss them. These two decisions helped us to limit the area of inquiry. Our job was to investigate the school by looking for matters that were important to participants in it in a collective way and/or the occasion of group conflict.

We did not concentrate equally on all participants but made the student our central concern and studied other aspects of the organization as they impinged on the student; we studied other participants as fully as was necessary to understand how they influenced students and why they acted in one way, rather than another, toward students.

Another theoretical choice further specified our task. We looked on the school as a social organism or system; that is, we expected the parts of it we separated analytically to be in fact connected and interdependent. Insofar as the school was a social system, we expected that the various phenomena we discovered in our research would have consequences for each other. For instance, we thought the nature of the relations between students would have effects on the relations between students and faculty and vice versa.

If we were going to look on the medical school as a social system, it seemed to us that a particular style of analysis was required. We would not be interested in establishing relationships between particular pairs or clusters of variables. Rather, we would be interested in discovering the systematic relationships between many kinds of

[3] For a more elaborate argument on the utility of studying tension and conflict see Alvin W. Gouldner, *Wildcat Strike* (Yellow Springs: Antioch Press, 1955), pp. 125–31.

phenomena and events considered simultaneously. Our analysis would proceed not by establishing correlations but by building tentative models of that set of systematic relationships and revising these models as new phenomena requiring incorporation came to our attention. We did not propose hypotheses and confirm or disprove them so much as we made provisional generalizations about aspects of the school and the students' experience in it and then revised these generalizations as "negative cases" — particular instances in which things were not as we had provisionally stated them to be — showed us further differentiations and elaborations required in our model.

The decision to look on the school as a social system (or, better, a complex of interwoven systems, for many systems could be found in the same data) led us to pay particular attention to those phenomena which were of interest to participants in the school and productive of tension or conflict which had the further characteristic of having demonstrable connections with many other observed phenomena. Such phenomena would aid us in building an over-all model of the organization we were studying, a model which would abstract from the mass of concrete events the recurring elements in that organization.

A final theoretical predilection should be noted. We concentrated less on the variations in attitudes and action to be found among students than what was common to all students except a few known deviants. We did this because we believed that before we could understand variations in student thought and action we needed to discover the relevant dimensions along which those thoughts and actions varied, the common elements which might be thought to differ from one student to another. This decision was later buttressed by our discovery during the field work of the tremendous homogeneity of the student body. Since the students were so homogeneous with respect to the problems we were studying, a focus on the variations between them would have yielded little.

Our theoretical commitments led us to adopt as our major method of investigation *participant observation*,[4] in which the researcher participates in the daily life of the people under study either openly, in

---

[4] For a general description of this method see William Foote Whyte, "Observational Field-Work Methods," in Marie Jahoda, Morton Deutsch, and Stuart W. Cook (eds.), *Research Methods in Social Relations*, II (New York: Dryden Press, 1951), 493–514, and *Street Corner Society* (enlarged edition; Chicago: University of Chicago Press, 1955), pp. 279–358.

the role of researcher, or covertly, in some disguised role, observing things that happen, listening to what is said, and questioning people over some length of time. Such a method afforded us the greatest opportunity to discover what things were of importance to the people we were studying and to follow up the interconnections of those phenomena. It allowed us to revise our model of the organization and the processes we were studying by furnishing us with instances of phenomena we had not yet made part of our over-all picture. It enabled us to return to the field for further evidence on these new problems. We shall describe later the specific observational techniques we used and the way we have tried to solve the problem of how to analyze systematically the large amount of data collected by this method. At this point we will discuss only certain major decisions we made about whom to observe and for how long.

In a study of the development of individuals as they move through an educational institution one faces the dilemma of intensive versus extensive study. Should we follow one group of students through four years of medical school or should we study different groups of students at different levels of the school for shorter periods of time? The arguments on both sides are well known. In the long-term study, one knows that the differences he detects between those entering and those leaving the school are not due to the fact that they are different people. On the other hand, he knows only one group, which may be atypical. During field work, we often heard about the vast differences, from the faculty's point of view, between one year's class and the next.

Since the major changes that concerned us were changes in attitudes and perspectives toward medicine and medical practice, and these seemed clearly tied to experiences in the medical school, we did not see the necessity of concentrating on one group of students. It was not likely that the development, let us say, of concrete attitudes about advantages and disadvantages of different specialties could be tied to extracurricular influences in such a way that the students would have developed these without the school experience. We took the risk that there would not be differing attitudes on the same subjects when successive classes were compared (as in fact there were not) and decided to sample extensively and not follow one group through four years. Considerations of time and efficiency also entered into the decision; we did not feel that the added safeguards would be worth the large amount of extra work that following one group would have entailed.

We still had to decide what students to observe and for how long. We will report in detail later on the students' academic schedule. Here we need only say that during the first two years they move through the school as a unit, all taking the same classes at the same time, while during the last two years they are divided into several groups, each of which takes the same group of courses but in a different sequence. Thus the decisions about whom to observe differ for the first and last half of school. Once we had made the general decisions discussed below, dictated by these differences in deployment of the classes, we found it necessary to make certain more specific decisions based on the knowledge of the rhythms of student life we acquired during our field work. We thus planned our later observations to include students at the time they entered school and at the time they were finishing school.

Our final decisions on the allocation of observation time were these: We started with the clinical years on the premise that these might more quickly reveal the ultimately decisive influences on the students. (Whether this was, in fact, true is hard to say; it is hard to single out "ultimately decisive" influences from others less decisive.) Juniors spend successive periods of three months in three main departments of the school; seniors have their year divided into four similar periods. We organized our observations so that we spent time with students in each of the departments in which they would receive training and saw something of each major training situation in the school. Furthermore, we usually (although not always) observed different groups of students in these different situations instead of following one group of students through the entire sequence of courses. We did this so that we could achieve extensive coverage of students as well as of situations, but for reasons of expediency as well; it took the students longer to finish their training in most fields than we wished to spend in those training situations.

We thought extensive coverage of both students and situations important. If we were to carry on our analysis by successive refinements of our theoretical models necessitated by the discovery of negative cases, we wanted to work in a way that would maximize our chances of discovering those new and unexpected phenomena whose assimilation into such models would enrich them and make them more faithful to the reality we had observed. By seeing many groups of students and many training situations we so maximized our chances of discovering negative cases.

With the freshmen and sophomores the academic schedule posed different problems for us. Skipping from group to group and situation to situation in the clinical years and looking at smaller groups instead of the entire class were dictated by the fragmented character of the clinical schedule, but the schedule of the basic science years was quite different and required us to think much more about the *class* (all the students in the same year) as a unit. In the first two years of medical school, and particularly in the first, the entire class moved together, did the same things at the same time in the same places, and reacted as more of a unit. (This was somewhat less true of the sophomore year when, although the general curriculum was the same for all, students were separated into smaller groups whose activities at particular times might differ.) Consequently, in our work with students in these years, and particularly with the freshmen, we made a greater effort to cover an entire class, to talk to every member about the major events in whose significance and effect we were interested.

Many observations of both the house staff (residents and interns) and the faculty were made during the field work with students, but these observations were limited to what could be seen while these persons were with the students. Because we wanted to see how activities with the students fitted into their perspectives, we carried on a three-month program of field work with the house staff. Unfortunately, we made no such intensive observations of the faculty.

We have explained why we decided to use participant observation as our basic technique and to analyze the data so gathered by attempting to build and progressively refine models of the school as a social organization and of the process of development of the student moving through that organization. We now turn to a description of just how we went about gathering data and analyzing it.

In participant observation, as we have said, the researcher participates in the daily lives of people he studies. We did this by attending school with the students, following them from class to laboratory to hospital ward. In studying the clinical years, we attached ourselves to one of the subgroups of the class assigned to a particular section of the hospital and followed the members through the entire day's activities. In studying students in the first two years, we did much the same thing, but since we were then attempting to study the entire class, we skipped from group to group in the class instead of remaining with one small group. We went with students to lectures and to the laboratories in which they studied the basic sciences, watched their activities, and engaged in casual conversation with them. We followed students to their fraternity houses and sat with them while they discussed their school experiences. We accompanied students on rounds with attending physicians, watched them examine patients on the wards and in the clinics, and sat in on discussion groups and oral exams. We had meals with the students and took night call with them.

We observed as participants in the daily activities of the school — which is to say that we were not hidden; our presence was known to everyone involved, to the students, their teachers, and their patients. Participating in the ordinary routine, we did so in the "pseudo-role" of student. Not that we posed as students, for it was made clear to everyone that we were not students: but rather that it was the students we participated with. When a lecture or class ended, we left with the students, not the teacher; we left the operating or delivery room when the student did, not when the patient or surgeon did, unless these happened to coincide. We went with the students wherever they went in the course of the day.

Since we were known to be observing participants,[5] the questions naturally arose for others as to who we were, what we were observing, why, and what effect this might have on the school. Students readily accepted our explanation that we were there to gather material for a book on medical education. The best evidence that our presence did not noticeably alter their behavior lies in the fact that they were willing to engage in behavior the faculty disapproved of while in our presence. On the other hand, we surely altered their behavior by our questions, at least in the sense that they became more self-conscious of certain aspects of their behavior. The faculty saw us in different ways; the clinical faculty often seemed almost unaware of our presence, while basic scientists were very likely to see us as potential judges of their teaching technique. In consequence, the science teachers seemed often extremely aware of our presence, while clinical men several times forgot who we were and asked us questions on medical subjects during class discussions. Neither students nor faculty gave evidence of concern about our presence. Both groups,

[5] Raymond L. Gold provides a useful classification of field work roles in "Roles in Sociological Field Observations," *Social Forces*, XXXVI (March, 1958), 217–23.

but the faculty much more so, saw in our study a possibility of improving medical education.

Two aspects of our participant observation are important: it was *continued* and it was *total*. When we observed a particular group of students, we observed them day after day, more or less continuously, for periods ranging from a week to two months; and we observed the total day's activities of such a group (so far as possible) rather than simply some segment of them. This latter was not always the case, for such a program of observation would leave little time for the recording and analysis of observations. After the first several days with a group we would leave parts of the day free, although often spending a full day now and again. (In saying "day," it should be understood that many of our days went on until late at night, when the students' day was of similar length, as with the hardworking freshmen or the students who delivered babies at night on obstetrics.)

We did not record every event we observed; encyclopedic recording is neither possible nor particularly useful. But this raises the question of how we recorded our observations and what we selected from the many possible things we had to record. We made it a rule to dictate an account of our day's observations as soon as possible after the observation period and to make this account fairly complete. The reader will get a more accurate impression than any quick summary can provide of the kind of thing we recorded and the detail in which we recorded it by noticing the character of the excerpts we quote from our field notes in the substantive sections of this book. We should, however, say that we typically included a detailed account of the activities students engaged in and observed, "verbatim" accounts of conversations we overheard or took part in which touched on topics of interest to us, and frequently our speculations or primitive analyses of various problems under study at the time.

We did leave things out. What was included or left out of our field notes depended very much on the problems we were pursuing at the time. We carried on a running analysis of the materials we gathered and as we became aware of certain problems made a greater effort to include materials which bore on those problems and tended to prove or disprove provisional hypotheses we were entertaining.[*] When a search for both positive and negative cases on some point was

[*] A general discussion of problems of analysis of field work data appears in Howard S. Becker, "Problems of Inference and Proof in Participant Observation," *American Sociological Review*, XXIII (December, 1958), 652–60.

thus occupying our attention, we were more likely to devote our major recording efforts to the materials so gathered. When we felt that we had sufficient evidence to substantiate some particular point we were likely to stop recording material bearing on it or to record it in a shorthand fashion, using some simple label to refer to an incident as an instance of something we had already described fully and simply noting that we had observed another instance of it. If the incident was a negative instance of our provisional hypothesis, we recorded it fully. Since we realized that our continuous revision of hypotheses might later call for information we had not considered relevant at the time of the earlier field work, we recorded many incidents of whose relevance we were not sure. In short, what appears in our field notes depended in part on the hypotheses we were attempting to explore, but our field notes also contain material not bearing on any hypotheses under consideration at the time, on the premise that we might later wish to construct hypotheses on points of which we were not yet aware. For example, we began recording the patterns freshmen fell into in seating themselves at lectures, although this bore on no hypotheses we were investigating at the time; later, the material so gathered suggested hypotheses and a more intensive search for positive and negative evidence was then made in the past field notes and in subsequent observations. We consider it some indication of the accuracy of our recordings that when we searched our previous notes for material on hypotheses constructed later we were able to find much evidence both positive and negative.

In addition to gathering data by participant observation, we also made use of two kinds of interview. We conducted many casual and informal interviews with individuals and groups during the course of our participant observation.[7] That is to say, our observation was not entirely passive; when the occasion presented itself, we asked questions of those we were observing, haphazardly on some points but in quite systematic fashion on others. For instance, we felt that it would be worthwhile to know something about the educational and social class backgrounds of those we observed, and we managed to find time for detailed conversations about this and about future professional plans with most of the students we observed. More haphazard interviewing occurred when some incident during the day's activities

<hr>

[7] Some problems of interviewing during field observation are discussed in Howard S. Becker, "Interviewing Medical Students," *American Journal of Sociology*, LXII (September, 1956), 199–201.

was made the topic of group conversation by the interviewer, who raised a series of questions to a group of students about it. This method of interviewing was also used in the field work with interns and residents.

We also made use of formal structured interviews with students and with faculty. The faculty interviews were exploratory and ranged freely over several areas: the faculty member's career, his aspirations, his attitude toward medical students in general and Kansas students in particular, his educational philosophy, and so on. The student interviews, following as they did a great deal of "exploratory" work, were much more structured, being designed to get information on particular points for a systematic analysis.[8] The sampling of the faculty was informal, the main consideration being to cover all departments and levels of rank. For the student interviews we used a random sample of fifteen students from each of the four years (although four additional freshmen were interviewed because we felt the random sampling had left out an important subgroup). We were unable to complete interviews with one sophomore and one senior.

We conducted the student interviews in a formal fashion, meeting the students in offices the medical school made available to us and recording the interviews on tape to give us a verbatim transcript of what transpired. We used an interview guide, asking each student 138 questions (the only exception being that some questions dealing with experiences in the clinical years were not asked of students who had not yet had those experiences). But we left much room for the free expression of all kinds of ideas and did not force the student to stick to the original list of questions or to answer in predetermined categories. Our intention was twofold. First, we wanted to check some of our major conclusions against a new body of data gathered in a different way. Second, we wished to make quantitative analyses of some points that lent themselves easily to that mode of analysis.

The reader will discover that we have made relatively little use of the interview materials in our later analyses. In part, this is because we asked some questions bearing on points we have decided not to treat in this monograph; for example, we asked many questions about how students decided to go into medicine but spend little time on this problem. In larger part, it is because the interview proved to be an unsatisfactory method of eliciting data on many of the problems we do deal with. (We intend to discuss the problem of the discrep-

[8] The schedule used in interviewing can be found in the appendix to this volume.

ancies between interview and field observational data in a separate publication.)[9]

We come now to the problem of the analysis of such a diverse and seemingly unsystematic mass of data as we collected during our two years of field work.[10] The records of our field notes and interviews occupy approximately 5,000 single-spaced typed pages. But, because we wished to use our data for a variety of purposes, they were not gathered in a form that lent itself to conventional techniques of analysis which depend on data gathered in a standardized way for systematic comparison and statistical tests. Use of such techniques is the most commonly accepted way of presenting evidence and testing hypotheses in present day social science. Since our data do not permit the use of these techniques we have necessarily turned to what is ordinarily vaguely referred to as "qualitative analysis." Qualitative analyses of field data are not new in social science; indeed, many classics of social research have been based on such analyses. But the methods of arriving at conclusions have not been systematized and such research has often been charged with being based on insight and intuition and thus not communicable or capable of replication.

We believe that the analysis of participant observation data can, and usually does, proceed in a careful way to test hypotheses in ways that can be communicated and replicated. However, it is usually true that the methods by which this is done are not described in research reports, so that a suspicious reader has some justification for his feeling that the research is not scientific. We think that the evidence for conclusions in field research is usually better than critics think. For that reason, we have attempted in this book to give a careful presentation of all the evidence we have on any given point, an assessment of that evidence in the light of relevant standards, and an explanation of why we consider particular items of evidence proof of particular propositions. We do not think our methods are new. But we do think it is a departure from conventional practice to make such systematic assessments of field data. From one point of view, our entire report is an experiment in being more explicit about the modes of proof involved in analysis of this kind.

[9] See the preliminary discussion in Howard S. Becker and Blanche Geer, "Participant Observation and Interviewing: A Comparison," *Human Organization*, XVI (Fall, 1957), 28–32. For an analysis of similar discrepancies found in another project see Lois Dean, "Interaction, Reported and Observed: The Case of One Local Union," *Human Organization*, XVII (Fall, 1958), 36–44.

[10] The following several paragraphs are adapted from Howard S. Becker, "Problems of Inference . . . ,"*op. cit.*

In this research, analysis was not a separate stage of the process which began after we had finished gathering our data. Rather, as some of our previous comments indicate, data-gathering and analysis went on simultaneously. This, of course, is a necessary consequence of our decision to proceed by making successive refinements of a model of the medical school and the professional development of students in it. It means, concretely, that much of our effort in the field was devoted to discovering relevant problems for study, building hypotheses that we supposed would provide a solution to these problems, and looking for valid indicators of the variables contained in those hypotheses. We have occasionally reported some of these preliminary steps of analysis by way of indicating to the reader the processes of inference which took place as we built our provisional models from incomplete field data.

Because we carried on a running analysis of our materials while we were in the field, we knew the general content of many of our major conclusions at the conclusion of the field work. To present evidence for these, however, we still had to work out modes of analysis and presentation.

In assessing the evidence for various kinds of conclusions we have taken a lesson from our colleagues in the field of statistics and have not begun with the premise that a conclusion is either true or false. The varying values of a correlation coefficient or of a significance figure indicate that a proposition is more or less likely to be an accurate statement of the facts, not that it is, or is not, correct. What we attempt in assessing hypotheses with our qualitative evidence is to say how likely it is that our final conclusions correctly state the relationships to be found in the medical school we studied.[11] Readers frequently suspect conclusions drawn from qualitative data because they are presented accompanied by some variation of the statement, "We have gone over our data and find it supports this conclusion," without being told just what the nature of the data or the process of "going over" were; such a statement provides no basis for assessing the degree of likelihood that the proposition is correct and leaves the reader in the uncomfortable position of having to accept the proposition essentially on faith.

We have tried to lessen our readers' dilemma by stating the nature

[11] Our thinking on problems of evidence and proof has been greatly influenced by George Polya, *Mathematics and Plausible Reasoning*, II. *Patterns of Plausible Inference* (Princeton: Princeton University Press, 1954).

and extent of our evidence on points under discussion in such a way that it will explain our own reasons for putting a certain degree of confidence in a conclusion, and give the reader ample opportunity to form his own judgment; that is, we describe all the items of evidence that bear on a given point (although usually in summary form) and the degree to which they seem to us to confirm our proposition. A technical problem arises in considering how one can be sure that all the items of evidence have been considered; it would clearly be impractical to search through 5,000 pages of notes every time one wished to check a proposition. To avoid this, we indexed our field notes and labeled each entry with code numbers referring to major topics under which the given item might be considered. These entries were then reassembled by code number so that we had in one place all the facts bearing on a given topic, thus making possible a relatively quick check of our data on any given point.

One specific technical innovation we have made is a form for demonstrating the customary and collective character of certain group perspectives. This form is described in some detail in the next chapter, where we discuss the specific concepts we have used in our analysis. It should be remembered that, although we started with no conception of the importance of the level and direction of students' efforts, this problem gradually came to dominate our thinking, so that what we ended with in the way of a theoretical position is somewhat different from what we started with.

Chapter 3 # Perspective, Culture, and Organization

In the last chapter we presented a simplified account of the theory and method we brought to our study. We made use of the opportunities our method gave us to shift the focus of our interest and attention and gradually came to center our analysis on the problem of the level and direction of students' academic effort. We had first the descriptive question: How much effort did students put forth and in what directions? Then we had the analytic question: Why were the students' level and direction of effort what they were and not any of the other things they might have been? Our final analysis of the data we gathered focuses on these questions.

Three concepts dominate our analysis. First, we are concerned with *group perspectives* — those of the faculty and, to a greater degree, those of the students. Perspectives, following the theory of George Herbert Mead,[1] are co-ordinated views and plans of action people follow in problematic situations. Group perspectives are perspectives held collectively by a group of people. We approach the problem of the level and direction of students' effort by searching for the perspectives which guide their behavior in situations in which academic effort is the appropriate activity.

Second, we note that the perspectives of students on the level and direction of academic effort are consistent and coherent. To deal with the consistency of perspectives with one another and with the relation

[1] *The Philosophy of the Act* (Chicago: University of Chicago Press, 1938), *passim*.

33

of the perspectives we studied to the role of student, we use the concept of *student culture*.[2]

Finally, we wanted to take account of the fact that students' actions occur in an institutional setting. Students occupy a defined position in the medical school and interact in ways that are specified by institutional rules with people occupying other socially defined positions in the school. We wanted to specify the ways problems arose for students out of this institutionally defined interaction. We wanted to investigate the restraints this institutional setting placed on the students' attempts to solve these problems. To these ends, we made use of the concept of *organization*.

Perspectives

We use the term *perspective* to refer to a co-ordinated set of ideas and actions a person uses in dealing with some problematic situation, to refer to a person's ordinary way of thinking and feeling about and acting in such a situation.[3] These thoughts and actions are co-ordinated in the sense that the actions flow reasonably, from the actor's point of view, from the ideas contained in the perspective. Similarly, the ideas can be seen by an observer to be one of the possible sets of ideas which might form the underlying rationale for the person's actions and are seen by the actor as providing a justification for acting as he does. Thus, one might believe that occupational security is very important and refuse to take jobs which had higher salaries and greater chances for advancement in order to hold on to a less advantageous position offering tenure. The actions flow from the beliefs and the beliefs justify the actions. Note that we avoid specifying either actions or beliefs as prior and causal. In some cases, the person may hold the beliefs and act so as to implement them. In others, he may take some

[2] We have discussed the concept of student culture at length in Howard S. Becker and Blanche Geer, "Student Culture in Medical School," *Harvard Educational Review*, XXVIII (Winter, 1958), 70–80.

[3] Our definition of perspective differs from earlier definitions in including actions as well as ideas and beliefs. Except for this point, our conception of perspectives is in fundamental accord with that of Karl Mannheim in *Ideology and Utopia* (London: Routledge and Kegan Paul, 1936), p. 239: ". . . the subject's whole mode of conceiving things as determined by his historical and social setting." Similarly, except for the fact that we include actions in perspectives, we essentially agree with the discussion by Tamotsu Shibutani in "Reference Groups as Perspectives," *American Journal of Sociology*, LX (May, 1955), 564: "A perspective is an ordered view of one's world — what is taken for granted about the attributes of various objects, events, and human nature. It is an order of things remembered and expected as well as things actually perceived, an organized conception of what is plausible and what is possible; it constitutes the matrix through which one perceives his environment."

actions and develop the ideas as an after-the-fact justification. In still others, ideas and actions may develop together as the person attempts to build a new approach to an unfamiliar situation. The person, of course, may not be aware of the connections between his thoughts and deeds that the observer perceives. This requires the analyst to give concrete and reasonable grounds for labeling any given act or idea as part of a given perspective.

Let us explain what we mean by a "problematic situation" and what we see as the relation between problematic situations and perspectives. A person develops and maintains a perspective when he faces a situation calling for action which is not given by his own prior beliefs or by situational imperatives. In other words, perspectives arise when people face choice points. In many crucial situations, the individual's prior perspectives allow him no choice, dictating that he can in these circumstances do only one thing. In many other situations, the range of possible and feasible alternatives is so limited by the physical and social environment that the individual has no choice about the action he must perform. But where the individual is called on to act, and his choices are not constrained, he will begin to develop a perspective. If a particular kind of situation recurs frequently, the perspective will probably become an established part of a person's way of dealing with the world.

Clearly, a situation will not present the same problem to all people. Some will have a way to act in the situation so that it calls for no thought at all; the situation is not problematic for them. Others will perceive the situation differently, depending on their prior perspectives. Choosing a college will, for example, be one kind of problem for a person who sees college as the gateway to a professional school, another kind of problem for one who intends to become a young executive, still another kind of problem for one who wants an all-around liberal education, and quite different still for a person who does not really want to go to college but is being forced to do so by his parents. In short, the immediate situation is problematic only in terms of the perspective the individual brings to bear upon it.

To take account of this, we distinguish in our analysis between immediate and long-range perspectives. Long-range perspectives are those which have brought the individual into the immediate situation: in this case, the would-be medical students' perspective that medical school is a good thing and that it is necessary to finish medical school in order to practice medicine. Given this perspective, the stu-

dent enters medical school and, in terms of his long-range perspectives, finds himself faced with a number of specific problems. In the
face of these, he develops an immediate short-run perspective. In
most of our analyses we are, as we shall see, concerned with the development of short-run situational perspectives and deal with long-
range perspectives primarily by way of specifying the conditions
under which a given immediate situational perspective comes into
being. Occasionally we are concerned with the way perspectives
formed in the immediate situation of medical school turn into long-
range perspectives on the students' future problems.

The perspectives in which we are most interested for purposes
of understanding and explaining students' level and direction of academic effort are group perspectives, those perspectives held in common by some group of people. Group perspectives are modes of
thought and action developed by a group which faces the same problematic situation. They are the customary ways members of the group
think about such situations and act in them. They are the ways of
thinking and acting which appear to group members as the natural
and legitimate ones to use in such situations.

We see group perspectives as arising when people see themselves
as being in the same boat and when they have an opportunity to interact with reference to their problems. Under these conditions, people
share their concerns and their provisional answers to questions about
the meaning of events and how one should respond to them. Individual and subgroup perspectives merge and are shared. Group perspectives gain strength and force in the individual's behavior by
virtue of being held in common with others. They have the prima
facie validity which accrues to those things "everybody knows" and
"everybody does."

Perhaps we can make clearer the meaning of perspective, as we
use this term, by distinguishing it from two somewhat similar concepts: attitude and value. Perspectives differ from values in being
situationally specific; they are patterns of thought and action which
have grown up in response to a specific set of institutional pressures
and serve as a solution to the problems those pressures create. Values,
on the other hand, are ordinarily thought of as being generalized and
abstract, capable of being applied to a great variety of situations.
Perspectives are related directly to dilemmas faced by the persons
who hold them, while values need have no such direct connection.
Perspectives contain definitions of the situation, as the actor sees

it, while values are essentially statements of the worth or "good-ness" of classes of things; perspectives contain such judgments, but also contain statements about the nature of the situation in which such judgments are to be applied. Finally, we include in perspectives actions as well as ideas; analyses of values ordinarily distinguish values from the actions presumed to flow from them.

Perspectives are distinguished from attitudes by the fact that they contain actions as well as ideas and dispositions to act. They are fur-ther distinguished from attitudes by their collective character. Studies of attitudes seldom deal with the degree to which ideas are shared or held collectively, except inferentially. In our analyses, how-ever, this characteristic of perspectives is of central importance.

Because· such a large part of this book is devoted to an analysis of those perspectives which affect students' level and direction of academic effort, we would like to explain in some detail the steps in such an analysis and the kinds of evidence we present. First, we present the situation in which the perspective arose as we observed this situation during our field work. Second, we formulate the con-tent of the perspective. This consists of a definition of the situation and the problems it presents as group members see them; an expres-sion of what members expect to achieve or get out of the situation (their goals); and the ideas and actions group members employ in dealing with the situation.

In formulating the content of a perspective, we worked with the incidents summarized and categorized in the index of our field notes mentioned in the last chapter. Each entry in this index summarized some observed statement or action of one or more students. Each entry was put in as many categories as it seemed to be relevant to. When it came time to analyze a given perspective or problem area we thus had available all the incidents in our field notes which might bear on that problem. After running through the incidents and re-viewing the tentative analyses made in the field, we formulated a general statement of the perspective as the students themselves might have put it. For example, in looking over the material on the students' relations with the faculty in teaching situations, we derived a tenta-tive statement of the students' perspective on this area of their lives. The coded incidents defined a problematic situation as the students saw it, stated what they wanted to get out of it, and described the actions they took to this end. The content of the perspective could be briefly characterized by saying that students felt they needed to

exert all their efforts to get along with a faculty which was in many
ways capricious and unpredictable and could vitally affect the students' professional futures.

We then prepared a more differentiated statement of the perspective by going through the field materials again, noting each different
kind of item which we regarded as a specific expression of the perspective in word or deed. For example, coming on this item:

5/25/6 (p. 6): Jones talks about Smith not having done well on the OB
[obstetrics] oral — says Smith is really smart but of course they can get you
in any oral, just by picking on something you don't know about.

we might jot down, "Student says faculty can get you on an oral by
picking on something you don't know"; and, coming on this item:

10/22/6 (p. 6): Brown says he failed to get the lab work on a patient and
got caught by Dr. Hackett. He copied the figures from the main lab, but
drew some blood too in case Hackett checked up on him.

we might note, "Student cheats in order to show faculty member he is
doing his work." Having accumulated a list of such notes, we then
formulated a systematic and more general statement of the kinds of
attitudes and actions which could be seen as expressing the basic
perspective. Many incidents had in common the fact that students
stated that it was necessary to please the faculty in order to get
through school. Other incidents, like the one about the faked lab
work, showed students acting in ways calculated to make a pleasing
impression on the faculty. Still other incidents, like the one about
the OB oral, had as a common theme the students' expressed belief
that it was impossible to tell what the faculty wanted of them. Each
category we formed had some underlying characteristic of this kind
which could be interpreted as an expression of the perspective; taken
together, the set of categories constituted the perspective.

Such a differentiated description of the perspective serves two purposes. On the one hand, it adds richness and detail to our description
of the perspective's content by spelling out the particular ways it is
seen to operate in actual situations. On the other hand, it describes
fully the kinds of items we use as evidence that the perspective is the
customary way students handle the problem of their relations with
faculty in teaching situations.

When preparing the final written presentation of the perspective,
each kind of item we have found to express it is described in terms
of the specific characteristics that do so. We find it useful to follow

the tradition of presenting illustrative quotations from our field notes; we depart from older practice in specifying exactly what it is about the quotation that is meaningful and in asserting that every item used in later analyses had the minimum characteristics, at least, of one of the kinds of items discussed. (In presenting quotations, we present certain facts about the situation and participants in summary form so that the reader will be able to make his own assessment of the representativeness of the sample of quotations given. In the material on the first-year class, we identify quotations by date and indicate which groups in the class are represented by the people quoted or described. In the material on the clinical years, we indicate date and the part of the hospital or school in which the material was gathered.)

Having described the content of the perspective in this way, we turn to establishing certain of its characteristics — its frequency, range, and collective character — in order to assess the extent to which it is the customary way students deal with the problem it refers to.

If the perspective is the students' customary way of dealing with a problem, it should occur frequently in our field notes. Actually, we become aware that a perspective exists from the frequent and continued repetition, in our field observations, of certain ideas by students. But we now want to demonstrate this point to our readers. So, we are first of all concerned with the ratio of positive to negative items in our field data. A positive item is some statement or observed activity of a student which expresses the perspective; a negative item is some student statement or activity in which the student uses some alternative perspective in dealing with the same problem. Because the final statement of the perspective was formulated after a great deal of field work and analysis in the field, there are usually relatively few negative cases. This fact lends some credence to the proposition that the perspective has a high relative frequency. If there should be a large number of negative cases, this would certainly require revision of any proposition that the perspective is in frequent use. In any event, a careful inspection of all negative instances is in order.

Aside from the question of negative instances, the major consideration with regard to the absolute number of incidents is that this number should be sizable. If it were very small, we would not be able to conclude that the perspective was used frequently; we might simply have seen a few odd cases in which it happened to be employed. But if the number of instances is as high, let us say, as 75 or 100 this could hardly be true. It would not be credible that so many instances should be observed if the null hypothesis that the perspective was not frequently used were true. The absolute number does not so much indicate that the perspective is frequent as negate the null hypothesis that it is not.

Since we seldom observed the entire student group at one time, it is legitimate to take into account the fact that the people we were not observing at any particular moment might well have been engaged in behavior that we would have counted as an instance in favor of our hypothesis had we been there to observe it. For instance, we typically observed from five to eight (and never more than fifteen) students at a time while we were in the teaching hospital. Yet there were always approximately two hundred students taking clinical work. We therefore consider it legitimate to estimate that probably ten times as many incidents as we observed to support our hypotheses probably occurred during the time we were making our observations and could, in principle, have been observed by us had there been enough observers to go around.

The number of items which consist of responses to direct queries by the observer must be considered in assessing the meaning of the absolute number of items from the data. If the percentage of items so directed by the observer is very large, this means that less meaning can be attached to the absolute number because it is now a function of the observer's activity rather than the students'. In short, no strict rule of interpretation can be stated, though the absolute number obviously has some meaning.

The second thing we took into account in checking on the characteristics of a perspective was how widely the items of data were distributed through the various observational situations. For example, we might observe student-faculty interaction in ten different places and find that the bulk of our items came from only one of these places. This might lead us to suspect that the perspective is a response to something unique in that particular situation. Similarly, the perspective might be used by students only with regard to one kind of activity or person and thus might not be so much widespread as a function of something connected with that activity or person.

Consequently, we made it a practice to list all the places in which observations of the problem we were considering were made and see in how many of them at least one instance of the perspective's use was observed. For example, students in the clinical years had some training in eighteen different departments of the hospital. It was a simple matter to check in how many of the eighteen some expression of the perspective was found. If no expression of it was found in observations made in some large proportion of these observational situations, we could not consider the perspective widespread. Similarly, where possible, we listed the kinds of activity the perspective might be relevant to and made a similar check to see that instances of it were observed in some sizable proportion of these activities.

Again, while this kind of check gives positive evidence that the perspective has a wide social range, it is also important in that it disproves the null hypothesis that the perspective was not widespread by showing that it occurred in many of the relevant situations.

We checked not only the situational range of the perspective but also its temporal range. Each example was dated; we inspected them to see how they were distributed over the period of observation. If most of the examples are confined to a short period of time, we consider the perspective ephemeral; if there is a relatively even spread, we conclude that it persists. Our confidence in its persistence, however, depends upon the length of the observation period. We are more satisfied that the perspective persists if we have had many opportunities to observe situations where it is likely to occur (and then find that it does) than if we have not.

Once we establish that the perspective is in frequent and widespread use by students, we want to demonstrate that it is collective, i.e., that it is shared by students and regarded by them as the legitimate way to think about and act in the area the perspective refers to. By shared, we mean that students not only use the perspective but use it with the knowledge that their fellow students also use it; by legitimate, we mean that students see the ideas and actions which make up the perspective as proper and necessary in this area of their lives.

The first point we considered in assessing the collective character of a perspective is whether or not expression of it is an artifact of the observer's techniques. If, for example, many instances consist in the observer's making a statement embodying the basic points of the perspective to students and asking them whether they agree or disagree, a high proportion of "agree" answers will have some value but is open to the criticism that while students may express agreement with this idea it is not one they themselves would ordinarily express.

Therefore, we classified each item according to whether it was *directed* by the observer's activities or was *volunteered* spontaneously by the students.

In classifying items as directed by the observer or volunteered by the students, we did not simply classify as directed any statement by a student made in response to something the observer said. In the field, we often made neutral remarks or asked neutral questions which brought out important items, but these were not classified as directed. Only those items in which we ourselves injected the points characteristic of the perspective were counted as directed.

In asking whether or not a perspective was collective, we also considered the degree to which the statements or actions expressing it occurred in public. In the course of participant observation there will be many occasions when one of the persons observed will be alone with the observer and talk at some length about his problems and aspirations. Material of this kind can be considered evidence that the individual involved in the conversation held this view (and was willing to express it, at least in private) but gives no clue as to whether the ideas expressed are held commonly or regarded as legitimate by all members of the group involved. It may, after all, be the case that many members of the group hold these opinions but hold them privately and neither express them nor act on them in the presence of their fellows.

To check this point, we classified all items according to whether they occurred in the presence of the observer alone or when other members of the student group were also present. If, for instance, we saw a student doing something in the presence of several other students who made no comment about it, we assumed that this kind of activity was legitimate enough to excite no comment from other members of the group. We did not make this inference if we saw the act performed when no one but the observer was present. Similarly, if a member of the group made a statement in conversation with other members of the group we regarded this as evidence of the perspective's legitimacy in a way we could not if the statement was made to us alone.

We also argued that when some of the terms of the perspective were used in everyday conversation among group members that this indicated that these people shared the perspective involved, for they could not use these terms to communicate unless the terms were mutually intelligible.

Finally, we took note of the proportion of items made up of observations of activity rather than statements. If all the items consisted of statements made by students, our conclusions would be affected by this disproportion. If all items were observations of activities and there were no statements on the subject, we would know nothing of students' views. Similarly, in the opposite case we might conclude that the perspective was "all talk," and unrelated to the students' behavior.

We have found it useful to present the findings of this kind of analysis in the following tabular form, presenting in each cell both frequencies and the appropriate percentages:

		Volunteered	Directed by the Observer	Total
Statements	To observer alone			
	To others in every-day conversation			
Activities	Individual			
	Group			
Total				

We have not developed any formulas for interpretation of a table of this kind, but we can state a few ground rules. In the first place, the number of directed statements should be small in comparison to the volunteered statements. Secondly, in the "volunteered" column, the proportion of items consisting of statements made to the observer alone should not be overwhelming. This, of course, begs the question of just what proportion would be large enough to cause us to doubt our proposition that the perspective is collective. We are inclined now to think that any proportion over 50 per cent would necessitate another look at the proposition, but we cannot state any rationale for this inclination. Third, there should be a reasonable proportion of activities as well as statements by students. Again, we cannot state any rigid formula, but we are inclined to think that somewhere in the neighborhood of 20 or 25 per cent would be an appropriate figure.

A table like this makes possible summary presentation of a great deal of material and is thus very useful. It gives the reader much of the grounds for concluding that the perspective is shared by students and regarded by them as legitimate, and allows him to see the basis on which that conclusion was formed.

The final step in our analysis of perspectives was a consideration of those cases found in the field notes which run counter to the proposition that the students shared a particular perspective. Because the statement of the perspective had been refashioned many times in the course of the field work and later analysis in order to take into account as many of the negative cases as possible,[4] this number was usually quite small. We considered each one carefully; whatever revisions it suggested were incorporated in the analysis. Two generic types of negative instances were noted, and we deal with each type differently. In one type, we found individuals not making use of the perspective because they had not yet learned it. Negative cases of this kind typically consisted of a student's taking action contrary to the perspective and being corrected by his fellows. Such an instance required no change in our proposition except to note that not everyone knows the perspective at first and that people acquire it in the course of their experience in the situation we were studying.

The second kind of negative case consisted of observations indicating that a few people had a perspective other than that which we postulated as the common one, or of cases in which students were observed to behave according to the perspective publicly but to deviate from it privately. In these cases, our most likely revision was to say that there apparently exists confirmed deviance in the social body or that there may be marginal areas in which the perspective is not necessarily applied, even though our evidence indicated that in most kinds of situations it was usual.

This second kind of negative case in fact afforded an opportunity for additional confirmation of the proposition that the perspective is a collective phenomenon. Where it could be shown that the person who acted on a different perspective was socially isolated from the group or that his deviant activities were regarded by others as improper, unnecessary, or foolish, we could then argue that these facts indicated use of the perspective by all but deviants, hence its collective character.

Through the kind of analysis just described, we demonstrate that students customarily operated in terms of a given perspective. Such a conclusion is, of course, descriptive. However, our analyses go a step

[4] We thus make use, in some sense, of the method of analytic induction. See Alfred R. Lindesmith, *Opiate Addiction* (Bloomington: Principia Press, 1947), especially pp. 5–20, and the subsequent literature cited in Ralph H. Turner, "The Quest for Universals in Sociological Research," *American Sociological Review*, XVIII (December, 1953), 604–11.

further, by suggesting the conditions under which given kinds of perspectives arise. Ordinarily, the propositions about the genesis of perspectives take this form: students with this kind of initial perspective, faced with this set of environmental problems under conditions allowing for mutual interaction, will develop this kind of perspective. We are not able to provide any demonstration for such propositions, other than the prima facie plausibility and reasonableness of the connections we postulate. The reason for our inability to provide any more conclusive assessment of the proposition is simple. Conclusive demonstration would require, at a minimum, comparison of at least two cases in which the postulated conditions varied and the perspectives developed by students also varied. But, as we shall see, the students we observed had remarkably similar initial perspectives and faced the same set of environmental problems. Thus, there were no alternative collective perspectives — only isolated cases of deviance — developed among the student body, and we had no opportunity for a systematic comparison. More compelling demonstration of these propositions on the genesis of perspectives of various kinds must necessarily wait on the study of more cases in which the consequences of differing conditions can be observed.[5]

Our report deals primarily with student perspectives. We have chosen, in the main, to deal with those perspectives which have a direct influence on students' level and direction of effort. Parts Two and Three of this volume deal with student perspectives in the freshman and clinical years of medical school. These parts, in effect, explain the ideas students hold and the actions they take with regard to the level and direction of academic effort with reference to these perspectives and suggest conditions under which these perspectives arise. Part Four deals with students' perspectives on the future of their professional careers: where they will practice and whom they will practice with; where they will serve their internships; whether they will go into a general or specialty practice and, if the latter, the criteria they use to assess specialties. This analysis of perspectives on the future allows us to consider the question of the effects of medical school on the prospective practitioner's professional orientations: to what degree is his view of the future colored by his school experience and perspectives?

[5] The preceding section first appeared in *Human Organization Research: Field Relations and Techniques*, edited by Richard N. Adams and Jack J. Preiss, (Homewood, Ill.: Dorsey Press), pp. 280–88.

Student Culture

In speaking of the perspectives which influence students' level and direction of effort, we often have occasion to use the term *student culture*. By this we mean the body of collective understandings among students about matters related to their roles as students. Our use of this phrase has several connotations.

In the first place, we mean to indicate that there is a substantial element of coherence and consistency among the perspectives we describe as making up student culture. In speaking of a group's culture, social scientists ordinarily mean to indicate that there is some such degree of coherence and consistency between the parts which make it up. We do not make this consistency a major focus of our analysis, but we do in various places indicate the connections between perspectives held by the students. In general, this consistency arises from the fact that the perspectives have in common certain assumptions students make, so that they may be said in a sense to have been derived from common premises.

The term student culture carries a second connotation as well. It is meant to emphasize that the perspectives held by the student body are related very much to the fact that these people occupy the position of student in an institution known as a school. As occupants of such a position, students have the rights and privileges, the duties and obligations, associated with that position. Because they all occupy the same institutional position, they tend to face the same kinds of problems, and these are problems which arise out of the character of the position. We might say that the important term in the phrase "medical student" is *student*. The opportunities and disabilities of the student·role are decisive in shaping the perspectives students hold.

This, by implication, brings out a third connotation of the term student culture. While it is true that students are preparing themselves and are being prepared for a career in medicine, the decisive influences on their perspectives are not medical. They do not develop their perspectives by simply taking over such aspects of the professional culture of medicine as are relevant and applicable to medicine. They do not act as young doctors might act, but rather act as students act. This overstates the case, for certainly students organize their actions with reference to a medical future. But what is important to remember is that this is a future and, while in school, they are not doctors, do not face the problems doctors face, and consequently cannot employ the perspectives and culture of doctors. We shall have occasion later to demonstrate this point directly, in the case of students' views of patients.

Likewise, by using the term student culture, we mean to indicate that students do not simply apply those perspectives which they bring with them from their previous experience in other institutional positions. Put another way, this is to say that elements in the students' background do not exert any decisive influence on how students behave in medical school. Such background factors may have indirect influence in many ways, but the problems of the student role are so pressing and the students' initial perspectives so similar that the perspectives developed are much more apt to reflect the pressures of the immediate school situation than of ideas associated with prior roles and experiences. We shall have occasion to deal with this point in more detail when we consider the perspectives freshmen develop on their school work.

We use student culture, then, as a kind of shorthand term for the organized sum of student perspectives relevant to the student role. This culture is characteristic of the occupants of a particular position in the organization of the medical school and has both roots in that organization and major consequences for its operation.

Organization

An organization, as we think of it, consists of defined groups of people who interact with one another regularly in patterned ways. It is a structured and recurring form of collective social action. In an organization, the relations between different kinds of people are governed by the consensus that arises as to what, under the circumstances, is the best form of the relation and by the rules that arise out of that consensus. To understand the behavior of any one category of people in the organization, we must see them in their relations with other persons with whom they come in contact.

We have stressed that people in an organization act as members of defined groups or categories. In an organizational setting we seldom see another person in his total human individuality; we treat him as a member of some category commonly used in the organization to distinguish different kinds of people. To be specific, in medical school people ordinarily distinguish these categories: students, faculty, residents and interns, patients, nurses, and auxiliary personnel. The student treats those he comes in contact with as members of one or another of these groups and is treated by them as a student.

Each of these groups has its own perspective on the problems that arise out of their mutual interaction. In this report, we have been most concerned with the perspectives of students and deal with those of other groups insofar as they present problems for students, place restraints on what kinds of perspectives students develop, or provide opportunities for development of student perspectives. In particular, we have concentrated on two other groups whose actions and ideas we think have the greatest effect on student perspectives: the faculty of the medical school and the residents and interns who work in the teaching hospital.

The ideas and actions of the faculty, residents, and interns affect the students, first of all, by setting the conditions under which students' problems arise. The rules the faculty makes, the way the faculty organizes and defines the situations in which students must perform, the way the faculty interprets and applies their rules and definitions — all these constitute a major part of the environment in which students act. The faculty and others in this way create the problems to which the perspectives of student culture comprise some kind of solution. (For this reason, in describing student perspectives, we have tried always to make clear the nature of the environment in which problems and perspectives arise.)

The ideas and actions of the faculty and house staff (i.e., residents and interns) affect the development of student perspectives in a second important way. Medical schools are, even more than other kinds of schools, organized in an "authoritarian" fashion: The faculty and administration have a tremendous amount of power over the students and, in principle, can control student activities very tightly and cause students to act in whatever fashion they (the faculty) want. To the degree that the faculty actually exercises such power, students will have no opportunity to build their own perspectives and will simply take over ideas forced on them by the faculty. Conversely, to the degree that the faculty cannot and will not exercise this kind of control, students will be able to build their own perspectives, and these may diverge considerably from those the faculty would want. Later in this volume, we consider the question of how much autonomy the medical students have in building their perspectives.

Chapter 4

The University of Kansas Medical School

A Brief Description

THE School of Medicine of the University of Kansas is, in many respects, like others in the United States and Canada. Its students, like nearly all medical students in the country, have graduated from colleges of arts and sciences. All applicants take the Medical College Admissions Test (MCAT), prepared by the Educational Testing Service for the Association of American Medical Colleges. The scores of all applicants are scaled; the schools to which a student applies know exactly how he stands in comparison with all applicants. Each school also knows how its accepted applicants compare with those accepted by other schools, but that knowledge is not made public. Each school sets its own standards of admission, according to the number and quality of applicants who, if chosen, will prefer it to some other school to which they have also applied. The Medical College Admissions Test is a great standardizing force.

The Association of American Medical Colleges works in various ways to improve medical education — by research, by exchange of information, conferences of medical educators, and by publication. The license to practice medicine is granted by the states, each for itself; but a national board sets examinations which are taken by all graduates of many medical schools and by numerous individuals from others. This also serves to standardize and elevate medical training.

The curricula of medical schools are similar in length and content. Two years are devoted to the sciences considered basic to medicine, to wit: anatomy, biochemistry, physiology, pathology, pharmacology, and microbiology. In the last two years, the students are taught the clinical specialties of medicine, psychiatry, surgery, pediatrics, obstetrics, and gynecology, as well as others. In these clinical years, the students learn by participating in the diagnosis and treatment of patients as well as from lectures, demonstrations, and reading. Some schools, or departments within schools, adjust their teaching to advances in scientific knowledge and the medical arts more quickly than do others. Some experiment with the curriculum and with methods of teaching; others are more conservative. In all of the several schools of which we have personal knowledge, a running argument goes on among the faculty over these matters. In spite of differences of opinion, most schools travel in the same direction of change, although at different rates.

All medical schools live in symbiosis with a general hospital and outpatient clinics. The whole generally constitutes a medical center which trains not only physicians and medical scientists but other medical personnel — the various auxiliaries to nursing, registered nurses, therapists, technicians, and perhaps even hospital administrators.

The medical center is more and more frequently a research center. The balance of the three activities — medical practice, education, and research — varies from one center to another, as do also the administrative and financial relations. The general trend is toward more emphasis upon research. At the University of Kansas the dean of the medical school is director of a comprehensive medical center.

Medical schools are nowadays nearly all affiliated with universities. Ours is an integral part of the state university and has never existed apart from it. Like most, however, its autonomy is rather great. Some medical schools are on the campus of the university; others are located at some distance, usually in a large city where clinical material is available for use in teaching and research. Even when the medical school is on the campus, the medical faculty is likely to be something of a body apart. In our case, the first year of medicine is on a small town campus, the rest is in a large city. It is all to be moved to the city.

The relations between the organized medical profession and a medical school vary. Physicians and medical associations appear to respect the quality of work done in medical schools. But they are watchful lest the medical centers where medicine is taught compete with private practice. University medical centers have been sued by state medical associations over this issue. There may also be strain between private practitioners and the schools over emphasis on specialties. All teachers of medicine are specialists; more and more of them have their whole careers in academic medical institutions. None is a rural general practitioner; few ever have been. These tensions and relations vary by state, region, and ownership of the school. State schools have to be especially sensitive to the local and state professional organizations; the latter may be listened to by the state legislators of their districts. Some state schools, ours among them, exert great influence over the standards of medical practice in their regions and promote and conduct active programs of postgraduate education for practitioners.

We have, thus far, noted some of the dimensions along which medical schools vary. There are certain basic relationships common to all schools. The intensity of the problems arising from them vary, but the problems themselves are to be found everywhere. We believe that the kinds of behavior, the conflicts, the understandings and misunderstandings we have observed in our school, are among those to be found everywhere. The burden of proof is on any institution which says "It couldn't happen here." The particular form and the degree will certainly vary. Those variations and their correlates are important; they call for careful study.

Before going on to further placing of our school among others, let it be clear that we do not evaluate it or any other school. The crucial evidence for evaluation would have to relate to the end product of medical education, the physician and the quality of his ministrations. We have no such evidence, nor have we sought it. Furthermore, the medical schools of the country are so few in number and are such complex entities that comparative evaluation would be a monumental statistical task — a task requiring immense knowledge and superlative wisdom. The reader, however, will want to place our school in relation to others in certain easily observable respects.

Kansas is the southwesternmost state of the North Central Region.[1]

[1] The North Central region includes Indiana, Illinois, Iowa, Kansas, Michigan, Minnesota, Missouri, Nebraska, North Dakota, Ohio, South Dakota, and Wisconsin. These states vary greatly in the proportion of urban and industrial population, wealth, level of education, and other features directly or indirectly related to the number and quality of applicants to medical school. The other regions are also heterogeneous.

The applicants from this region accepted by medical schools in 1958 ranked, on the average, somewhat lower on the Medical College Admissions Test than did those of the Northeast Region; about the same as did those of the West Region; and significantly higher than did those of the South Region. Klinger and Gee,[2] in their report on applicants for 1958, conclude that the admission practices of medical schools in the North Central Region are near the national average in the weight given to MCAT scores and age.

In 1958, 156 residents of Kansas applied for admission to medical schools; of these, 97 were accepted by one or more schools. With 7.58 applications per 100,000 of population, Kansas was the twenty-ninth state in rate of applications and in the modal group of eighteen states with between 7 and 8 applications per 100,000. With 4.71 accepted applicants per 100,000 of population, Kansas was the twenty-first state in this respect, as it was in the modal group of twenty states with between 4 and 5 successful applicants per 100,000 of population.

With 62 per cent of its applicants accepted, Kansas was tied with Michigan for the twelfth and thirteenth place in this regard. Eleven states showed higher rates of acceptance; the percentage for the whole country was 55 per cent.[3] Kansas is one of twenty states which have one or more publicly owned medical schools but no private medical schools. In 1958 the median rate of acceptance of applicants for such states was 59; for states with both public and private schools it was slightly lower (58); for states without a public medical school or with no medical school at all, the rate was distinctly lower (52 and 53 per cent). According to Klinger and Gee, "The presence of a publicly owned medical school in the state appreciably enhances the probability that an applicant will be accepted." Kansas is, in this regard, typical of states which have a public medical school and no other. In 1958 Kansas ranked eighth among the states in the number of residents in first-year classes of schools of medicine and osteopathy per 100,000 population of the age of twenty; the rate was just above

[2] Eric Klinger and Helen H. Gee, "The Study of Applicants, 1958–1959," *The Journal of Medical Education.* XXXV (February, 1960), 120–33. Most of the facts reported in this section are from this article and from *Physicians for a Growing America,* Report of the Surgeon General's Consultant Group on Medical Education, U.S. Dept. of Health, Education and Welfare (Washington, D.C., 1959). (The latter is known as the Bane Report and in subsequent notes will be so designated.)

[3] Facts thus far presented are computed from Klinger and Gee, *op. cit.,* Tables 10, 3, A2, and 7.

five, that of the country just about four.[4] The rate of attendance at medical schools by residents of a state is strongly related to the number of bachelor's degrees granted to residents, to the number of places available in medical schools in the state, and to the number of physicians per 100,000 population. In bachelor's degrees, Kansas is well above the average. In 1957, with 102.4 active non-federal doctors of medicine per 100,000 of population, the state was well below the national rate of 118.4, but probably above other states equally rural (Bane Report, Appendix Table 4).

Kansas was one of the eleven states which supported medical education in 1958 with more than $0.25, but less than $0.40, per $1,000 of personal income. Eight states spent more than $0.40; twenty-nine spent less than $0.25. Kansas is in the modal group and in the upper half (Bane Report, Chart 17). All of this support presumably went to the University of Kansas Medical School, the only such school in the state.

The 156 Kansas residents who applied for admission to medical schools in 1958 placed 359 applications, or 2.3 each. Applicants from New York, Connecticut, and California placed 5.8 or more applications each. The Kansas applicant was not only fairly likely to be accepted but also to get into the school he wanted, or at least into the school of his second choice (Klinger and Gee, Table A 2).

The Medical School

Most of the students at the University of Kansas Medical School are residents of the state, and most medical students who are residents of Kansas attend it. It is distinctly a Kansas institution. In 1958, 94 new students entered the first year of the school. Ninety-seven from Kansas were in that year accepted by one or more medical schools. If 80 per cent of the new first-year students, 75 in number, were Kansans, then 22 Kansans presumably went out of the state to enter medical school; if, as is more likely, 90 per cent, 84 in number, were Kansans, then only 13 Kansans went out of the state to enter medical

[4] Bane Report. Chart 8. Although the Missouri-Iowa-Kansas region is the home of osteopathy, and although Missouri has two schools of osteopathy very close to Kansas, there is no evidence that Kansans are especially likely to study osteopathy. With 9.5 active osteopaths per 100,000 of population, Kansas was tied with Vermont for tenth and eleventh place in the country, and was above the rate for the whole country (7.6 per 100,000), but far below Missouri (27.1) and Maine (23.2). Osteopathy is far from as popular in Kansas as in the neighboring states of Colorado, Oklahoma, Missouri and Iowa. Cf. Bane Report, Appendix Table 4. There is one osteopath for every ten active, non-federal doctors in Kansas.

school.[5] The Bane Report (Appendix Table I) shows that in 1958 Kansas had fewer first-year places in medical school than the number of Kansas residents in such places. Those 16 are evidently attending schools outside the state. It seems clear that the medical students of the University of Kansas are predominantly residents of Kansas and that only a handful of Kansans go elsewhere to study medicine. The Bane Report states that average Medical College Admissions Test scores for first-year classes in 1957 and 1958 tended to be lower in schools with fewer out-of-state students than those with more such students, that schools with fewest out-of-state students had a higher proportion of withdrawals as the result of poor academic standing. A combination of less than 10 per cent of students from out-of-state with total expenditures of less than $2,000,000 for basic operations and research was associated with very low MCAT scores of the students. In a six-cell table[6] classifying medical schools into three categories according to expenditures and into two categories according as they have less than 10 per cent of students or 10 per cent or more from out of state, higher expenditures combined with more than 10 per cent of out-of-state students are favorably related with MCAT scores of students in all cells except one. Schools which spend more than $3,500,000 per annum have better students even though they have less than 10 per cent of students from outside the state. Our school falls into the middle category on expenditures, with a total of nearly $3,000,000 for 1958–59. It falls into the upper category with respect to out-of-state students, with 16 per cent from out of state.

Most public medical schools draw the overwhelming majority of their students from the supporting state. Of the 91 medical schools in the United States (including Puerto Rico) and Canada in 1956, 54 got 76 per cent or more of their students from among residents of the home state, province, or territory. Kansas is among that 54 per cent, but not among the schools which have an extremely high proportion of local students. Some states require that all students of the medical school be residents; others require nearly all to be local. Kansas is again somewhere in the middle, but probably unusually liberal in comparison with other state schools. It is generally believed, although

[5] Computed from Klinger and Gee, op. cit., Tables A 1 and A 2. There are, no doubt, minor errors in the figures given by Klinger and Gee, due to the dates on which reports are made and to varying practices of states and medical schools in reporting to the Association of American Medical Colleges. The Bane Report may also deviate slightly from the Klinger and Gee report.

[6] Bane Report. Table 9, p. 16.

it has not been proved, that residents of the state are more likely to remain within the state to practice. In contrast to the state schools, and some private schools, eight of the leading private medical schools show only 42 per cent of their entering students from the states in which the schools are situated.[7]

It does not follow that the students of state schools are academically poorer than those of private schools. It follows even less that the students of any particular state school are poorer than those of any particular private school. The medical schools of the country vary greatly in the quality of their students, as measured by MCAT scores and by the performance of the graduates in the national board examinations. Some 22 schools have students whose mean MCAT scores are 550 or above; the students of about 23 schools fall below 500. The other 40 schools fall between. Results of the national board examinations, for the graduates of 30 schools from which 90 to 100 per cent took them in 1959, range from a mean score of 85.6 with 35.6 graduates making honors and none failing from one school, to an average of 76 (barely above the failing point) with almost none making honors and 35.3 per cent failing from another.[8]

The quality of students attracted to and admitted by a school is correlated with many other variables, but the relationships are gross. Certainly some of the more famous medical schools, although none of the half-dozen most famous, are public. The proportion of medical school graduates from public schools becomes greater year by year. In 1931, only 35 per cent graduated from public schools; in 1958, 47 per cent. In the same interval, the number of graduates of public schools has increased by 94 per cent; of private schools, by 18 per cent. Approximately one-fourth of all medical graduates in 1958 were from public schools in states which, like Kansas, have no private schools.[9]

[7] Figures are computed from Klinger and Gee, op. cit., the Bane Report, from a report in the Journal of the American Medical Association, CLXXI (November 14, 1959) 1538–39, other reports, and privately given information. One must be very sceptical of the comparisons of expenditures because of various ways of calculating them. The percentage of students from in or out of the state is also a complex figure affected not only by policy but by the demographic characteristics of states. States with great cities produce many medical students for export to other states. They are also likely, as in the case of New York and Chicago, to have several medical schools which absorb many outside students as well as a large number of local applicants. We must insist that the comparisons made here are, at best, generalizations.

[8] John P. Hubbard and William V. Clemans, "A Comparative Evaluation of Medical Schools," Journal of Medical Education. XXXV (February, 1960), 134–41.

[9] Bane Report. Appendix Table 10, and other sources.

It is evident that the publicly owned schools will produce an ever greater share of the nation's physicians. If they continue to restrict enrolment rather closely to residents of the state, the trend to public schools might reduce nationwide competition for the best students. But there are many trends which work toward general increase in the quality of medical students and education. For one thing, the public schools will probably have more money available for basic operations and research. Medical curricula and pedagogy are the object of greater attention than ever, and many improvements are being made. However that may be, the medical school of the University of Kansas is, in most of the characteristics that are easily measured, a standard school, one of many and of a type which will become even more numerous. Its students compare well with those in the majority of the good medical schools of the country. There is no reason to believe that their conduct in medical school differs markedly from that of other medical students.

We have thus far said little about this school as a particular enterprise.

When proprietary medical schools flourished elsewhere, they also flourished, although rather uncertainly, in Kansas. Like population and cities, they were concentrated in the northeastern corner of the state in the neighborhood of Kansas City, Missouri, and its satellite, Kansas City, Kansas. Eventually a two-year school of medical sciences was established in the small, proud university town of Lawrence, about forty miles from Kansas City. Later, in 1905, a clinical school was founded in a hospital in Rosedale, adjacent to Kansas City, Kansas. Two schools in Kansas City, Missouri, joined in the forming of the new university school.[10]

The then chancellor of the university declared that it was time for Kansas to build the best medical school between Chicago and San Francisco. His view was not shared by many of the physicians of Topeka and Wichita, the two cities of such size as to consider themselves fit centers for the state medical school.[11] As Thomas N. Bonner

[10] For history of the school, we rely largely on Thomas N. Bonner, *The Kansas Doctor: A Century of Pioneering* (Lawrence, Kansas: University of Kansas Press, 1959).

[11] The region of which Kansas City, Missouri, is the dominant center extends only a short way east into Missouri but for many hundreds of miles west and southwest through Kansas and other states. St. Louis has been the center of medical education in Missouri, with two private medical schools. When the state of Missouri finally established a four-year medical school, the chosen site was neither of its two contending

says in his history of medicine in Kansas, the physicians of the state did not relish the knowledge that three-fourths of the faculty of the new state school lived in Missouri.

When, in 1911, Abraham Flexner made his famous grand rounds of medical schools, he reported that the University of Kansas had two half-schools, a competent scientific school in Lawrence and an inadequate, isolated clinical school in Rosedale. He commented that "No administration, let alone a divided one, could exert authority over unsalaried practitioners who gave only a small fraction of their time to the school." [12]

In the twenties, an energetic dean moved the clinical part of the school to the present site where it has grown into a major medical center. He also brought in a consultant who, after study, recommended new buildings, a long-range plan for unifying the school in Kansas City, and "continuance of the policy of hiring the best clinical men available, whether resident in Kansas or Missouri." But that dean was soon fired by the governor of Kansas, apparently in a new outburst of reaction to the interstate character of the staff and to the new policy of paying salaries to clinical men when there were many willing to give their time free. Bonner reports that in 1929–30 half of the Kansas residents who studied medicine still did so outside the state.

Thus did our school suffer the ills and struggles characteristic of nearly all which have survived into this new day of medical education. Progress continued to be made in spite of the setback of the twenties. A great renaissance came with the appointment of Dr. Franklin D. Murphy [13] as dean in the late forties. Since then the physical plant has doubled in size as has also the number of patients annually treated at the center. The full-time staff has been multiplied by more than five; it consists more and more of promising medical scientists and clinicians picked competitively in the national market.

large cities but the small university town of Columbia in the middle of the state. State patriotism and the tension between cities and the country enter a good deal into medical, as into other, politics. In the case of Kansas, the matter is complicated further by the fact that a large and growing number of the upper-middle-class suburbs of Kansas City lie in Kansas. A considerable proportion of the students of the state university of this predominantly and self-consciously rural state are children of business and professional people whose work is in Missouri.

[12] Ibid., p. 147.

[13] Dr. Murphy was appointed chancellor of the university a few years later. His successor, Dr. W. Clark Wescoe, has continued the march toward progress with great energy, and has lately succeeded Dr. Murphy as chancellor. Dr. C. Arden Miller is the new dean. We are indebted to all of them for their support of this study.

The regular faculty has been put on "geographic full-time." Those
who are clinicians may and do have private, paying patients; but the
patients must be referred by physicians or agencies outside. The staff
physician has no office outside, and all of his cases are teaching cases.
Staff members have no competing practice outside the medical school
and center. Those staff members who are primarily medical scientists
are on salary and do all of their work in the laboratories and clinics
of the center.

These very changes have, oddly enough, brought the school closer
than it has ever been to the practitioners out in the state. For these
changes include a plan of training for general practice, which uses
selected general practitioners in rural communities, and a vigorous
program of postgraduate education both at the center and out in the
state.

The Faculty

In 1956–57, the faculty consisted of 332 persons, of whom 118 were
full-time. As in most medical schools, a large part-time staff, consisting of physicians practicing elsewhere in the city, participated in
various ways in the teaching program. They gave occasional lectures
or participated in small discussion-conferences with students. Most
frequently, they served in the hospital's outpatient departments,
supervising the work of the students in the clinics.

The full-time faculty, who spend most time with the students and
have control over the curriculum, differ from the part-time faculty
in several ways. Most of the part-time faculty were trained at the
University of Kansas, at Washington University in St. Louis, or at
one of the other schools nearby; they are men of the region who have
taken their places in its indigenous medical system. The full-time
faculty also contain men of this type; some of the most distinguished
members were trained in Kansas. But a sizable proportion of the
faculty, particularly the new department chairmen and the younger
men they have brought into their departments, are of the newer
breed of academic medical men who may move from one medical
center to another.

The full-time faculty, almost to a man, differ radically from the
part-time faculty (and from most other medical practitioners) in having had little experience of the practice of medicine outside teaching
institutions. While most medical practice in the region is carried on in
conventional style — an individual practitioner or group of practi-

tioners practicing apart from an institutional setting — few members of the full-time faculty have ever engaged in this kind of practice. The majority of the faculty, after completing their residencies, immediately began an association with medical schools which has been interrupted only by service in the armed forces.

One segment of the faculty differs even more radically from the average medical practitioner of the region (and in this Kansas resembles all other medical schools). The basic sciences of the first two years, excepting pathology, are taught almost entirely by nonmedical people, by scientists with Ph.D. degrees rather than physicians with M.D. degrees.

Members of the faculty have many responsibilities. In addition to teaching, many engage in research. The clinical teachers, who are physicians, train residents; the scientists train graduate students. The physicians also treat patients. All sections of the full-time faculty co-operate in setting up the formal rules by which the school is run. As members of committees on admissions, curriculum, and the like, they work out the series of courses students will take, the order in which they will be taken, and so on. A good deal of discretion is left to the departments as to how individual sections of the curriculum will be taught; neither the dean, his staff, nor the various faculty committees intervene in the internal operations of the departments, beyond organizing a basic schedule and curriculum and setting up a standard form in which grades are reported for individual students.

The Students

The medical students of the University of Kansas are a homogeneous body. To say that they are young, white, male, Protestant, small-town native Kansans who are married describes a very sizable majority of the entire student body. They are what they are not because of any policy other than that of taking most of each class from the state. In what follows we quantify this description somewhat, giving simple percentages based on a random sample of 62 medical students who were interviewed.

Most of the students are in their early twenties; the median age of the freshmen was twenty-three, that of the seniors twenty-five. About 20 per cent of the students in each class are older, in their very late twenties or early thirties. (The school will ordinarily not accept as a freshman anyone over the age of thirty.) The students' youth is again indicated by the fact that the education of 41 of the 62 interviewees had not been interrupted by military service or by work; these students had gone straight from college into medical school.

The overwhelming majority of students are men, but each class contains a number of women, ordinarily around five. Similarly, the overwhelming majority of students are native-born and white. Each class will contain a few students from such faraway places as Central America or Africa, as well as a small number of American Negroes, possibly four or five. The small numbers of women and Negroes do not reflect any intent to discriminate. The school gets very few applicants of either category.

The religious affiliations of the students accurately reflect those of the population of the state of Kansas. Our sample of 62 students included one Jew, five Catholics, and one who admitted to no religion at all. The remaining 55 students were Protestants. Of these, five belonged to such sectarian groups as the Mennonites; the others belonged to more conventional denominations.

Forty-five of the 62 students had been raised in the state of Kansas; seven more came from nearby Missouri. Only ten came from elsewhere, and of these about half came from neighboring plains states and half from the east or west coasts. Thirty-three of the 62 students had been raised in rural areas; but of the 29 raised in urban areas, many came from small towns in Kansas, Missouri, and neighboring states, towns of perhaps 10,000–20,000 people.

Thirty-nine of our 62 interviewees were married and, as might be expected, the proportion increases with each succeeding year in school. Eight of 19 freshmen interviewed and 13 of 14 seniors were married. Though the percentage varies from year to year, 85 to 90 per cent of each graduating class is married.

Tables I and II, giving the education and occupations of students' fathers, indicate that students come from predominantly middle-class homes. But these tables also show that the fathers of 17 students did not complete high school and that 18 fathers were laborers, skilled workmen, or farmers. We cannot say that the students are entirely of middle-class origin.

Nevertheless, the students are quite homogeneous in their present, and will be more so in their future, social class affiliations. Though they may have come from lowly origins — the industrial slums of a large metropolitan area or a subsistence farm in Kansas — they have all graduated from college and, furthermore, are all on their way to one of the most prestigeful occupational statuses in American society.

TABLE I

EDUCATION OF STUDENTS' FATHERS

EDUCATION	NUMBER OF FATHERS	TOTAL
	N 62	
Don't know	1	
Some grade school	6	
Grade school graduate	3	
Some high school	7	
High school graduate..........	9	
Some college	7	
		33
College graduate	6	
Some graduate work	1	
M.A.	3	
Ph.D.	2	
M.D.	12*	
Other professional degree......	5	
		29
Total		62

* One also has an M.A.

TABLE II

OCCUPATIONS OF STUDENTS' FATHERS

OCCUPATIONS	NUMBER OF FATHERS
	N 62
Medicine	12*
Other professions	10†
Farmer	11
Executive	3
Self-employed businessman	7
White-collar worker	8
Salesman	4
Skilled worker	3
Laborer	4
Total	62

* One also teaches.
† One also farms during the summer.

Their college experience has taught them middle-class ways, and they look forward to the upper-middle-class existence of the successful physician.

Kansas students are perhaps more likely to enter the middle class in this way than students who have lived their lives in such a giant metropolis as New York or Chicago. In these enormous urban centers, it is possible for a student to attend college and medical school while continuing to live his extracurricular life in a lower-class or ethnic enclave. Such a student is shaped by his origins far more than the Kansas student who leaves his family behind to attend the state university.

Kansas students are also provincial, particularly with respect to their educational backgrounds. They have had little experience or knowledge of the world of higher education beyond their immediate geographical region. Forty-four of our 62 interviewees got their college training in an institution supported by the state of Kansas. Twenty-five went to the University of Kansas; seven attended Kansas State University (the land-grant institution), and twelve more came from the smaller state institutions which were once teachers' colleges. Fifteen students got their training in the small colleges so characteristic of the region: private institutions, often affiliated closely with some Protestant denomination, serving from 200 to 800 or 900 students. Only three of our interviewees went to "eastern" schools; two of these men were from the east coast themselves.

This educational provinciality shows up in another striking statistic. College students who want to go to medical school often apply to a great many schools and to schools of many different kinds. They may apply to several of the best-known schools, to two or three in their immediate vicinity, and to a few whose standards are supposed to be lower. In this way they aim for the best but take out insurance in the form of applications to more accessible schools. Students whose grades are not outstanding may not bother to apply to the "best" schools but will scatter their applications among several schools where they think they might have a chance. The number and kinds of schools to which students apply may fairly be said to give some indication of the breadth of their horizons.

Thirty-five of our 62 interviewees applied only to the University of Kansas Medical School. Of the remaining 27 students, nine had applied to one or more neighboring state schools. Only 18 considered applying to any of the more nationally known schools, and even these choices tended (though not completely) to be restricted to such nearby schools as Washington University at St. Louis.

Kansas students also had a constricted view of the possible professional futures open to them. With few exceptions, they had no intention of going into any kind of scientific or clinical research career and showed no interest in the academic side of the medical profession. Only three of our interviewees expressed any interest in a research career, and only five would consider a full-time position in a medical school. In short, the only kind of career they envision for themselves is in the private practice of medicine. Within this area, they are very likely to think of themselves as general practitioners. When we asked our interviewees what kind of practice they thought they would enter, 24 of the 62 said general practice; four did not know; and only a few of the 34 who thought they would have a specialty practice could specify which specialty they had in mind. The point is that, having no clear view of the kind of medicine they would practice, students (as we shall see in some detail in the next section of this book) had no easy way of deciding what knowledge was important for them to acquire. To say that one intends to have a general practice means that one must learn everything he possibly can, for no one can tell what a general practitioner may be called on to treat. Similarly, to say that one will specialize without knowing in what area that specialization will be also means that one must learn everything. In contrast, we might suppose that a student who entered school with a firm intention to become a cardiologist, let us say, would be better able to pick and choose what he would need to know, using as a criterion the relevance of any bit of knowledge to the practice of cardiology. Because this vagueness about the future is most often expressed in the intention to become a general practitioner, we might refer to it as the "prospective G.P." perspective.

We are to describe the perspectives on their study, their future work, and their careers developed by a group of intelligent, provincial young Kansans homogeneous as to background and alike in purpose. They attend a medical school which, although closely bound to its state and region, aspires to high standards and a wider reputation; a school whose faculty consists of men, all specialists and many of them trained in the best-known schools of the country, who are not fully familiar with the kind of practice towards which most of the students are headed. We write in the conviction that the way in which these young men develop their perspectives on their present and future is, in its essentials, like that in which other medical students develop theirs.

Part Two:

STUDENT CULTURE
IN THE FRESHMAN YEAR

Chapter 5

The Long-Range Perspective

"Best of All Professions"

Eᴠᴇʀʏ group has choices and decisions to make in a new environment. Its members go through a learning process in which they define their situation sufficiently, although often inaccurately, to be able to adopt what seems to them appropriate behavior. In some instances there may be little definition beyond a glancing recognition that the new situation is similar to an old one and previously learned behavior will suffice. At other times, beginners may find the new environment so different from any they have experienced before that the understanding necessary to deal with it comes slowly or not at all.

If we shift our focus from the entrants to the social system being entered, we call those features of the system which entrants see as demanding choices on their part or new forms of behavior, "problems." This usage of the word does not carry any implication that either the social system or its entrants are at fault, but simply points to the fact that beginning involves choices and changes in behavior. Thus, when we began our study of the freshmen we expected them, no matter how well-prepared or well-oriented, to have problems.

In later chapters in this section on the freshmen we present the perspectives, the co-ordinated patterns of ideas and actions, that students develop in attempting to solve the problems they see in their new environment. We learn about these perspectives from what the students tell us and from what we see them do. As observers, present on the scene while students are developing and using these perspectives, we can also describe the social system the students enter and the general environment it provides them with, as well as some of the particular situations they encounter. Thus, we present each perspective in its situational context, for we think that much of the instrumental behavior a group displays is best understood in relation to the immediate social setting in which it takes place.

While an effort to explore the relationship between perspective and situation has been one of our chief concerns in this study, and we are thus most often concerned with what Mead calls the "knife-edge" present, immediate situations are easier to understand when we know something of their relation to the larger environment provided by the social system of which they are a part. Similarly, our understanding of the behavior of a group is enhanced by knowledge of its antecedents and the purposes and expectations its members hold in common. Thus, we preface our findings on the students' situational perspectives with what data we have on their attitudes toward medicine and the medical profession, their long-range perspective, in the first chapter of this section; and describe the medical school environment in a second chapter. The social background of the student body has already been discussed.

With the exception of these introductory chapters which contain material applicable to subsequent chapters, our analysis of the freshman year takes a narrative form. It is divided into three parts: the initial perspective characteristic of the period from the beginning of school until shortly before the first major examinations, a provisional perspective characteristic of the period just before and during the examinations, and a final perspective in use for the remainder of the year. The three perspectives are successive attempts of the students to solve one central and persistent problem: the proper level and direction of effort in academic work.

Although we were studying a school, we did not anticipate that the freshmen's major problem would be their academic work, and that their concern about studying would be so great as to overshadow all other problems. Since we were committed to theory and methodology that required us to focus our interest on the students' major concerns rather than our own, we followed the students' lead. The data that forced our choice appears in the chapters to come.

One further note: although we make some use of interviews with a random sample of students, nineteen of whom were freshmen of the class observed, data for these chapters were collected largely by participant observation. We began the day the freshmen arrived and continued almost daily through the first two months of the fall semester. Thereafter, we observed for periods of two or three days during November, January, February, and March, and September of the following year. These visits were timed to coincide with major examinations, the change of semester, and other events of the school year we thought might prove important to an understanding of student perspectives.

It may not be immediately apparent why we choose to call the general notions about medicine and the medical profession that freshmen bring to medical school their "long-range perspective." Ordinarily, such general notions are called values, attitudes, orientations, motives, or other terms. When social scientists question people about these things it is usually without reference to behavior in actual situations; but a direct relationship, often a causal one, between values and action is suggested or predicted. Since for the moment we want to put aside questions about the relationship of values to action, we use the term "long-range perspective" because it does not imply causality and is reasonably accurate shorthand for our subject matter.

When students pause to take up a mental stance outside the present knife-edge of their experience and think of medicine, the medical profession, and their goals within it, their mental vision embraces the social space of the medical school and the even wider reaches of the profession beyond. They use a wide-angle lens. Similarly, their thought refers to many years which they lump together in time. The wideness of their vision and their lack of experience with what they are thinking about preclude detail. Their long-range perspective may be emotionally intense, but it is necessarily vague. Thus, according to our definition, a long-range perspective is the mental process of describing a relatively broad area of social space (an entire profession or school career) extending over an indefinite period of time, usually several years. The description is general; it has little detail. It is accompanied by a goal which the thinker wishes to reach over time within the social space he describes, but it does not specify in detail the kind of action necessary to achieve the goal. The long-range perspective that we deal with in this book is part of the collective behavior of a group.

Such a perspective has another property, not always apparent to its possessors but frequently of interest to people outside the group: it can be called idealistic, cynical, or pragmatic. There are undoubtedly other evaluative adjectives applied by one group to another's long-range perspective, but we confine ourselves to these since they came up frequently when the medical school faculty discussed students with us.

At first glance, it may appear axiomatic for students to begin medical training in an idealistic frame of mind. Americans commonly approve of high ideals in novices and expect people embarking on a long and difficult course of action that entails deferred satisfaction to justify their choice high-mindedly. Nevertheless, a self-seeking perspective may exist, although it may be more difficult to maintain if the social system being entered is commonly thought of as requiring idealism of its members. For example, students might have a long-range perspective defining medicine as primarily a get-rich profession and take money-making as their goal. Or, they might see medicine as a field for research rather than for practice, and want the M.D. to get prestige or access to hospital resources. We can think of other long-range perspectives that would not be idealistic about the practice of medicine. Thus, while we may expect the long-range perspective of the freshmen to be vague by definition, we can have no expectation as to whether it may be characterized as idealistic, cynical, or pragmatic (by us or any other group) without reference to the student group itself and the influences to which it is exposed before coming to school or early in the freshman year.

What about the entering students? Are they likely to be idealistic about medicine or to view it from some other standpoint less consonant with current notions of what is proper for members of the service professions? From the data given in Part I on the social characteristics of the student body, we know that typically they are native Midwesterners raised in small towns or rural areas, whose origins and present status are middle class. Their educational experience and horizons are largely confined to Kansas and neighboring states. It is an homogeneous group which, if not provincial, is scarcely cosmopolitan. The students mirror the local population accurately. Given this similarity, can we expect the freshmen to have the diffuse and idealistic views of medicine current in the general population?

If the freshmen can be shown *not* to have sources of information about medicine more detailed than those of the layman, the answer to this question is "yes." From our interviews with a random sample of students in all years, nineteen of whom were freshmen of the year observed, we find that 48 per cent have parents or other relatives who practice medicine and 23 per cent have been friendly with their family doctor or have friends who are physicians. Thus, 71 per cent of the sample have had some contact with members of the profession. But in answer to the question: Have you learned anything about what medicine is really like from talking to such people? 68 per cent answer "little or nothing," and of the twenty students (32%) who answer "yes," three gained their knowledge from working in a hospital before coming to school. Thus, according to the students themselves, the knowledge they have before entrance is of the general nature people pick up from being patients, reading books, and seeing movies.

At the beginning of our study we thought that advanced students might provide freshmen with another source of information. This turned out not to be the case, not only because students take the first year on the university campus forty miles from the medical center where the others are, but also because the freshmen report that information from other students is seldom useful; that it is either too general, and thus not much more helpful than that from the lay culture, or refers to situations students have not as yet met.

In later chapters, we will see that freshmen make use of their experience in college in solving some of the immediate problems of getting along in medical school, particularly in dealing with the faculty. (Everyone learns techniques for this in the course of sixteen years of schooling.) But college does not provide courses in what occupations or professional schools are like. Training in basic science does not supply this lack as it is oriented toward research rather than medicine. Rightly or wrongly, a college education probably gives premedical students little more knowledge of what it is to be a doctor than the lay culture. If we thus rule out the possible sources of detailed information, we may conclude that freshmen at the school we studied are likely to have an unspecific picture in their minds of what is before them, a picture not very different from that held by laymen. We thus expect the freshmen to share the popular notion that although some doctors are said to be more interested in fees than they should be, most physicians are the idealistic benefactors of humanity, both hard-working and selfless in their efforts to help the sick.

In our field work we found this was indeed the case: the long-range perspective of the freshmen is both unspecific and idealistic. Their images of the future are peopled with featureless patients, occasionally with other physicians, but most frequently with the student himself in the role of the ideal physician he hopes to become. They do not often put the perspective into words or act on it directly, but, in spite of the difficulties of observation, we were constantly, if somewhat indistinctly, aware of the idealism of the students' definition of medicine and the medical profession, of their goals for themselves as physicians, and of their approach to the first months of medical school.

We present the content of the long-range perspective first in brief summary and illustrate it with excerpts from our field notes. We then present what evidence we have that students held these idealistic long-range views.

We find in our field notes a number of statements of the long-range perspective made by the students. We summarize their statements as follows:

1. Medicine is the best of all professions.

2. When we begin to practice, we want to help people, have enjoyable and satisfying work while upholding medical ideals. We want to earn enough money to lead comfortable lives, but this is not our primary concern. (Note that this implies an unquestioned assumption by the students that they will practice, rather than enter research.)

In the following pages we present a few of the incidents recorded in our field notes from which we derive this summary. In the first excerpt, a student speaks of medicine as a peerless profession, one so high in prestige that to do any other sort of work is necessarily to come down in the world:

After anatomy lab I stayed with Harvey Stone while he was scrubbing up. Harvey said, "You know we were talking it over at the [fraternity] house last night. We were wondering what it would be like to flunk out of medical school. I just can't imagine it because if you went back home everybody would say you had failed." I said, "Do you think it is more important than flunking out of other schools?" Harvey said, "Oh, yes. You know medical school is a kind of little plateau; it's the very tops in most people's minds. . . . I think it would be harder to go back and face all those people talking about you than it would be to stick it out here even if you were pretty unhappy here. I don't think many people have the guts to take social pressure of that kind. We've got so much at stake here it really isn't funny."

(October 2, 1956. Married fraternity man.)

Although there may be one or two students in each class merely "trying on" medicine, most of the freshmen arrive firmly committed to it as a career and expecting to go into practice. They see themselves as having offices and patients when they graduate. As we shall see, this definition of their future remains with them through school and influences their other perspectives.

In the next excerpt a student makes this point in different words, adding an image of the medical profession, or rather of his life as student and future physician, as continuous and arduous achievement:

At dinner at his fraternity house Sam Watson said he liked to test his concepts by making pictures of them in his mind. I asked him how he would feel if he flunked out. He said, "Oh, I guess I would be very angry." Then he began to think about it and said, "Well, I guess it would be pretty hard to go back home and face the people. I think that would be very difficult." I said, "Do you think it would be more difficult than flunking out of any other school?" Sam said, "Yes, I do. You see medical school is like a dream. Now if you were in law school and flunked out you could very easily go into some business course and make out just as well, but once you started in medicine you couldn't work in any small part of medicine because you never would be satisfied. I have a picture for that. Medical school is like a stairway and I am standing on a stair and it is about three feet high and I am normal size, but I just look at this one stair. I can see the ones above but the thing I have to do is get up this step right now — this one step, and I can't really do anything about the ones above me. I think all of life is a stairway and I hope there will never be anytime when you come out on any platform at the top. I like to think that we could always look upward and never have to look down. I think we do. I think when you get to the top when you get your degree, you don't look back on what you have done, you look ahead again."

(October 2, 1956. Single fraternity man.)

If the student of the first excerpt saw medicine as a great plateau high above all other professions, this one sees himself standing at the bottom of a grand stairway with such high steps he can barely clamber up; the next step is above his head; he must devote all his energies to the one he is on. He thinks this harrowing process will be endlessly repeated, but there are great rewards: to climb two steps is to become someone unimaginably accomplished.

In both of these illustrations students speak to the first point we made in our summary — medicine is the best of all professions. In our next excerpts from the field notes, students talk about medical practice with equal idealism:

I walked back from the Union to Haworth Hall with Al Jones. He told me he had done work in a hospital with pre-op cases. He said he had not gotten to do a great deal in surgery beyond getting instruments for the doctor and preparing patients physically and mentally for their operations. I said, "Does this mean you want to be a surgeon?" He replied, "Well, I'm very idealistic about medicine. I feel very strongly about medical ethics. I don't know yet because I haven't seen enough, but I don't want to be a surgeon if I'm going to mess up anything. I've seen some of these guys in hospitals messing things up. Money is the worst thing in medicine, if you want to know what I think."

(September 14, 1956. Married independent.)

The student takes it for granted that he will practice. He will be idealistic about it and only do what he knows he can do, even if it means passing up good money. This attitude toward money comes up frequently in the students' talk. They are uncomfortably aware that many people think doctors are only out for a fee. The following incident in class later provoked several students into voicing their ideals:

In his opening lecture Brown, a preclinical teacher, wound up by defending his subject. He said that the human body is a wonderful thing and expatiated on this. Then he asked for questions; there were none. He said, "Now any time you don't understand something I say, raise your hand. It's no reflection on you; it's a reflection on me. It means Brown is not doing his job. We're trying to give you the things applicable to the practice of medicine. This is your job as future physicians. I'm not up here making apologies for what I'm saying. The human body *is* a wonderful thing. It puts rocks in your pockets, for instance, when you're sitting up there in New York in your office on the sixteenth floor."

(September 19, 1956.)

This was intended as a joke but some of the students took offense:

I was with three students, Hap Garrett, Al Jones, and Ken Thomas, who were arguing about whether or not the faculty should give grades. Hap said, "I don't think the guys would work without competition. Lots of them just want to learn enough to get through and they need more than that to be a successful physician." I said, "What is a successful physician?" Hap said, "Well, I *don't* mean what Brown said about rocks in your pockets. Guys I know can't stand him for saying that. For me it's to know enough to handle my practice, but of course, I don't know what that is yet." Al said vehemently, "It's to be dedicated to the practice of medicine."

(October 1, 1956. Three married independents.)

It is clear that the students are not using the word "successful" here in a worldly sense; "ideal" is closer to their meaning. They think practicing medicine will take even more knowledge than school requires of them.

We asked students in different living-groups about their idea of the successful physician:

Having coffee in the basement of Strong with Phil Lee and Dick Porter, I said, "Yesterday some of the guys were talking about their ideas of a successful physician. Have you got any ideas about that?" Phil said, "Gee, that is a good question." Dick said, "Boy, it sure is. I haven't thought about that. I don't think it's money though. I don't think that is the only thing." Phil said, "I don't think money has anything to do with it." Dick said, "I thing it's more of a matter of whether you can use all your knowledge, your medical knowledge, in your practice." Phil said, "Well, I think being in the position to help people is important too, but it's hard for us to say about this now."

(October 2, 1956. Two single fraternity men.)

At the Union I had coffee with Tom Arnold, Bud Jansen, and Harold Murphy. I asked them the question about the successful physician. Tom said, "Gee, I don't know what I think about that." Bud shook his head over it too but presently said, "I don't think it's the question of money but I just want enough to live on." Harold said, "You can make enough to live on in some other job. You don't have to come in to medicine for that." Bud said, "Sure, but I wouldn't be happy digging ditches, for instance. I think you have to have some kind of work that is satisfying. I think a physician's work should be self-satisfying to him; I mean he ought to enjoy what he's doing." Harold said, "I feel the same way; I think these guys that go into ditchdigging didn't really want to do that, but once they get in it they haven't much complaint. They might as well do that as something else. The thing I don't like is having to punch a timecard." Tom said, "I know one thing, I wouldn't want to drive a truck for a living, although you can make a lot of money and it's exciting sometimes."

(October 16, 1956. One married independent, two fraternity men.)

In addition to endeavoring to refute the popular image of the physician as money-grubbing, these students talk about serving people, the satisfaction of using knowledge, and enjoying their work. They think practicing medicine will give them the freedom to do their best. If we use the word "idealistic" in its common, everyday sense, all these images of themselves as future physicians are idealistic. Although the students' expression of the long-range perspective varies in detail and articulateness, they always take it for granted that they will practice.

What evidence do we have that this idealistic view of medicine and future practice is characteristic of medical students as they begin the first year? Table III shows the number of statements students made expressing the long-range perspective and the circumstances under which we obtained them. We distinguish between statements volunteered to the observer and those made in answer to the observer's question, since it is more likely that the former express the student point of view. We also distinguish statements made to the observer alone from those made in the presence of other students. The former may express personal views not shared by other students, but the latter, by the very fact that students felt free to make them in the presence of their fellows and what was said was understood and not questioned, carry more weight as expressions of a perspective students share.

TABLE III

STATEMENTS OF THE LONG-RANGE PERSPECTIVE CLASSIFIED BY
THOSE PRESENT AND WHETHER VOLUNTEERED OR DIRECTED
(First Semester, 1956)

STATEMENTS	VOLUNTEERED	DIRECTED	TOTAL
To observer alone..........	6	0	6
To others in every-day conversation..........	5	6	11
Total	11	6	17

We have altogether only seventeen expressions of the perspective. Six students speak to the observer alone, eleven speak in the presence of other students who tacitly accept what is said by making no objections. The statements are not confined to any group or groups in the class.

Seventeen items, however, from a class of 104 students is not enough to be convincing. Why then were the observers convinced that the students were idealistic, that no other general perspective on medicine was characteristic of them?

In answer to this question, what must be least acceptable to a critic was most convincing to the observers in the field: a piling up of detailed experiences with students that made it difficult to think of them as not having an idealistic long-range perspective. They communicated it by gesture and tone of voice and the innumerable other nuances of human interaction impossible to record or quantify.

Furthermore, the lack of explicit expression of the long-range perspective does not necessarily mean that it was not widely held by members of the class. In the first place, the homogeneity of the student body in background, religion, and many other factors mentioned in Part I suggests that an hypothesis that students entered with similar long-range views of medicine is likely. In the 1956 freshman class we studied, 87 per cent of the students were from the Midwest area, nearly all of these from Kansas or adjacent states. Seventy-four per cent of this group were from towns of less than 10,000 people. In the second place, students were so overwhelmed with work they seldom stopped to talk about general things; they were fully occupied with the task at hand. Interested at the time in discovering what students talked about most as an indication of what was important to them, the observers were afraid of influencing the students and asked few general questions. It is therefore not surprising that there are so few expressions of the long-range perspective. The fact that both students and observer were most concerned with immediate events is enough to explain it. It is also true that no student expressed a long-range perspective that was other than idealistic.

In addition to the field data, we have material from interviews with a random sample of students, nineteen of them freshmen. We asked two questions bearing on the degree of commitment to medicine. Table IV shows during what years in school students decide to go

TABLE IV
How Did You Happen to Choose Medicine?
(Random Sample of 62 Students: Spring, 1957)

RESPONSE	NUMBER	PER CENT
"As a child," "long ago," in grammar school	20	32.3
In junior high school or high school	25	40.3
In college or later	17	27.4
	62	100.0

into medicine. Seventy-three per cent decide on medicine before leaving high school. Table V shows how many students would make the same decision again. All nineteen freshmen in the sample answered affirmatively. Taken together the two tables suggest that most of the medical students we studied are committed to their profession. Freshmen in the sample, the class we did the field work on, do not differ from the other classes.

TABLE V

IF YOU HAD IT TO DO OVER AGAIN AND KNEW WHAT YOU KNOW NOW,
WOULD YOU GO TO MEDICAL SCHOOL?
(Random Sample of 62 Students: Spring, 1957)

RESPONSE	NUMBER	PER CENT
Yes	57	93.4
Unsure	2	3.3
No	2*	3.3
	61†	100.0

* Both seniors.
† One student not asked through oversight.

The interviews also provide data on how the students characterize the successful physician. Table VI gives the answers of students who entered school in the fall of 1956.

TABLE VI

WHAT IS YOUR IDEA OF A SUCCESSFUL PHYSICIAN?
(Random Sample of 19 Freshmen: Spring, 1957)

RESPONSE	NUMBER	PER CENT *
Medical skill and knowledge	17	89
Money secondary	4	21
Respect from communitiy or patients	3	16
Personal satisfaction	2	10
Getting along with patients	2	10
A large practice	2	10
A comfortable living	2	10
Miscellaneous	3	16

* Since nearly every student gave more than one answer, these figures total more than 100.

If we consider only the first two characteristics idealistic, eighteen students give at least one answer consistent with the long-range perspective. Seventeen say medical skill or knowledge is necessary to success. Of the four who say money is secondary, three also give the first characteristic, the fourth does not, but since the unimportance of money is one of the major propositions of the perspective, we consider this student idealistic.

Of those who speak of medical skill and knowledge, five mention curing people or helping them. One thinks a successful physician is one who contributes to medicine. Two speak of realizing one's limitations and not wasting the patient's money, that is, not attempting for reasons of pride or money to do things for a patient that cannot be done or that another physician, probably a specialist, could do better. A successful physician does the best possible job medically; he does not make mistakes. Seven simply say the successful practitioner has medical skill and knowledge, without going into details. One says such a man has the respect of his colleagues, and we may presume that this is because he is skilled. These are all idealistic notions, surprisingly similar to those of the advanced students we interviewed, although much less detailed.

The interviews indicate that the freshmen held an idealistic long-range perspective on medicine. But we did the interviews in the spring, and they cannot be used to show that freshmen were idealistic on entering school. We have no reason to suppose they changed their views, however, and every reason, as we shall see in the next chapters, to think they might have been less idealistic in the spring than in the fall.

With data from the interviews thus supporting the field work, we conclude that freshmen enter medical school full of enthusiasm, pride, and idealism about the medical profession. For many it is the realization of a dream, a day they have been looking forward to since childhood. They have worked hard to get in, are proud to have been accepted, and find it difficult to imagine themselves anything else but future practitioners.

Chapter 6 # The Work of the Freshman Year

IN this chapter we describe the salient features of the
school environment to which entering medical students bring their
idealistic long-range perspective. Following Homans, we use the term
environment in a broad way, including in it physical, technical, and
social dimensions. The physical environment of the medical school
includes buildings, classrooms, laboratories, and the campus. The
technical environment comprises all the apparatus of teaching and
learning: cadavers, books, schedules, courses, and knowledge. The
social environment consists of whatever groups work in the medical
school: faculty, graduate assistants, and students.

We try to keep faculty and student perspectives out of our description — to put things down solely from the observer's viewpoint. To do
so may give the environment a static quality that we do not intend,
since it plays such an active part in the perspectives the students
develop after they begin school. The environment, and the particular
situations within it, forces on students certain choices of perspective
and suggests others. It thus sets part of the conditions necessary for
the development of student culture. We believe, for instance, that
quite a different student culture would arise in a liberal arts college
where students follow a variety of academic programs from the one
we observed in the medical school where all students take the same
work. But when we look at the way the medical school environment
is structured and talk about the demands on the students made by its
particular form of organization and the constraints it puts on their
behavior, we must remember that the environment does not exist for

any of the groups engaged with it in the abstract way we describe it. Instead, it is always seen through the eyes of a specific group. The faculty, with its own set of perspectives or culture, understands it in one way, the students, with their idealistic long-range perspective, in another.

The first year studies are preclinical; all the work is in the sciences basic to medicine. Students take an integrated course in the morphology and function of the normal human body. The subjects covered are anatomy, neurology, physiology, biochemistry, and introductory psychiatry. During the year students dissect a cadaver, perform chemical and animal experiments, and study textbooks, but they have no hospital training or experiences with patients.

The student gets an over-all view of what he is going to do from an outline of the year given out during Orientation Week.[1] At the same time he receives a detailed schedule of the first semester. This gives him lecture topics, exactly what is to be covered in laboratory periods, and the dates of examinations. There are no electives; the entire class follows a schedule of lectures and labs from 8:00 A.M. until 5:00 P.M., five days a week. The day begins with a lecture lasting an hour or two; the actual time is up to the instructor. Lecture content is usually related to the lab which follows immediately after it and lasts until noon. From noon until 1:00 P.M. students are free for lunch, then the schedule repeats itself with a lecture and a lab period until 5:00 P.M. Occasionally there is no afternoon lab, but in this case the time is filled with another lecture. Figure 1 gives a typical page of the schedule.

Morphological studies dominate the first semester. Two full days of the week are devoted to gross anatomy, three mornings to microanatomy, and the remaining three afternoons to neuroanatomy, neurophysiology, and psychiatry. Students spend more time on gross anatomy than any other subject; it consumes sixteen of the forty hours of classes and labs scheduled each week.

A day of gross anatomy begins with a formal lecture. Students take notes and may ask questions at the end. There is usually a short "break" for them to go out for a smoke. Content of the lectures closely follows one of several anatomy texts. Most of the material is factual, but there are references to research findings and clinical practice as well as advice about dissection. Students are given a list of several

[1] We use the present tense throughout for immediacy although the freshman program has since been changed.

FRESHMAN MEDICAL SCHEDULE
1956–57

Week: 3   Dates: Sept. 24–28
Lectures at 8:00 A. M. and 1:00 P.M. in Room 103 Haworth unless otherwise designated. Laboratories immediately follow lectures.

A.M. 8–12	P.M. 1–5
Mon. Microanatomy	Neurology [a]
Lecture: Cartilage, bone	Lecture: Physiology of Muscle
Lab: Cartilage, bone, p. 22, Par. 4, 5.	Lab: Stimulus-response relationship in skeletal muscle.
Tues. Gross Anatomy	Gross Anatomy
Lecture: Lymphatics	Lecture: Nervous System I
Lab: Through p. 8	Lab: Complete sect. on lower extremity.
Wed. Microanatomy	Neurology
Lecture: Integument & mammary gland	Lecture: Physiology of skeletal muscle
Lab: Integument, p. 38, mammary gland p. 48, Par. 6.	3–5 Psychiatry: Outline of personality development.
Thurs. Gross Anatomy	Gross Anatomy
Lecture: Nervous System II	Lecture: Homologies of the extremities [b]
Lab: Upper extremity to bottom of p. 9.	Lab: To Par. 3; p. 11.
Fri. Microanatomy	Neurology
Lecture: Early development	Lab: Effects of some environmental changes on skeletal muscle.
Lab: 33-hr. chick, p. 5 through Par. 4, p. 6.	

[a] In this particular week Neurology labs and lectures were given by the Physiology Department.
[b] An unannounced quiz took the place of this lecture.

Fig. 1. — FRESHMAN MEDICAL SCHEDULE

anatomy textbooks to choose from; most of them use Morris,[2] a very detailed book of nearly 2,000 pages.

There are two gross anatomy laboratories — long rooms with a row of shallow metal tanks for the cadavers. The tanks contain preserving fluid into which the body is lowered after dissecting periods. Each tank rests on a frame which puts it about table height for convenience in dissection, but the tanks are so close together that students at adjacent ones must plan their work so that they will not get in each others' way.

Each lab has an instructor and several graduate assistants. The faculty assigns students in groups of four to a cadaver. Assignment is not alphabetical. Students pair up within the fours, and each pair

[2] Sir Henry Morris, *Morris's Human Anatomy*, edited by J. P. Schaeffer (11th ed., New York: Blakiston, 1953).

divides the dissection of half of the cadaver between them. The lab instructor tells them they may not change partners without permission, and then only if they can persuade another student to make an exchange. Each student has a detailed lab manual which tells him what and how to dissect; he also brings his text to lab. The instructor suggests that one partner dissect while the other reads out directions about what to do from the lab manual and, as the dissection proceeds, identifies structures in the cadaver with the help of his textbook.

Aside from the difficulties of learning to recognize and name the thousands of structures of the body, their function and clinical significance, students of gross anatomy have certain technical problems. There is so much variation from the "normal" in cadavers that identification of structures is often difficult. A part may be missing, oddly placed or so distorted by use during life that it bears little resemblance to the idealized diagrams of the textbook. A student may also destroy the very structure he is trying to study. If peripheral nerves and blood vessels are to be preserved, initial skinning and reflection of subcutaneous fat must be done with great care. It is a laborious process. Even on deeper levels of dissection, if the student is not careful he will accidentally cut muscles, nerves, or blood vessels. If he cuts more than one such structure, he is faced with an identification problem. For example, a student ordinarily recognizes a muscle by its position in relation to adjacent structures, or by tracing it out to its junction with other structures — its origin and insertion. If he has cut a muscle, he often cannot determine its proper relation to other structures, and unless he can fit the two ends together with some certainty he can no longer identify it by its origin and insertion. Problems of this sort can sometimes be solved by looking at other cadavers.

Dissection is time-consuming as well. More than half the student's time is spent pulling or cutting away skin and fat to expose muscles and nerves and in untangling vessels and ligaments. Much of this work is preliminary and affords little opportunity for study. Furthermore, as dissection proceeds the outer layers of the body are destroyed in exposing the inner ones. This makes it difficult for the student to use his cadaver for review; he must learn as he goes along.

Of necessity, dissection is done by regions of the body. This poses a problem of integration. It is impractical, for instance, to trace all the nerves at one time. Students work first on the extremities, starting with the skin, and down through the layers of muscles and deeper vessels to the bone; they then go on to another region, where the process is repeated. This approach differs from that of the textbooks, which take up the entire nervous system or musculature of the body at one time. It is therefore necessary for the student to skip about in his textbook in order to find material on the region he is studying. In reviewing he must integrate the firsthand knowledge of a region that he gains by dissection with his book-knowledge of body systems.

At the end of the labs scheduled for dissection of a given body region, the faculty sets an examination students call a "block."[3] There are three blocks during the semester. Between them students may get unscheduled examinations which they call "shotguns."

In addition to his problems with anomalies in his cadaver and the difficult and time-consuming nature of dissection, the student has certain minor worries. His fingers become temporarily numb from long immersion in the preservative fluids in the dissecting tank. He has long hours of standing, and it is difficult to reach many areas of the body without bending over it. He must tolerate the firm if somewhat greasy feel of the cadaver. The disinfectant smell is strong although comparable to other laboratory odors, unless discarded fat has been allowed to disintegrate in the tank. The student is told there is little or no chance of infection, but that cuts must be carefully tended.

During lab students bring up questions of two sorts. They may, for example, expose a blood vessel they cannot name. Or, the manual may have directed them to expose a given blood vessel lateral to this or that muscle, and they cannot find it or distinguish it from other vessels in the area. If they want help, they raise their hands or otherwise attract the attention of the instructor or his assistant. Instructors have two methods of helping. They may use a Socratic style of questioning until the student can solve his own problem, or simply make an identification for him. If a given structure cannot be found, the instructor may help the student by further dissection or establish that it is missing by naming adjacent structures.

The faculty recommends that students read relevant material in their texts before each lecture. Topics are given in the student's outline of the semester. After hearing the material in the lecture and doing related dissection during the day, students should review. This

---

[3] The term "block" probably refers to a block of time or subject matter. The students use it to refer to a major examination.

means that each student who follows these suggestions will have been through the material on any given topic four times.

The teaching of microanatomy (histology and embryology) proceeds in much the same way as in gross. Twelve hours a week are devoted to it. There are three morning lectures followed by labs. Because it is a rapidly developing field, whereas research in gross anatomy has been largely completed, micro lectures contain many more references to recent experimental work and research.

In the laboratory each student works alone at his own microscope, examining a series of prepared slides in the order set forth in a laboratory manual. As in gross, he must learn to recognize and identify normal structures of the body (in this case cells and tissue) and understand their function and clinical significance by reading his textbook. Instructors and graduate assistants are there in the lab to answer questions and give demonstrations.

Although learning to recognize tissue is often difficult and using a microscope is initially a problem for those students who have had little science, there are two ways in which microanatomy is easier for students than gross anatomy. In gross the student must "discover" for himself what he is to study; that is, he spends a lot of time uncovering and locating a given muscle or organ to study it. In micro he is given a prepared slide. And where the lab manual in gross contains only directions for dissection, the micro manual has explanatory material and references to a textbook. This means that the student does not have to search for reading relevant to his lab work. The material is organized for him.

The faculty schedules two examinations in microanatomy. One, written and practical, comes at the time of the first gross anatomy examination; the second, written only, comes at the end of the semester.

Twelve hours a week are devoted to the general subject of neurology, which includes neuroanatomy, neurophysiology, and psychiatry. Lectures are given three afternoons a week on an irregular schedule. With the exception of psychiatry, the topics covered relate to the work in gross anatomy. For example, in the same week that the student dissects the muscles of the extremities, there are lectures and labs on the physiology of muscle.

Lectures in neuroanatomy are of the same type as in gross and micro, but many neuroanatomy lectures closely follow a manual written by the instructor rather than a text. The students follow the lecture word by word in the manual and mark points the instructor emphasizes. Lab periods entail work with microscopes and dissection of the brain. The only major neuro examination is a written one at the end of the semester. Lesser examinations are announced.

Neurophysiology is taught by members of the physiology department. Lectures emphasize theoretical material and experimental work. The style of lecturing entails discussion and questioning of the students. In the laboratory students perform classical experiments, with animals or themselves as subjects, and watch demonstrations by the faculty. There is no lab manual, and lab periods are scheduled at irregular intervals. Usually directions for experiments are handed out during lectures. The faculty gives announced tests.

Staff members and visiting physicians of the psychiatry department at the medical center give a series of informal lectures throughout the first semester. Whereas most of the Lawrence faculty are scientists with Ph.D.s, these men are M.D.s with practices. They frequently tell students about patients seen earlier in the day. There are movies and discussion periods, but readings are suggested rather than assigned. Instead of an emphasis on facts, as in anatomy, or research and theory in physiology, there is an attempt to introduce the student to the bearing of psychiatry on his own adjustment to medical school and to the place of psychiatry in the treatment of patients. Questions on psychiatry appear on the examinations at the end of the semester.

During the second semester, freshmen spend all their time on biochemistry, physiology, and psychiatry. Of these, biochemistry and physiology are the most important, but more attention is given to psychiatry than during the first semester.

The semester begins with three weeks of biochemistry. This is a period of review of college work and is called in the students' outline "Foundations of Biochemistry." After this, biochemistry and physiology are integrated. Faculty from both departments lecture on topics in the following sequence:

Intake, digestion, and absorption of food.................. four weeks
Circulation and respiration................................ four weeks
Energy metabolism... one week
          Spring vacation................................. one week
Intermediary metabolism, regulation of
          the composition of body fluids................. three weeks
Integrated functions of endocrines........................ one week
Final examinations .... May 20

Unlike the first semester, when the students are given detailed schedules of what they are to cover each day, during the second semester schedules are handed out at the beginning of each block of work. The student's day begins with lectures from 8:00 to approximately 10:00 A.M. The lectures are followed by lab until noon, and a long lab from 1:00 to 5:00 in the afternoon. Tuesday afternoon is free, but the staff remains on hand in the medical building to help students who feel they need it. All day Thursday is given over to psychiatry. Examinations, lab, or lectures are frequently scheduled on Saturday morning.

Although this schedule sounds as rigorous as that of the first semester, some students feel that they have more free time. This is particularly true in biochemistry, which many students have had in college; they find they need not spend as much time in the afternoon lab as they did in anatomy. Physiology lab, where students work with live animals, involves preparation and cleaning up that often takes longer than the assigned time. Thursday afternoon is generally free, as the psychiatry conferences do not take up the whole day.

In biochemistry instruction proceeds by lectures in which there is a good deal of drill work — question and answer in rapid fire between instructor and student. They are given mathematical problems to work out at home but are not required to hand them in. In the lab, they are assigned desks alphabetically and divided into three sections (for the three laboratories), each in the charge of a graduate assistant. Most of the lab work consists in following a lab manual which directs them to combine certain chemicals and note the reaction. At the end of a week or two weeks, an examination in unknowns is given. Each student receives several small bottles and is expected to find out what is in them by process of elimination. The unknowns are the same substances they have been working on.

In physiology the students may choose their own lab partners. The lab work is of two kinds: procedures which they try out on themselves or each other, taking blood pressure, putting down gastric tubes, and so on; and operations on dogs or other small animals, which demonstrate various living functions. They learn a little surgery, how to slit the trachea to put a tube in it, for example, and make use of their anatomy in identifying the proper nerve to stimulate or finding a certain area of the heart. They learn to anesthetize the animals and put up with their whimpering until the anesthetic works. Frequently the animal dies before the experiment is concluded, and there is some competition between students to see how many experiments they can manage to get through without killing off the dog. As in anatomy, the students help each other in these experiments. One records data, another does the actual operating, and the third acts as assistant to the surgeon by holding hemostats and mopping up blood. There is opportunity for a student who does not like to operate to avoid it by being an especially helpful recorder or helper. In physiology labs are more informal than in biochemistry; there is confusion and a good deal of pressure to get through, whereas the biochemistry lab period is characterized by long periods of waiting in line for chemicals someone else is using.

The system of frequent examinations, one every week or two, which began between Christmas and the end of the first semester, is continued into the second. Students are notified when they do not pass these examinations by "pink slips" sent to them by mail. Such a student is then called in to be counseled or, in their phrase, "chewed out."

Psychiatry is given on Thursday morning. There is a lecture followed by conferences in which the class is split up into small groups of fifteen or so. In these conferences the psychiatrist attempts to orient students toward medicine and their work in it. He also discusses questions which the students bring up from the lectures. The sessions sometimes degenerate into wrangles about psychiatry in which the students' resentment of the subject, developed late in the first semester, is barely kept under cover.

The academic environment of the freshman year provides two of the three conditions, in a rather extreme form, that make it possible for a group to create the immediate, situational perspectives characteristic of an autonomous subculture. The students have pressing common problems which they face in relative isolation. We consider the third condition, group consensus, in a later chapter.

The environment of the first year is so structured that freshmen are virtually isolated from everyone but their own classmates and faculty. All freshmen follow a uniform schedule and curriculum. Each student does the same thing at the same time and in the same place, except when lab sections are in different rooms. The class is together in the medical school building, except during lunch hour, from eight in the morning until five in the afternoon. Students attend few university functions; they have virtually no student government or other extracurricular activities. Since lectures are of indefinite length (there is no system of bells to keep the faculty in line) and labs begin immediately afterward, students have little chance to see anyone but class-mates during the day. They seldom see medical students from other classes. Sophomores, juniors, and seniors are at the medical center forty miles from the university, and freshmen get there as a group only about once or twice a year. Evenings and many hours of the weekend are filled with preparation and review of daily work. With the exception of brief vacations, the schedule continues without pause.

The size of the class (about one hundred students) and the formal lecture system minimizes interaction between students and faculty. Although students ask questions after lectures and during labs, there is insufficient time and staff for much individual attention. Each student is assigned a faculty adviser, who calls him in if he is in danger of failing, and whom he may see at other times if he wishes, but not many students take advantage of this. Students are photographed at the beginning of the year and wear their names on their lab coats, but even at the end of the first semester instructors have trouble fitting names and faces. Attendance is not taken. Since faculty mem-bers hold Ph.D.s in the preclinical sciences rather than medical de-grees, and lab assistants are graduate students in these disciplines, neither serve as career models for the freshmen, except for the rare individual (one in the class we studied) who intends to leave medical school after the first year to take a basic science degree.

The uniformity of the medical school schedule insures that, al-though a student may have his own troubles, there are many problems the class as a whole has in common. Unlike college or high school, where students have different daily schedules and an examination period of a week or more, the medical school schedule is continuous. All students have the problem of "keeping up"; they must learn every-thing as they go along. By lessening each student's chance of individ-ual help, the size of the class prevents enterprising individuals or groups from obtaining advantages unavailable to the whole class.

Examinations are a major common problem. They must be passed if the student is to stay in school as they are the faculty's chief means of assessing freshman work. Students are very frightened of them, but they are, after all, an expected feature of school life. The new and most pressing problem faced by all students in the freshman year is the tremendous amount of material to be learned — the "overload."

In describing the coming year to the freshmen during Orientation Week lectures, the faculty hints at the overload as follows:

Start work immediately because there will be no time to catch up. Perhaps for some of you, even if you are caught up, there will not be time enough. We want to keep the tension down for you. Doctors are always anxious. There are 5,000 names of parts of the body you will have to learn. . . . The one thing you want to remember is to really work hard the first part of the year.

(September 5, 1956.)

Now as to the way we run the [anatomy] lab. There will be no breaks; you are expected to be there all the time. You can go out for a smoke if you think you can afford it. It will be necessary to work after hours, however, in order to get your dissection done. There is not enough time to get it all done in the lab. *It is your responsibility to learn as much as you have capacity for in the time you have.* . . . Sure, go ahead and make drawings if you wish. There is not much time, however.

(September 10, 1956.)

These statements informed both the freshmen and the participant observer that in the eyes of the staff the students faced a year of hard work, more work than some of them would be able to do in the time available. But warnings of this kind are usual at the beginning of a school year. There is no comment in the field notes to indicate that either the participant observer or the students considered the admonitions of particular interest.

No doubt we should have paid attention, for such statements are likely to be meaningful when made by those in authority. The faculty of a professional school often believes there is a more or less standardized body of knowledge that graduates must know in order to practice the profession.[4] In medicine, as in many other fields, this body of knowledge is being constantly augmented by the findings of new research which some faculty members feel must be incorporated into courses. Instructors with this perspective may feel they are not responsible for the amount students have to know; the subject matter itself forces an overload.

Whether or not students sympathize with this point of view, such a situation presents them with a major common problem which under certain circumstances may become virtually insoluble. Whatever its source, an overload exists when people believe there may be more work to be done than they can do in the time available. A potential overload may be even more difficult to deal with than a real one.

[4] See Renée C. Fox, "Training for Uncertainty," in *The Student-Physician*, Robert K. Merton, George G. Reader, M.D., Patricia L. Kendall (eds.), (Cambridge, Mass.: Harvard University Press, 1957), p. 207.

For many people subject to direction or authority, overload is easily recognized; it is simply a matter of how much work is required. Hours of work are fixed, and workers bargain only about the amount they are asked to do. For students the situation is less well-defined. Their hours of work are not fixed. They must choose between study and leisure and often between study and sleep. Thus, even without an overload, students confront the problem of deciding how much to study.

The decision is made more difficult by the indefinable nature of students' work. They must know certain things, but what things and in what detail? In the simplest school situations, students use faculty requirements to decide. In medical school, however, while instructors direct freshmen to keep up with dissection and turn in certain lab reports, they do not require attendance at lectures, reports on reading, or term papers. Thus, the daily requirements of the faculty are minimal. Students can not use them to determine the level or direction of their efforts.

Teachers often make informal suggestions about methods of work which students use in making decisions about what and how much to study. In the medical school, as we have seen, instructors suggest a four-way exposure to each topic: reading, attending lecture, doing lab work, and review. Each night the student has the dual task of reviewing his day's work and reading about the topic scheduled for the following day. In following this suggestion, a student may involve himself in many hours of study or cover the material quickly by skimming and using outlines. Since the student is not questioned or graded on daily work, the decision as to whether he is doing enough remains with him at least until examination time.

The prospect of major examinations does not immediately solve the students' problem, however, for there is no necessary relationship between the fact of having to pass them and the amount there is to be learned. The two are related only if it is known that the faculty or some other agency sets or grades examinations in such a way that a large body of knowledge, more than the students think they have time to learn, is needed to pass. Thus, when faculty requirements are not specific, students, and particularly those cut off from upperclassmen who might be of help, face the problem of overload alone. It is the students' solution to this problem as it affects the level and direction of their effort in school that chiefly concerns us in subsequent chapters.

Chapter 7 The Initial Perspective

An Effort to "Learn It All"

During Orientation Week, when they are not listening to talks by the faculty about the coming year or visiting the medical center in Kansas City, freshmen buy lab coats, books, microscopes, and dissecting tools. Married students settle in trailers and apartments; single ones in rooms or in one of the three medical fraternity houses. At the beginning of the next week they start the daily round of lectures, labs, and study.

For the participant observer, orientation continued through the first weeks of classes. We learned about courses and schedules and began the process of getting to know the students. Table VII shows that by the end of Orientation Week we knew almost half the students well enough to be able to identify them and carry on a casual conversation. A little over three weeks later we were on this footing with the entire class. We knew in most cases which students lived in fraternity houses, in rooms near the campus, in trailer camps and apartments. We knew who was single and who married. These were

TABLE VII

Timetable of Observer's Identification of Students

Week and Event	Number of Students Identified[*]
September 5–8 (Orientation Week)	49
September 10–14	87
September 17–21	93
September 24–28	93
September 27 ("Shotgun" examination in anatomy)	104

[*] Of 104.

92

important matters, since differences in residence and marital status were initially the chief barriers to interaction in the class.

When the students start classes, one major theme emerges from nearly everything they say and do. It occupies so much of their time and attention that we began to see our task as one of explaining it, and the theme itself as central to an understanding of the freshman year. Briefly, the students' concern is their work: how much to study and to what end. While it is true that they have other concerns, such as becoming accustomed to handling the cadaver, these problems are short-lived in comparison with their continuing concern about academic work.

This concern is expressed in a co-ordinated set of ideas and activities which we call the initial perspective. In line with the idealism of their long-range views of medicine, the initial perspective students bring to medical school embraces a high level of effort directed towards learning everything.

If the long-range perspective and the initial perspective are similarly idealistic in content, they differ in other respects. The initial perspective is immediate and situational. It consists of the students' definition of their present situation, the goals they set for themselves in it, and the activities they undertake in it. It is because these three elements are so closely bound up together, each relating to the external situation in the same way, that we consider them together under the term situational perspective.

With the long-range perspective no such immediacy of thought and action is possible. Students define medicine as the best profession and their goal is to become an ideal physician. Definition is diffuse, for the student has not experienced what he is talking about and must depend on the opinions of others who are often not intimately acquainted with medicine. His goal may be unrealistic because it is unchecked by knowledge of the problems involved. Immediate action is not possible, for students may not practice medicine until after they graduate.

Now, if the long-range perspective is as vague as this, what use can students make of it while they are in medical school? As upperclassmen they use it to guide their choice of situational perspective when the environment permits. At the beginning of school students are not familiar enough with their new environment for it to influence their choice of perspective very much. The initial perspective is simply an application of their ideals to the medical school situation.

In the following pages we first let the students state the initial perspective in their own words, then summarize the data that lead us to believe it characteristic of students during the first few weeks of the freshman year.

We find many instances in our field notes in which students exhibit in speech and action a high level of academic effort directed toward learning everything. These indicate that students in their first weeks of schools use a perspective we summarize as follows:

1. We want to learn everything, as we will need it when we become physicians.

2. There is a tremendous amount to learn.

3. We have to work very hard — that is, many hours.

4. If our present hours of work are not enough for us to get everything, we'll do whatever we can to increase them — but how?

Partly from lay concepts of the many things a physician must know, but more concretely from immediate experience with the heavy first-semester schedule, the students define their situation in medical school as one in which there is an almost overwhelming amount of material to be learned. Their goal is to "learn it all" (and thus become good physicians) by working hard. In the next few pages we describe the initial perspective in greater detail by quoting from our field notes representative instances in which students express it in words or actions.

Expressions of the initial perspective fall roughly into three types, each including one or more of the points listed above. In the first and most numerous type, students talk about the number of hours they have studied or intend to study. In the more complex statements of the second type they point to the tremendous amount there is to learn as their chief problem. The emphasis is still on amount: it is not that the work is difficult but that there is so much of it. In the third type of statement students speak of their desire to learn it all, connecting this goal with the hours necessary to achieve it. In a subtype, of which we have only a few examples, students justify their initial perspective by means of their long-range ideals.

Our field notes contain a great many statements about long hours of study. The following examples illustrate the matter-of-fact way students talk about doing a lot of work. They show no hesitation in speaking like this before each other:

The observer said to Dick Porter, "What are you going to do this week-end?" Dick answered, "Well, I'm going to study all the time but I'm going out Saturday night. I think you have to do that."

During dinner at his fraternity house, the same man said to other students at his table, "We really don't know it [anatomy]. I plan to study Saturday morning and all day Sunday."

(September 21, 1956. Single fraternity man.)

When such minor sacrifices do not suffice, students take further steps to increase study time:

I went out for a break with two students. Cal Jordan said, "How is your study coming? I don't feel any different now than when I came except I study more." Dick Porter said, "I know I'm different because I just called up and put off a date for this weekend." Jordan said, "Say, I did too. We can't afford to go out with any chicks this weekend."

(October 2, 1956. Two single fraternity men.)

They set up special schedules to get more done:

I asked Vic Morse how much he had studied over the weekend and he said, "Well, every Friday I go home and sleep after supper until 1 A.M., and then I get up and work until 7 A.M. Saturday morning we went over to the anatomy lab. In the afternoon I took off and Saturday evening we had a slide session. I went to church Sunday morning and in the afternoon I studied again."

(October 1, 1956. Single fraternity man.)

In talk of this kind, students are doing several things for each other. First, they are exchanging information about the means of reaching their goal: they say in effect, to learn it all you must work *this* many hours a night. Second, they are setting up a hierarchy of activities: studying comes before dating; time off is redefined as necessary recreation in order to study well.

When people in a group exchange information of this sort, they are setting norms: in this case, maxima. For instance, those who study two or three hours a night say, "I *only* studied two or three hours," meaning, this is not very much. They often excuse themselves by saying they did not study because their parents came or a friend was being married. But studying four to six hours a night is spoken of matter of factly; although, if we remember that students are in class from eight A.M. to five P.M., four to six hours of study after supper means a twelve- to fourteen-hour working day. We may state these maximal norms as follows:

1. You ought to spend four to six hours a night studying.

2. You ought to study five to seven hours a day over the week-end.

3. You ought to return to the anatomy lab one night a week to review or finish up assignments.

4. You ought not to go out on a date more than one night a week.

There are further norms, so much taken for granted that they are not mentioned by the students but were observed to hold true:

5. You ought to attend every lecture.

6. You ought not to cut lab except just before a block (i.e., major examination).

When his eight-hour-day of lectures and labs is included, a student following this schedule works seventy-seven hours a week.

Students express the initial perspective in activities as well as words. Our field notes contain references to large numbers of students who returned to work in the anatomy lab at night. Here are a few examples of this kind of data:

September 19: Nineteen students worked in anatomy lab at night.[1]

September 24: Eight students working in anatomy lab right after supper, 6:30 P.M.

The observer went to supper at a fraternity house on Friday night and saw that a majority of the members went off to study; only a few were out on dates.

We consider such items evidence of the initial perspective.

Students express another proposition of the initial perspective when they speak of the tremendous amount there is to learn. The problem is not one of the difficulty of the work but of time to do it.

The observer asked John Trent how the first few weeks had gone. He replied, "Well, you know, I've always wanted to do this ever since I was a little boy. It's very hard. Just about as I expected, but it's not so much hard as it is that we have so much to do. They just keep us busy all the time. It's not difficult to understand once you get there."

(September 24, 1956. Married fraternity man.)

This statement expresses both the long-range and initial perspective: a strong commitment to medicine and expectations of hard work in medical school from the former; a recognition of the amount of work there is to do from the latter.

---

[1] The field notes contain the names of these students.

Signs of increasing strain are evident in the next example:

In the course of a conversation, Al Cowper said to the observer, "This week they really have thrown the book at us, and I'm now getting a little behind in everything, and I can't see any prospect of catching up. It kind of gets you."

(September 18, 1956. Married independent.)

For some students there is desperation:

Coming down the stairs from a lecture Al Jones said to the observer, "You know, what you ought to do is to come and see us in the evening. You just don't really know what it's like until you come in the evening. Last night we got out our books and got all ready to study, and then it came to us how much there was to do and we were so scared we couldn't do any-thing. We had to get up and make coffee and walk around . . . You should have been there."

(September 13, 1956. Married independent.)

When they think of how much work they are doing, students are bewildered by the fact that they are still not getting it all done to their satisfaction. A few blame the faculty for "loading it on," as in the ex-ample below. Being "behind on Monday" becomes a standard joke. Uncritical learning, memorizing really, presents itself as a way of cov-ering the work when there isn't time to think about it:

As we left physiology lecture this afternoon, there were general expres-sions from the students of lack of comprehension and anger. Fred Brown said in a loud voice, "I'm getting near my excitation point. . . . I'm going to boil over." (The lecture had been on excitation points in muscle.) There was general laughter at this by the students going down the stairs. Bob Simpson said, "I am beginning to think it's true. You haven't got time to think about anything in your first year; you just learn it." Fred agreed with this. He said, "It's only Monday, and I'm behind all ready." Al Jones who was also there said, "Well, it's just the tradition to load all this stuff on us."

(October 1, 1956. Three married independents.)

In the third and last type of item that expresses the perspective, students frequently connect learning everything with their ideas about how much they should study. They connect level with direc-tion of effort. The two boys in the conversation below cannot see how the girl can "really know all this stuff" if she only works an hour and a half a night:

Many students went down to get a coke after the lecture and I went with

them. Jane Matson joined me. Jim Peters and Eddie Cawley came up.
Eddie asked Jane how much studying she had been doing. She said she'd
been doing "hardly any, only two or three hours." She thought the work
so far was easy and couldn't understand why some people were so worried.
(Jane has a rather off-hand, laughing manner about all this.) Eddie looked
at her in disbelief and so did Jim. Eddie said, "Well, I've been studying
until very late at night and I mean to study all weekend and come in Saturday and go over my anatomy." The boys kept questioning Jane about how
much she had actually studied. She said she skimmed over the material
before each lecture and then read it more carefully at night, but it did not
take her very long. They asked her how long it had taken her to read the
thirty pages of neurology, and she said, "Oh, about an hour and a half."
Jim said, "Come study with us some time, and we'll give you a quiz and
see whether you really know all this stuff."

> (September 14, 1956. A married fraternity man,
> a married independent, a girl independent.)

In another item of the third type, a student relates his present notions about working hard to the long-range perspective. He says he
works much harder in medical school than he did in college, and explains that he is now idealistic because he is studying for his own
future benefit:

I talked to Bud Janson as he was packing up to leave the lab. He said,
"You know, this studying is very different from undergraduate school.
When I was an undergraduate I didn't do much of anything. Maybe I
studied Monday, Tuesday, and Wednesday but Thursday night I went
out and I didn't do much after that. I'm real idealistic about this now. I
really want to learn it to use later."

> (September 17, 1956. Single independent.)

There are not many items of this type in our field notes; we did not
ask students about the relation between their present perspectives
and their long-range views, and in the rush of daily work they seldom
volunteered it. But, although students are explicit about the direction
of their efforts in only a few items, we believe the notion of learning
it all is implicit in all their statements about studying a lot. We
can't say more than this here; in the next chapter, when, as we shall
see, the students redefine the situation and alter their goals and activities, the nature of their revision makes it clear that the direction of
their effort in the initial perspective was toward learning everything.[2]

Taken together these excerpts from the field notes give the con-

[2] See p. 111.

tent of the initial perspective. But to convince ourselves that this perspective is the students' customary approach to medical school work, we must do more than describe it. Even though freshmen act out the perspective or tell us about it in their own words, we are not convinced it is customary behavior until we know something of the range and frequency of its use. We ask the question: How confident can we be that a high level of effort directed toward learning everything is customary among freshmen during the first four weeks of school?

We answer this question in part with three tables showing to what extent the initial perspective is in frequent, widespread, and legitimate use in the freshman class. Table VIII gives the number of student statements and activities by weeks, starting with the first week of classes, classified as to whether they express the initial perspective or not.

TABLE VIII

FREQUENCY OF OBSERVED WORK ACTIVITIES AND STATEMENTS ABOUT WORK WITH (+) AND WITHOUT (−) INITIAL PERSPECTIVE
(September 10 – October 3, 1956)

WEEK OF SCHOOL	STATEMENTS		ACTIVITIES		TOTAL OBSERVATIONS
	+	−	+	−	
September 10–14	16	1	0	2	19
September 17–21	29	3	20	5	56
September 24–28	25	6	8	5	41
October 1–3*	16	2	18	0	36
Total	86 (57%)	12 (8%)	46 (30%)	8 (5%)	152 (100%)

* The observer did not go to the medical school October 4–5.

The proportion of observations expressing the perspective, 132 out of a total of 152, assures us that students exhibit a high level of effort directed toward learning everything, much more frequently than other perspectives on their work. We also conclude that the perspective is of more than momentary concern as it persists over a period of three weeks.

The negative cases in this table deserve comment here. In most of them students speak of taking time off to go hunting or not having done much over the weekend. Although we have little reason to believe such statements refer to more than occasional interruptions of effort, we consider them negative instances. The activities counted as negative cases are also occasional rather than recurrent behavior. They are instances of students leaving lab early or failing to attend. We might say they provide evidence for the perspective rather than against it, since if two students were noted absent on any given day, 102 were present.

The time periods covered by successive perspectives of the freshman year are not clearly distinguishable; there is much overlapping. Some students continue to try to learn everything until the first major examination. Others question the initial perspective as early as September 25 and begin to look for a new one. We shall consider the seventeen forerunners in the next chapter.

While Table VIII indicates the basis for our confidence that the initial perspective is the students' dominant way of dealing with their academic work, we also want to know what confidence we can have that it is not confined to any group or groups in the class. Table IX answers this in part by showing the distribution of items counted as expressing the perspective among various groups in the class. Our reasons for dividing the class into these particular groups are unimportant here; it is enough to say that they are, to a large extent, residential groups whose members see more of each other than of other students.

Table IX demonstrates that the initial perspective is not confined to any group or combination of groups in the class.

In another check on the collective nature of the initial perspective, we ask to what extent it is part of the legitimate everyday behavior of the students. If all our observations were of students matter-of-

TABLE IX

DISTRIBUTION OF OBSERVED INSTANCES OF USE OF THE
INITIAL PERSPECTIVE BY STUDENTS IN DIFFERENT GROUPS
(September 10 – October 3, 1956)

STUDENT GROUP	NUMBER		PER CENT
Fraternity Men:	83		63
Alphas		34	
Betas		6	
Gammas		43	
Independents:	49		37
Married Men		27	
Single Men		9	
Girls		13	
Total	132*		100

* The twenty negative cases are evenly scattered among the groups.

factly stating the perspective in the presence of other students or acting it out in the course of their daily activities, we could feel confident that students consider it a legitimate thing to say or do. Again, when an instance of the perspective is obtained by questioning, we wonder if it reflects the observer's interests rather than the students'. If only the informant is present, we wonder if what the student says or does reflects interests peculiar to him which other students might consider improper behavior. Table X classifies the 132 items carrying the initial perspective according to whether they are volunteered or directed by the observer and whether students other than the informant are present.

TABLE X

STATEMENTS AND ACTIVITIES EXPRESSING THE INITIAL PERSPECTIVE
CLASSIFIED BY THOSE PRESENT AND WHETHER VOLUNTEERED OR DIRECTED
(September 10 – October 3, 1956)

		VOLUNTEERED	DIRECTED	TOTAL
Statements	To observer alone	23 (17%)	17 (13%)	40
	To others in everyday conversation	41 (31%)	5 (4%)	46
Activities	Individual: not seen by other students	1 (1%)		1
	Group: other students present	45 (34%)		45
	Total	110 (83%)	22 (17%)	132 (100%)

We see that 83 per cent of the items in Table X are volunteered and may thus be presumed to reflect the students' concerns and not the observer's.

Were Table X divided into weeks, it would show no directed statements until the second week of school. A check of the field notes indicates that although the observer collected nineteen instances of the perspective in the first week, they went unrecognized as an important concern of the students. Thus the perspective is not an artifact of the observer's interests. The presence of directed items after the first week assures us that the observer was making an attempt to find negative cases by pursuing the topic with various types of students.

We note in Table X that nearly all observed activities and more than half (64%) the volunteered statements occur with more than one student present. As students do not challenge the statements or remark on the activities as unusual, we conclude they accept these expressions of the perspective as proper, legitimate behavior for students. With somewhat less confidence, we may extend this conclusion to expressions of the perspective occurring when only the observer is present, and to ones directed by the observer if, as is the case, examination reveals little difference in content and style between volunteered and directed, public and individual behavior.

We have presented three tables that summarize the data in our field notes which lead us to have confidence that the initial perspective is the customary way for freshmen to deal with their academic work. By customary we mean the perspective is frequently used by groups then visible in the class and that students not only use it themselves but accept it as proper behavior in fellow students.

Thus students repeatedly make the point that in spite of the fact that they work very hard, there is still an overwhelming amount to learn. Although they begin to refer to the faculty as "they" and sometimes blame them for "loading it on," they are not making the common student complaint about long assignments. We might translate their phrase "learn it all" with the words "learning medicine." They feel this is their responsibility; the faculty acts as an intermediary, scheduling greater or lesser amounts to be learned in a given period of time. In this sense they are the most idealistic of students — those who learn to satisfy themselves. Their chief problem, as the first weeks of school go by, is that they cannot find time to learn more.

At the beginning of this chapter we spoke of the initial perspective as the major concern of freshmen in the first four weeks of school. But the evidence we have presented thus far points only to their concern about studying; we have said nothing to substantiate our statement that the initial perspective dominates them to such an extent that, as students, they have virtually no other collective concern.

While laymen and novelists often recognize that medical students strive desperately to master their studies, it is often taken for granted that getting used to dissecting is a major problem for freshmen, that first contact with dead bodies must be a difficult, if not traumatic, experience. Such experiences are said to have lasting effect on students and central importance in the process of becoming a doctor. In fact, novelists have a well-developed theory of student behavior which, if it is correct, contradicts our belief that students' chief concern is their work.[3]

[3] In preparing ourselves to do this study, we read many popular novels about medi-

Novels picture medical students hardening themselves to face suffering and death. Some students, although seldom the hero, become cynical and parade their lack of feeling by continual obscene joking. In anatomy, fictional medical students harass the girls in the class by gags with the sex organs of cadavers or profane the lab by throwing around the detritus of dissection. They wear filthy lab coats and use obscene rhymes as mnemonic devices. The novels explain this cynical and obscene behavior as the result of the trauma of contact with death.

We cannot say much about the psychological aspects of this theory because we studied students' daily behavior, and we made no attempt to get at their inner experience. But, if the overt behavior stressed in the novels does not occur frequently among the freshmen we observed, the rest of the novelists' theory becomes open to question.

We found this to be the case. Prepared by the lay literature, we looked for evidences of trauma, but they were so startlingly rare that we tried to stir things up a bit ourselves by telling dirty jokes, getting little in return except a few smutty stories, not about medical school, that were currently going the rounds. If students had any standing joke, and repetition of the same kind of joke seems essential to the theory, it is the one we quoted earlier in this chapter: "It's only Monday and I'm behind already."

We observed no instances of harassed girl students; and, although we went to the anatomy lab at night, when instructors were not there, we saw only one instance of "profaning" the lab. With few exceptions, freshmen had their lab coats washed often, and did not use dirty rhymes as mnemonic devices.

Evidence of this kind, however, is negative and not very convincing. When we began analysis of our data, we wondered if there might not be positive evidence, in addition to the one hundred or more instances of the initial perspective, of schoolwork as the chief concern of the students. In sociological literature, it is suggested that underlying tension often reveals itself in jokes.[4] According to this hypothesis, we expect student jokes to be about their work, if work is a source of serious tension. The joke about being behind on Monday is a case in point.

cal students and doctors. We also asked the 62 students we interviewed what they had read about medicine before coming to medical school. With one exception, if they had read anything, it was these novels.

[4] See particularly Renée C. Fox, *Experiment Perilous* (Glencoe, Ill.: Free Press, 1959), pp. 76–82, 170–77.

The students have a standard joke about their troubles with seeing things on slides:

Sam Watson started out the histology lab by complaining in a gentle way that he didn't see anything or understand anything and that all he had in his microscope field was "a big blob."

After awhile he said to his desk partner with heavy irony, "Fascinating! Say, Bill, look what I got, I found a cloacal membrane." Bill got up and looked at it and said, "Well, I don't see anything." Sam said, "You have to use your imagination."

(October 8, 1956. Two single fraternity men.)

Jokes of this kind may be complaints about not having a good slide, but they have a wry implication that the student himself is stupid and can't see anything, but says he does anyway so as not to look foolish. In the chapters on the clinical years, we describe similar jokes about something equally difficult for beginning students: hearing heart murmurs.

Occasionally, the students persuaded an instructor to look for non-existent muscles in a cadaver; if he went along with their trick, they repeated the story with endless delight. But the most common kind of humor is the mock-serious kidding they employ, particularly before examinations:

Two days before the block, I went to the anatomy lab at night. Nels Thompson was looking in his cadaver for some structure that he had cut, accidentally or according to directions in the lab manual, and now could not trace. He yelled, "I'll never cut another anything!"

(October 9, 1956. Married fraternity man.)

On the same night, the boys were having a big discussion at one of the tanks. Max Bender said, "If you see anything you don't know, cut it out." He meant that the faculty couldn't tag anything in a cadaver for the coming practical examination if it wasn't there to tag.

(October 9, 1956. Single fraternity man.)

A good deal of the conversation that evening went as follows:

"What's this?" a student would say, putting his probe under a very small ligament. His partner said, "They wouldn't ask that. It's too small a detail." The first replied, "Oh, wouldn't they?"

(October 9, 1956.)

Another kind of joke involved the word "trauma" itself. Freshmen pick up the word early in the year and use it frequently with deliberate irony. The following quotation is apparently a joke, but like the students' kidding it has undertones of misunderstanding between students and faculty:

Scott said to me with a smile, "Well, you saw our first trauma today." I said, "What was that?" He said, "Oh, old Green keeping us so late [in class]."

(September 7, 1956. Single fraternity man.)

Thus we have a little positive evidence from jokes that students are tense about schoolwork. We thought dreams might also indicate underlying tension. There are five in the field notes, three that happened on the night of the first day of dissection; two from later in the first semester. The first three are undoubtedly trauma dreams. One of them is about a cadaver sitting up in the tank, another about a body that opens the pet cock of its tank and drains out the phenol. Later dreams are of a different kind; here is one of them:

During supper at the Union, Betsy Holloway was telling me about her studying. She said, "When I'm doing one thing I can't really concentrate on it because there're all these other things to do. I haven't been able to really concentrate since I got here; and I don't sleep well — I have these nightmares every night. One night I dreamt that I was a nerve and I was lying in the cadaver and somebody was coming in to cut me. There were other nerves around but I didn't have any relationship with them."

(September 27, 1956. Girl independent.)

The reference here to cutting a nerve that is out of relation to other nerves recalls the recurrent problem students have with dissection mentioned in Chapter 6. If a structure is cut before it has been identified, it is very difficult for the student to discover what it is; and, since identification often depends upon relationship to other structures, errors like this are cumulative. A failure to identify one thing leads to difficulties in identifying the next ones a student uncovers, and there is no way of retrieving the error. He has wasted the hours he spent on the painfully slow process of reflecting skin and fat, and cannot use this part of his cadaver for study or review.

The girl in the example says she has so much to do she cannot concentrate on anything; she dreams about a mistake that would further confuse her and hamper her work. It is a kind of "academic trauma."

Our interviews with a random sample of sixty-two students provide a check on the occurrence of a traumatic reaction to academic work. Table XI shows that of the nineteen freshmen in the sample, five say

TABLE XI

CAN YOU THINK OF ANY PARTICULAR THINGS THAT
HAVE BEEN TRAUMATIC?
(Random Sample of 19 Freshmen: Spring, 1957)

RESPONSE	NUMBER	PER CENT
None	12	63.0
Examinations	4	26.0
Generalized academic fears	1	
Disappointment with instruction	1	5.5
Physiology experiments	1	5.5
Total	19	100.0

academic matters have been traumatic. None mention the cadaver as traumatic, although one freshman speaks of experiments on dogs in physiology. Twelve say they had no trauma at all. While Table XI does not provide convincing evidence that freshmen are traumatized by academic work, it does suggest they are not very concerned about the trauma of death.

Of course, it may be argued that students are emotionally bothered by the cadaver in ways not apparent to our observation of their daily activities. There were certainly one or two students in the class of whom this seemed to be true, and it is possible that others might have had such a concern without bringing it to the surface. Such a contention is impossible to refute; indeed, for the purposes of this study, we need not refute it. It is sufficient to be able to say that freshmen have no co-ordinated set of ideas and activities, no continuing perspective on death or the cadaver that cannot be subsumed in their perspective on academic work.

Chapter 8   The Provisional Perspective

"You Can't Do it All"

Unlike the long-range or initial perspectives, the situational perspective we present in this chapter is not something each individual student brought with him to medical school, but a collective development. The idealistic perspectives of the first weeks of school belonged to an aggregate of students who did not know each other well and could in no sense, except nominally, be called a group. We explain the similarity of the freshmen's views at this time by the fact that the students came from similar backgrounds in a region of rather limited horizons and were embarked on the same career. But as they continued in school, all facing the same problems and subject to the same environmental constraints, the freshmen began to get to know each other and collectively develop a group perspective that solved the problems presented by their situation.

Although they made progress in both respects during the period we deal with in this chapter, September 24 to October 12, the freshmen neither became a unified group nor attained a final perspective on their work. They did reach a provisional perspective, between their initial perspective and their final one, part of which differed in two major groups in the class; that is, while all of them agreed on a definition of the chief problem in their situation, some students took one way of solving the problem, other students another. We reserve discussion of how the class became one group for the next chapter, and discuss the provisional perspective here.

We saw in Chapter 7 that the freshmen set themselves an idealistically high level of effort when they first got to school and that the direction of this effort was toward learning everything. They defined medical school as quite different from college, where what they learned often had little direct application to their lives. In medical school, they thought, everything taught them would be relevant to the clinical years and to medical practice upon leaving school. This initial perspective was characteristic of freshmen during the first weeks of school, a period we somewhat arbitrarily end on October 3, about a week before the first major examinations.

By assigning this date we do not mean, of course, that the class abruptly abandoned trying to learn everything and took up a new perspective, but that up until that time the initial perspective predominated. Toward the end of the period, although no one questioned the necessity of a high level of effort, a few students began to discuss with each other a change in the direction of their efforts; after October 3 this change of perspective became dominant. We explain how the time periods of the two perspectives overlap in greater detail when we discuss the data.

Several events influenced the change or partial change in the students' perspective. Figure 2 shows the sequence of these events.

September 27 — Unannounced quiz in gross anatomy: "shotgun."
October 5 — Shotgun grades given out.
October 11–12 — The block: examinations in gross anatomy and
    microanatomy.

Fig. 2. — EVENTS OF THE PERIOD OF THE PROVISIONAL PERSPECTIVE (September 24 to October 12, 1956)

Getting their papers back from the shotgun and the approach of the examinations precipitated discussion among the students about how well they were doing. The block itself provoked more discussion and self-examination. This "traumatic" event, to use the students' word, consisted of four tests: a written and a practical in both gross and microanatomy. The written examination in gross anatomy was of the essay type, calling for thoughtful, organized answers on a few topics. The practical exam took place in the lab and was conducted as follows: Each student was given a clip board and an answer sheet. At the ringing of the bell, he moved from one tank to another in sequence around the room. Each cadaver had one or more structures tagged, and the student had two minutes to find this tag, identify the structure, and name it on his answer sheet. There were about fifty questions.

If his performance on an examination was borderline or unsatisfactory, a student received a "pink slip" in his mail box. He got some idea of how well he did when the instructor went over the examination in class. The faculty also conducted what the students called "chewing out sessions," in which borderline students were called out of lab for personal interviews.

The microanatomy examinations also consisted of a written and a practical. The practical was conducted in the same way as in gross except that the student moved at the bell from one microscope to another. In the two minutes he had to adjust the instrument to his eyes, identify the tissue, and name it.

While some students prepared themselves for the examinations alone, others held bull sessions or returned to the lab at night in a group to review on a particularly well-dissected cadaver. Another way students prepared in gross was by "tank hopping": touring the lab to look at other students' dissection or spot cadavers with anomalies. This was encouraged by the instructors, as it is often quite difficult to recognize a structure in another cadaver. As for the anomalies, some students were convinced that many of these would appear on the practical, while others scoffed at this, saying it would not be "fair"; the faculty could not demand such detail.

The large number of items on the practical exam encouraged some students in the belief that the faculty would be "out to get them" with trick questions, anomalies, or minutiae, since there were not, in the students' view, as many as fifty prominent structures in the dissected region. They therefore decided that the faculty in making up the test might have to resort to questions on small things little emphasized in texts or lectures. Thus, students regarded the practical very much as they would a paper-and-pencil objective or short-answer test and studied for it by memorizing, often emphasizing things they considered unimportant. This is in direct contrast to studying for an essay examination, where students reason that if there are only a few questions, these will be on important topics.

Studying for microanatomy entailed fewer problems of this sort because the lab manual in this course directed students' attention to what was important in the text and on the slides. Graduate assistants and instructors helped students prepare for the microanatomy examinations with slide sessions in the lab at night. Fraternity houses also held slide sessions, using a projector and screen to show enlarged pictures of tissue which the students could identify together.

In addition to the two opposed ways of studying suggested to students by the different demands of essay examinations and practicals, the two courses, gross anatomy and microanatomy, demanded different things of them in a wider sense. These courses typify alternative styles of preclinical teaching. One type, as in gross, presents students with a mass of material, detailed texts, big projects in lab: the subject in all of its ramifications. While lectures organize major topics in this material for the student, there is a lot left for him to deal with himself. Students call such courses "big," "tough," "important." The other type presents material in organized form from the beginning, as in microanatomy, where students had a manual that co-ordinates reading and lab work. Both students and faculty argue among themselves about the relative merits of these two types of teaching, using the term "spoon-feeding" to describe extremes of the latter if they oppose it.

Faculty proponents of spoon-feeding say there is so much for students to learn that this is the only economical way to teach them. Those who favor the detailed style believe that students must be taught to think and that having them organize a mass of material for themselves is the way to do it. On the whole students developed perspectives to solve the problems arising in the "big" course. What they do, and what is so disturbing to some members of the faculty, is to devise the most economical ways of studying. The faculty often sees their methods as ways of avoiding thought.

Let us make it clear at the outset that as sociologists rather than medical educators we take no side in the "thinking" versus "spoon-feeding" controversy; nor do we, because we looked more closely at students than faculty in our study, take sides for or against faculty or students in the argument that now begins between them and continues in various forms through the four years of school. It is a timeless argument, after all, present in most educational institutions and seldom solved. Students see things one way; faculty another.

What we do want to make clear is what perspectives the students had and how these relate to their environment.

While it is true that the major events of this period in which the students changed their perspective were the examinations, by describing them at such length above we are not suggesting them as causes of the change. They provided a focus for student discussion and an occasion for self-assessment; but, as we saw in the illustrations of the initial perspective, many students were already discouraged with their attempts to learn everything. No matter how hard they tried, they were not succeeding in the effort to learn it all. Thus, the pressure for change arose directly from the difficulties they encountered in carrying out the initial perspective under the environmental conditions of a heavy, continuous schedule of large amounts of work described in Chapter 6. This student puts the dilemma well:

I said, "Has it been the same as you expected it would be?" Harry Singleton said, "Well, no. It really is different. I expected that medical school would be different than college and that you would really learn everything there was to know about things, so that you would remember it for later. But you can't learn all this and get it in your head so you never forget it. I guess you just have to learn for the test . . . I guess these subjects that we have the first year are not as important as I thought they were. You just learn them so you can refresh your mind later and look it up in a book when you have to. You'll forget it all after the test, there is so much. It has been a real shock to me."

(October 9, 1956. Married independent.)

There is too much to learn, this student says. His solution, and we shall see that this is one of the alternatives students saw during this transitional period, is to learn for the test. But he is disillusioned; he thought medical school would be a place he could learn for himself; it is not. There is a hint in what he says that he thinks perhaps next year, when he gets to the hospital, he will be able to return to his idealistic initial perspective and learn everything because everything will be relevant to practice.

We find many other instances in our field notes in which students show that they have given up their initial perspective and developed a new perspective, which may be summarized as follows:

1. In spite of all our efforts, we cannot learn everything in the time available.

2. We will work just as hard as ever, but now we will study in only the most effective and economical ways, and learn only the things that are important.

3. Some students said: We will decide whether something is important according to whether it is important in medical practice.

Other students said: We will decide whether something is important according to whether it is what the faculty wants us to know.

We call this the provisional perspective because it is a bridge between their initial perspective and their final views. While all students agree in the provisional phase that there is more than they can learn in the time available to them, and that they must therefore *select* what is important and study that, they are not agreed about the proper criterion for making this selection. Some students think they can decide what is important according to whether it is important for practice; others think the best criterion is what will be on the examinations. Students with the former view ask themselves: Will I have to know about this when I am in practice? Those with the latter view ask: How can I find out what the faculty wants us to know?

In presenting the incidents from our field notes as illustrations, we argue that each incident expresses one or more points of the provisional perspective outlined above. There are four types of items. In the first type students admit there is more to learn than they can master and describe their decision to give up trying to learn it all. They usually give a general plan of what to emphasize when studying and what to leave out. In the other types of items students take for granted the necessity of selecting the important things.

In the second type of item students discuss the most effective and economical ways of learning. In type three, they make judgments about areas of knowledge they consider important or a waste of time, by which they mean work to be emphasized or relatively neglected. In the last type, students use one criterion or the other (practice or the faculty) to decide what to review for the block and to criticize the examinations after they have taken them.

Early indication that a few students were beginning to adopt a new perspective as to the direction of their efforts came as the result of the observer's asking an irrelevant question:

I asked Howie Newell if the boys studied in groups at his fraternity house. He replied, "Well, some . . . but all the guys now are trying to find out what it is they want us to know; I think it stands to reason that lectures are important and you don't have to learn it all yourself."

(September 25, 1956. Single fraternity man.)

The next day the same student took the observer aside and explained himself in greater detail. This student has clearly given up trying to do everything. There is not enough time. His problem is now one of selection:

During a coffee break Newell came up to the observer and took her off a little way from the rest of the students. He said, "I have a theory worked out about this studying. I think that the most important thing is the lectures. . . . I think that if you take very good notes at the lectures and use your textbook to fill in parts you don't understand, you will get through very well. I think these guys who sleep through the lectures have got the wrong end of this. You know, it just stands to reason there isn't time to go home and figure it all out in your books the way Vic Morse (his fraternity brother) does. We just couldn't get through if we did that. Now, just think about how much time we have. We are in class eight hours a day and then we go home and study four or five hours. Now, that chapter on bones took four hours to read. If you did that you wouldn't have time to read up on the things that you did during the day. That would be only two hours reviewing and two hours preparation, so I think the thing to do is to just skim through the chapters so you are familiar with spelling and then go to the lecture and take very good notes and after the lecture just pick up the parts you don't know.

I think this week there's been a big change in us. I think most of the guys are trying to figure out what to do, that is, a system to study by, but you know, I think there are an awful lot of them who don't know what they are doing at all. Now in our house — this is confidential, of course — we've been trying to figure out . . . everyone is trying to figure out a system. I think I'm the only one who is working on mine but I think I'm right — I hope I am. I think I'm just about an average guy in this class . . . but I don't think I'm good enough to get all this stuff by myself."

(September 26, 1956. Single fraternity man.)

In selecting among the various ways of studying, this student chooses to emphasize lectures; he thinks they will give him the most information about what the faculty wants. What he means, of course, is that he thinks the examinations will be based on the lectures; and, if this is true, reading and figuring things out for himself, at least things not in the lectures, is not very important. He is thus departing from faculty advice, mentioned in Chapter 6, that students follow a fourfold program of study: reading, attending lecture, working in lab, and reviewing.

We note that other students in his fraternity house are also trying to decide what is important and that they discuss it with each other.

The girl in the next example makes much the same point: there is not time enough to follow the fourfold program. (This pretentious term is ours; the students did not use it.)

The observer had supper with Betsy Holloway. She said, "The trouble is, of course, that you should review this [dissection] every night, but then you don't get a chance to prepare for the next day; so, I haven't been doing the reviewing. If I had been I think I would have done all right on this quiz [anatomy shotgun]. It really has made me feel a lot better to have taken it. I'm not so frightened of the block any more, but I think we'll really find out then what they want. It's so hard to tell what they want. Of course, they say that you are supposed to go as far as you can on each subject, but when the instructors come around, they don't tell us anything. They won't answer any questions about that. They just say, 'Do the best you can,' and it really makes me feel very insecure. I wish they would give us assignments and chapters to read so that we knew how much to do. The way it is this way, you read and read and you don't know whether you've done enough and you always feel that you haven't."

(September 27, 1956. Girl independent.)

This girl is also selecting, but she has chosen to emphasize the preparatory reading and skimp review. She makes it very clear that her criterion is "what the faculty wants." But a rebellious note is sounded which might have become a dominant part of the provisional perspective; indeed, some of the staff were afraid it would. She is upset when she asks the faculty what she should know and they answer: "Do the best you can." In common with many students using the criterion of "what the faculty wants you to know," she is resentful when they do not uphold their part of the bargain and explain what they want in concrete terms.

In one of the illustrations of the initial perspective used in Chapter 7, a student suggested that one way of dealing with the tremendous workload was to memorize, as it takes less time than "thinking." This is a kind of selection; a discouraging one to faculty who feel that thinking is important. In the incident below, two students have a rather confused conversation in which one of them advocates memorizing. The observer then brings up physiology, since in this course the instructor had been making special efforts to get the students to think. The students complain that they made a mistake, or "goofed," by going into the assignment on too deep a level:

The observer joined Al Cowper and George O'Day, married students who live in the same trailer camp, who were sitting outside the building and talking. Al said to George, "You know, I think that anatomy is the easiest subject for me — it's just a question of memorizing. I have a very hard time with the other subjects because you have to recognize your cells." The observer said, "How did you like physiology lab on Monday?" Al replied, "Oh, I enjoyed that very much. I think that's one of the most interesting things we've done so far. There are some things about it that weren't good, though. We certainly goofed on it, didn't we, George?" George said, "Yeah, we spent three hours Sunday afternoon reading up on that darned thing and then when we got to the lab we discovered that they hadn't wanted us to do that at all. All they wanted us to do was to be able to set up the experiment." Al explained, "You see, what happened was they didn't tell us what to do, so we went in much deeper than we had to. As a matter of fact Professor Z explained all that to us in his lecture and what happened was that we went over to the library late and the other guys had taken out all the recent books. We had these books going back into the thirties and twenties, giving the theories that are no longer any good, and we worked on that stuff and then we found out that it had all been a waste of time." The observer said, "Well, which way would you rather study — that way or the way it is in the other courses?" Al said, "Oh, I think the only thing for us here is to have them tell us what to do. There's so much work to be done that we don't have time to think about it."

(September 27, 1956. Two married independents.)

When it is a question of how deeply to go into a subject, these students want the faculty to tell them; they think they do not have time to figure it out for themselves.

Then they were joined by a fraternity man with quite another idea:

Jim Hampton came up and stood listening to this conversation. He said, "Well, I don't see how you can tell what level to be on in anatomy." Al said, "What do you mean?" The fraternity boy replied, "Well, how do you know how much they want you to know?" Al said, "I don't think it's a question of how much they want you to know. I think everyone has to go in there — at least this is the way I figure it — and learn all he possibly can. I don't think we'll have time to learn that extra something and know completely all about it, but I think you have to try to do the best you can and hope that that will come out all right." The observer said, "How can you tell when you're on the right level or not?" Al replied, "Well, that's the trouble, you can't. There isn't any way of telling."

(September 27, 1956. Two married independents,
one single fraternity man.)

The fraternity man takes it for granted that it is up to him to find out what the faculty wants. The other boys disagree. They are not willing to give up learning the subject and start "learning the faculty." Although they agree with the first proposition of our summary of the transitional perspective, "We can't learn it all," they want to continue trying to do all they can, hoping the faculty will help them, rather than making any selection of what to learn on their own. We count such statements as negative cases because they are unwilling to select.

The incident illustrates a division between fraternity members and independents which we discuss in the next chapter.

Once a student has changed the direction of his effort from trying to learn everything to a more limited perspective, and even before he has quite made this decision, he begins to distinguish certain activities as a "waste of time" and others as "important." Those that waste his time he skimps or shirks; he puts his time on important ones. Putting aside for the moment the question of whether his criterion for such judgments is importance for practice or examinations, what activities does he think waste his time, what is or is not important?

Students use the phrase "a waste of time" about physiology lab experiments and certain stages of dissection — peripheral nerves and vessels or deep areas such as the axillary. They think the information they get from such activities could be more easily and quickly learned from a textbook. They also consider they have wasted their time if they read material not subsequently covered in lectures. This notion implies an assumption on their part that only material covered in lectures is likely to appear on examinations.

In this example a student followed faculty advice and read up on the lecture topic before coming to class:

During a break from psychiatry lecture with Al Jones, Hap Garrett, and Ken Thomas, Ken said, "I think they should give us more definite assignments. Remember that lecture on early development we had last week? I read the chapter corresponding to it and he didn't talk about it so I wasted my time and we don't have time to waste."

(October 1, 1956. Three married independents.)

Students who disregard instructions in the lab manual usually say it is to save time:

At tank 2D two partners, Downing and Boas, discussed how far they would go in the dissection of the axillary area, an extremely complex part of the body. One of them said to the other, "I'm not going to dissect any more in this axillary area. It's not worth it. You can pull them [nerves, blood vessels, and lymph nodes] out and look at them, and we don't have time to do it [dissect further]."

(September 27, 1956. Two single fraternity men.)

Sometimes students do things they think the faculty might consider cheating but which they regard as sensible short cuts. In the following example, one student teaches another how to take such a short cut, explaining his action as he does it:

I watched Joe Field and Tom Gordon doing a physiology experiment with a frog. The experiment consisted of dipping one of the frog's toes into acids of increasing strength and noting the muscular contraction. Mimeographed instructions directed the student to put the toe of the frog into the acid at just the same level each time and directed them to keep track of the time that the frog left his toe in the acid before he drew it out. Tom made quite a fuss over trying to get the toe into the acid at just the right depth, but Joe really was not making any effort to keep track of the time period. He just wrote down approximately what it was, although he did time the rest periods in between the dipping carefully with his watch. He said, "I think redoing these old classical experiments is a waste of time. I did this one in college and all you have to do is look up the results in a textbook and you'll find out a lot more clearly than we are here." The directions, which I had read, asked the students to explain why various reactions took place, in the light of the lecture they had been given on the topic. The students did not discuss any of this. Joe just wrote down a few times on a sheet of paper. Tom came over and copied down the results. (They had been told to do this experiment separately) Joe observed that I was watching this maneuver and said, "We want to have this look all right, you know."

(October 12, 1956. Two fraternity men, one married, one single.)

The students' perspective in incidents of this type is one of saving time and using what seems to them the clearest and most authoritative source of knowledge. In almost all cases this quick, clear source is the textbook, provided the text readings are also covered in lectures. Although there is a division of opinion among the students, and some of them believe lab work is valuable because "it gives you a feel for things," selecting the textbook as the most economical and effective way to learn is very common. On the whole, the faculty oppose it, as they do memorizing, but do little about it. Thus, the students reason from their definition of the situation: if there is more to do than can be done in the time available, we can solve the problem by taking short cuts in the *way* we learn.

Although there is no hard and fast division, fraternity men are more apt to be concerned about way of learning than independents are.

In addition to deciding on the way to study, students developing the provisional perspective also define entire courses or areas of subject matter as relatively unimportant and hence worthy of less effort. Their criteria for making such judgments are drawn from notions about what doctors actually do in practice, or from clues provided by the faculty: scheduling and grading. Sometimes, as in the first example below, a student makes use of both criteria:

Before supper at the Gamma house several students were talking about their courses. Larry Horton said, "Anatomy is our most important course; I don't think histology is so important. Anatomy is important because it's half our points and besides this will really be practical. You have to know it to set broken bones."

(October 9, 1956. Single fraternity man.)

Students not in a fraternity are more apt to cling to the idealistic criterion of utility for practice:

During a break from the lecture I talked to Hap Garrett and two friends. Hap spoke of an incident which had just occurred in the physiology lecture and then said, "I don't get this physiology anyway. I can't see any application."

(October 12, 1956. Three married independents.)

The basic sciences taught in the freshman year, with the exception of gross anatomy, are now undergoing a period of rapid change; research scientists publish new concepts and revolutionary findings frequently. Lawrence faculty members, most of them themselves engaged in research, include new findings and theory in their lectures. But in spite of faculty emphasis, some students have little use for research and slight courses in which it is presented:

After embryology lecture I joined Al Jones and asked him what he thought about the test (the first quiz in anatomy). He said that he thought it was very fair and had been well marked. He began to talk with considerable violence about some of the other teaching, however. He said, "A lot of this stuff is just belly wash. All this recent research stuff is of no use to us."

(October 8, 1956. Married independent.)

The student in the next example makes the same point, somewhat less colorfully, but is contradicted by a man from last year's freshman class returned to do research:

During his discussion with the last year's student, Phil Corliss said that he thought they ought to have more time in the anatomy lab rather than attending the other lectures. "We need more time on the anatomy. These other things are too scientific. I think science has to do with mathematics and statistics and doctors don't have anything to do with this." The student from last year cut in at this point and said, "Well, I think things are changing about that."

(October 12, 1956. A single independent, a student from the '55–56 freshman class.)

This is the only case of interaction between the freshmen and upperclassmen we observed.

Although these students are using criteria from the provisional perspective to assess the importance of research so that we can use their statements as illustrations of the perspective, their bias against research is not entirely situational. As we mentioned in Part One, many freshmen entered with an anti-research bias brought from the lay culture. They defend their decision to practice medicine rather than go into research by saying that they like to work with people (in research, they think, you work with animals) and are not bright enough (they think research scientists must be exceptionally brilliant). When the demands of their academic situation make it necessary to study only the important things, they incorporate this general bias against research into the provisional perspective that guides their choices.

Within the provisional perspective itself students who use medical practice as a criterion for deciding what is important to study draw heavily on the lay culture for their ideas about what practice is like. With the exception of the psychiatrists and one other person, of whom they see little, their teachers are not M.D.'s but Ph.D.'s, expert in their own scientific discipline but with no clinical training. In the freshman year the students learn little of what physicians actually do. This lack of knowledge handicaps them when they try to decide what to study, but they make up for their vagueness by a rather literal-minded use of what ideas they have. They have been in doctors' offices, for example, and know that it is the technician and not the doctor who uses a microscope. This leads them to the conclusion that courses like histology which involve use of the microscope will be less useful to them in practice than anatomy since both student and physician deal with the human body.[1] Notions of this kind are not likely to be good predictors of what will be on the test.

But if freshmen inflate the importance of anatomy and fail to see the "application" of physiology, they do it with what knowledge they

[1] In a curious inversion of the history of medical research, one student labeled histology "ancient history."

have at the time. That many of them change this opinion in the clinical years does not point so much to any failing on the part of the first-year faculty or lack of understanding on the part of the students as it does to a perennial problem in education: the articulation of subject matter. We will return to this point later. At first glance one might say it could be easily solved by integration of clinical and preclinical courses, but rapid advances in medical knowledge make it difficult for faculty as well as students to know "what is important."

While students using the practice criterion are handicapped in deciding what to study because of their limited knowledge of practice, students who try to decide what the faculty wants them to know also have problems. They are, perforce, more catholic in their judgments, since they can not define a course in the curriculum upon which they will be examined as unimportant. Nevertheless, in their efforts to get things straight in their heads for the test, they lose patience with knowledge which is not both easily grasped and concrete. Research and theory often come into these categories. The two may contradict each other. Both may be at odds with fact; established fact, that is, of the sort found in the textbook. Students reason that whatever else the faculty demands, a passing grade on the test surely requires a knowledge of well-established fact, so that they should study these first. By this reasoning students rank research as something to be reviewed "if we have time." Theory that is difficult to understand may also fall by the wayside in the drive for economical and effective learning. Thus, although they arrive at their conclusions by different paths, students using both criteria of the provisional perspective slight research and theory and make their main effort in anatomy ("practical" to one group and "factual" to the other), while relatively neglecting their other courses.

Similarly, students using the two criteria often have a meeting of minds over exactly what to review for examinations. Among the students who have decided that the best criterion for limiting their work load is what the faculty wants them to know, studying for an examination becomes a matter of prediction. In the following example, students advance various reasons for their guesses about what will be on the test. These range from such objective matters as faculty tips, old examinations, and emphasis in texts or lectures to notions of the importance of a structure in medical practice. In the last instance students straddle the fence as far as their criterion goes: in predicting what will be on the test, they assume faculty choices are based on medical practice.

Some of the students got into a discussion about what would be on the examination. Sam Watson said, "Well, I think we ought to know the collateral circulation. Dr. N told us we should, and I have seen it on the exams from last year." Phil Lee put in, "There's the lymph nodes. I'm sure we will have to know those because N was talking about them in lectures too." Rod Wilson said, "I don't see how he can ask any questions on that. There isn't enough to it. It just goes from here to there." Sam said, "Well, I can think of a good question they might ask, although I think we are getting too test-wise. I don't like to see us doing that. They might ask a question on mastectomy. When they do that they have to remove all the lymph nodes in the axillary area, and down around the sternum too, and under the mammary gland, and I think they take off the skin too." Phil said, "How can they do that [ask such a question]? I don't see how they can." Rod replied, "I don't think they'll ask a question like that." Sam said, "Well, it's all in Morris, and I think they might." Rod said, "I think they'll ask us about the peripheral nerves. I think that's very important. You can get it all out of Morris." Sam said, "Well, I don't see why that's important." Phil agreed with him, but Rod began to be interested in the question and said, "Suppose someone came in with a gash across his wrist here . . . what would you do?" "Well," Phil said, "Hell, that's no problem. You just sew it up and the nerves don't regenerate anyway." Sam said, "Well, suppose someone came in and his thumb and forefinger were numb. They didn't have any sensation. Which nerve would it be?" They argued for some time about this and Sam said that he was interested in it because it was clinical.

(October 9, 1956. Three fraternity boys.)

The students in the incident above are certainly "test-wise," although one of them is sorry to be that way. They give four reasons for thinking something will on the exam: it was in a lecture, on last year's exam, in Morris (their textbook), or if there is enough to say about a structure for it to appear as a discussion question.

This last point reveals why students want to know how many questions there will be on a test. They assume that if there are many questions on an essay examination, some of them may be relatively small points about which there is little to say; but if there are only a few questions, they will be on topics that can be discussed at length. Thus when students ask the question that so often annoys teachers: How many questions will there be on the test? they are looking for a principle with which to organize their review. If they are told there will be six questions, they match wits with the faculty as to which six topics in the subject are important enough to be on the examination. Misunderstandings arise, and the teacher is called unfair, when students and faculty have different criteria for determining what is important.

In the next example, a student describes how he prepared for the block (and illustrates our point very well):

I talked to Al Jones in front of the building after the examination. He said, "I don't like to say it in front of the other guys, but I think the practical [examination] was very easy. I knew just about everything on it, I think. It was a good exam, but I think the written part was lousy." He pulled the exam out of his pocket and began to go over the questions with me, telling me which ones he thought he had done well in. "Now this second one, this is the one on collateral circulation. I just happened to hit that by luck. The night before the exam I was going thru the book and I saw this thing about the subscapular artery and a couple of pages on I saw there was whole network of little vessels in there and I got interested and I started to study it. So really that was just luck, but that's all we can do I guess. First we study the things that we think are important and then we study the things that we think they think are important. Only it's hard to get them all in. There isn't time."

(October 11, 1956. Married independent.)

Thus the examinations provide students with a test of their principles of selection. When a student says a question is unfair because it could not have happened in practice, we can take it that he used medical practice as a criterion in selecting what to study. (The next incident takes place immediately after the one above.)

At this point Chuck Dodge came up to join us. He looked rather grim. He broke in on the conversation between me and Al and said he thought the second question was terrible. "It isn't important in practice what happens under the subscapular," he said. "We'll never see anything like that." I said, "What do you mean you won't see anything like that?" "Well," he said, "in practice. Of course, I don't know much about it. But people come in with broken arms and legs. They don't come in with broken subscapulars." [This was a misreading of the question which referred to an embolus in the subscapular region.]

(October 11, 1956. Married fraternity man.)

Conversely, the student who complains that the faculty has unfairly based the examination on Morris rather than on the lectures has been using the criterion of "what the faculty wants."

Jim Hampton came out and joined Al, Chuck, and me, saying, "Well, that certainly was a fouled up thing. There wasn't a single good question on there. They were all unfair. This isn't the kind of thing to do us any good." I asked Jim what he meant but he seemed unwilling to explain or unable to. I think probably one of the reasons for this was the presence of the two other students who are not part of Jim's group. Jim took out the examination paper, however, and started to go over the questions. He said, "Well, the first one was a very good question. I expected something like that. I thought it was excellent." The other students disagreed with him and there was a good deal of discussion in which Jim took no part. At the end of this Jim said, "Last year's exam was much more on the lecture notes than this one. This is really all out of Morris." He went off in quite a high state of anger.

(October 11, 1956. Single fraternity man.)

The two examination questions mentioned in this incident, the question on the subscapular region and the first one on the wrist, were much discussed by the students. The observer was repeatedly told that students had heard, first or second hand, that the instructor said in lab that these areas were not "important." Students using both the practice criterion and the "faculty-wants" criterion neglected the areas in review:

I went out for a break with Eddie Cawley and he told me his mark on the anatomy practical. He said, "I think they were fair tests except maybe the written anatomy. That was on questions we didn't have in dissection. Remember the question on the scapula? And then there was the one about the wrist. I heard that N [instructor in the course] said that the wrist was not important, so I didn't study it. Then on that scapula business, we didn't dissect under there at our tank; I heard N tell somebody that it wasn't important. I don't think that test covered what I knew. When I went into the exam I thought I knew a great deal. I had a lot of knowledge stored up and the test didn't use it. I think a lot of guys felt that way. These things are important to know when you get to be a doctor." He took hold of his forearm and said, "I studied the collateral circulation in the forearm and the lower leg. That's important. I knew it cold. You have to know that when you are a doctor."

(October 12, 1956. Married fraternity man.)

This incident shows a student extending his own criterion to the faculty. He is not above using faculty "tips" before the examination because he thinks that an instructor who says it is not important to dissect a certain area is really saying that the area is not important in medical practice and thus will not appear on the examinations. In other words, the student is so sure his basis of selection is correct that it never crosses his mind that his instructors do not share it. Misunderstandings of this sort between students and faculty are most apt to arise just before examinations when students think almost any utterance of the faculty refers to the test.

Students who study by trying to find out what the faculty wants also think the examination unfair:

After the anatomy examination I talked to Howie Newell (the boy who first discussed this matter of study systems with me before the test). He said, "I had all the wrong leads. There was even a boy from last year who gave me an outline of everything I ought to know for the first test, and it was all wrong. Another thing I found out was that it was wrong . . . the way I was studying. I'm never going to listen to another thing that the lab instructors say to you. They tell you things that they are interested in, but which have nothing to do with us. You know, things that are interesting for them and we don't care. Then I made another mistake; I thought embryo was most important, so I studied that very carefully, but it was only half the exam and I hadn't studied the histology at all because I thought anatomy was the big course here, and it wasn't necessary." Howie got more and more excited and it was difficult to follow him as he jumped from subject to subject, or rather from complaint to complaint. "I think it is wrong to have us study by regions and get all those details and then to ask us general questions on the test. You have to work everything backward, and that isn't fair."

(October 12, 1956. Single fraternity man.)

This is an angry student. He has worked out an elaborate system to find out what the faculty wants, but they have played him false by not following his system.

At this time, students' anger at the faculty for not making up the examination according to one or the other of their criteria was approaching a peak. Some students even suggested that the lab instructor had given them a false tip deliberately and took this as evidence that he was "out to get them." No doubt they felt uneasy about these extreme feelings, for several of them sought out the observer to express more moderate views. Students using the criterion of what comes up in practice justify the faculty as follows:

Hap Garrett, Paul Inkles, and Bob Warren came up to me after the histology practical. Bob said, "I used to teach school and I know it is hard for students to understand what you are getting at sometimes. Now that anatomy exam [yesterday] *was* practical. Remember the question on the wrist and the question on collateral circulation? Those are practical questions. They are things that might really happen."

(October 12, 1956. Three married independents.)

But a student in the other camp blames himself for not having followed his criterion (what the faculty wants) well enough. Indirectly he justifies the faculty:

In the lab I watched Joe Field and Tom Gordon do their experiment. As he worked on his frog, Joe said, "I thought the anatomy practical was good, and both the histology tests were good, but I didn't like the anatomy written. I didn't expect the questions they gave. Of course they have a right to ask anything they want to. I understand that and I think they should. Perhaps it was just because I hadn't figured out that they would ask those particular questions."

(October 12, 1956. Two fraternity men.)

Note that, as in other examples, it is an independent who speaks for the practice criterion, a fraternity man who believes he should select what to study according to what the faculty wants.

In the preceding illustrations we have described the major themes of the provisional perspective. Before summarizing these themes and relating them to the demands and constraints of the students' situation, we present evidence for our contention that the perspective is the customary behavior of students during the period immediately preceding and including the first block. We do this by showing to what extent the perspective was in frequent, widespread, and legitimate use. Table XII shows the frequency with which students use the provisional perspective as recorded in our field notes.

TABLE XII

FREQUENCY OF OBSERVED WORK ACTIVITIES AND STATEMENTS ABOUT WORK
WITH (+) AND WITHOUT (−) PROVISIONAL PERSPECTIVE
(September 24–October 12, 1956)

WEEK OF SCHOOL	STATEMENTS		ACTIVITIES		TOTAL OBSERVATIONS
	+	−	+	−	
September 24– October 3....	17	2	0	0	19
October 8–12...	31	3	6	0	40
Total	48 (81%)	5 (9%)	6 (10%)	0	59 (100%)

Table XII probably underestimates the number of freshmen who agreed to statements of the perspective. Several students were often present when one expressed it, and we counted only the speaker. As the others made no comment or objection, they might well have been counted too.

It is quite clear from Table XII that many more students express the provisional perspective in their statements or acts than do not. Ninety-one per cent of the total (the sum of the positive columns) believe that there is more work to be done than they can do in the time available and solve this problem by taking short cuts to effective learning and studying only those things they consider important. Even the students who are not trying to be selective, the five negative cases in the table, agree they can not learn it all. Their words echo faculty admonitions during Orientation Week:

Vic Morse, after telling me (in answer to my question) about his study schedule, went on. . . . . "I think I have figured out their philosophy. They are giving us more than we can possibly do, but they want us to work up to our own capacity."
(October 1, 1956. Single fraternity man.)

On the way home I asked Dan Hogarth, "What do you think of the curriculum for the first year?" He said, "I think it's fine. After all these guys know what they are doing. I know there are some kids in high school who think they know so much they would like to reorganize all their studies, but I'm not that kind. I think they [the faculty] know what they are doing. I just try to do the best I can. I know they give us more than we can do, but I figure there are a lot of boys brighter than I am and they have to give it to them so that they will have enough to do."
(October 10, 1956. Married independent.)

These students solve the problem of the heavy work load by relying on the limits of their own abilities.

While the number of students who use the provisional perspective is much greater than those who do not, we may wonder if a total of fifty-four instances is meaningful when there are over one hundred students in the class. There can be no very clear answer to this, since the number of observations is related to the fact that there was only one observer in the field and that this observer could not be with more than a few students at a time. Forty observations on the topic in one week (October 8–12) compares favorably with weekly totals for the initial perspective;[2] and we might well argue that had the observer been able to be with more students in the class during the period, more instances of the perspective would have been found.

There is another problem about this total of fifty-four cases, an artifact of our methods of analysis. Since consensus comes about slowly in a large group and is possible only under certain conditions (we discuss these in the next chapter), separating the period of time in which the provisional perspective predominates from earlier and later periods is difficult if not impossible. But to see process and understand it, we must arrest its passage, even if in doing so we create new problems.

We made October 3 the end of the initial perspective because after that date students no longer spoke of trying to "learn it all." They did continue to work hard and expressed feelings of panic as the examinations approached (29 cases, 10/8–10/12). We do not consider these negative instances of the provisional perspective, as they concern level, not direction, of effort. They are additional evidence that students' level of effort remained high in spite of its new direction in the provisional perspective.

In Chapter 7 we mentioned seventeen instances of the provisional perspective in the last two weeks of the period of the initial perspective. These we counted as negative cases. In this chapter we use them as illustrations of the provisional perspective. They are particularly revealing, since they show students thinking out the change from one perspective to the next. There is no doubt that they should be counted in the provisional perspective. From the point of view of time, however, the cases do not represent the behavior of this whole class; the students who express them are forerunners. Nevertheless, we include them in the tables on the provisional perspective, since we have every reason to believe the forerunners kept their views and acted on them during the week of examinations in which the provisional perspective predominates.[3]

Table XIII shows the overlap between the two perspectives.

In answering the question as to whether or not we can consider the provisional perspective customary behavior among the freshmen, we

[2] See p. 99. A total of forty observations in one week, of course, does not represent the total observations on all points during that time. The observations on other points, however, could not be considered collective or recurrent.

[3] On subsequent brief trips to the medical school, the observer checked the stability of the perspective by seeking out students who had spoken freely about the provisional perspective and ascertaining their later views.

TABLE XIII

FREQUENCY OF OBSERVED EXPRESSIONS OF INITIAL PERSPECTIVE
AND PROVISIONAL PERSPECTIVE
(September 24–October 12, 1956)

| | SEPTEMBER 24–OCTOBER 3 | | OCTOBER 8–12 | |
	Statements	Acts	Statements	Acts
Initial Perspective	41	26	8	21
Provisional Perspective........	17	0	31	6

want to know not only whether it is frequently expressed but also whether it is expressed by members of all groups in the class. We have mentioned the division in the class between fraternity members and independents as to the criterion they used in deciding what to study. The observer recorded the interaction of approximately equal numbers of fraternity men and independents throughout the period of field work.[4] But in Chapter 9 we will show there was reason to divide up the class into still smaller groups, based on residence: each of the three fraternities, married men, single men, and girl students being considered separately. Table XIV shows the distribution of the provisional perspective among these groups. The fact that the provisional perspective is expressed in each of the groups assures us that it is widespread.

The variation in the number of expressions of the perspective from

TABLE XIV

DISTRIBUTION OF OBSERVED INSTANCES OF USE OF THE PROVISIONAL PERSPECTIVE BY STUDENTS IN DIFFERENT GROUPS
(September 24–October 12, 1956)

STUDENT GROUP	NUMBER		PER CENT
Fraternity Men:...........	40		74
Alphas		12	
Betas		1	
Gammas		27	
Independents:	14		26
Married men...........		10	
Single men............		2	
Girls		2	
Total	54		100

[4] See Table XVIII, p. 149. The ratio of all recorded interaction (including such matters as sitting next to each other in class) and the number of students in the group is 358/60 for fraternity man and 174/42 for independents. Two members of the class who were identical twins are omitted because the observer could not distinguish between them at this time.

one group to another need not concern us here; the groups are not equal in size, and they are too small for the totals to be meaningful. That 74 per cent of the expressions of the perspective came from fraternity men is a point we discuss in the next chapter. The negative cases (not shown in Table XIV) are evenly distributed: three from fraternity men, two from independents.

Still another way of estimating how much confidence we can have that the provisional perspective is customary behavior among the freshmen is to ask who is present when it is expressed. If in a large percentage of instances only the observer is present when a student states or acts out a perspective, one could argue that they are expressions of individual students and not in any sense collective behavior. If, however, other students are there and tacitly agree to the perspective by making no objections, verbal or otherwise, we can be confident that freshmen consider the perspective a legitimate thing for students to say or do, and in this sense share it.

In asking how confident we can be that the perspective is legitimate, we must also distinguish those situations in which the observer elicits an expression of it from a student by direct questioning from those expressions that students offer spontaneously. Clearly, the latter carry much more weight. Table XV shows how many expressions of the provisional perspective are volunteered and how many are directed. Since all expressions of the perspective are volunteered, and 76 per cent (combining statements and activities) take place with other students present, we conclude the perspective is a legitimate form of behavior among the freshmen.

If we now combine the information from Tables XII, XIV, and XV, we conclude that, although the absolute number of instances is small, as might be expected in so short a period of observation, we

TABLE XV

STATEMENTS AND ACTIVITIES EXPRESSING THE PROVISIONAL PERSPECTIVE
CLASSIFIED BY THOSE PRESENT AND WHETHER VOLUNTEERED OR DIRECTED
(September 24–October 12, 1956)

		VOLUNTEERED	DIRECTED	TOTAL
Statements	To observer alone	13 (24%)	0	13
	To others in everyday conversation	35 (65%)	0	35
Activities	Individual	0	0	0
	Group	6 (11%)	0	6
	Total	54 (100%)	0	54 (100%)

know the provisional perspective is relatively frequent because positive far outnumber negative cases. The fact that at least one member
of every residential group in the class expresses it gives us confidence
that it is widespread. That students volunteer it and feel free to express it before other students whose understanding they take for
granted suggests that the freshmen consider the perspective legitimate behavior. Taken together, these findings lead us to conclude
that the provisional perspective, during the period just before and
including the first examinations, is customary among the freshmen.
The students define their situation as one in which they can not learn
everything in the time available. They continue to work hard but now
select only important things to study. The perspective is provisional
in that some students select what to study according to its importance
in medical practice and others by whether it is "what the faculty
wants us to know." We devote the next chapter to the conditions
which make it possible for the class to reach final consensus.

In thus defining the overload as their chief problem and agreeing
on selection of what is important as the proper solution, the freshmen
display a surprising amount of autonomy. Their behavior does not
fit the conventional model of the proper relationship between teacher
and pupil, for we ordinarily think of students as individuals, not as a
group capable of consensus or of setting their own level and direction
of effort. According to the popular conception, teaching is a dyadic
transaction, an act involving two people with the more experienced
person helping and judging the less experienced. Both have the same
goal: that the pupil should learn. But Mark Hopkins' ideal is not often
realized.

Among themselves, teachers speak of classes as units: this class
is bright, that one slow, a third rebellious. Most of us can remember
ganging up on a teacher in grammar school to sabotage lessons with
fits of giggling, epidemics of shoelace-tying, paper airplane barrages,
squeaking chalk, or clouds of choking eraser dust. But teachers and
children have no common goal; it seems natural enough for children
to combine against a teacher who wants them to read when they want
to have fun.

Some educators explain such outbreaks of concerted action among
students as lack of motivation. If only students wanted to learn, the
educators think, the dyadic model would work. Teachers of this per-
suasion make every effort to prevent students from helping each other
with homework, passing notes, or prompting each other in class, for

the dyadic model assumes that knowledge should be transmitted only from teacher to pupil. Schools reinforce this principle by the grading system, since a child's desire to help his friends can be pointed out to him as "unfair" if the friends get good grades for work they have not done. Even in classrooms where there is an attempt to break down the dyadic model by asking students to report to the class rather than recite to the teacher, the dyad remains the model for examinations.

In these days when co-operativeness and friendliness are so much desired, we understand the teacher's difficulties in maintaining the dyadic relationship. He can probably only do so by punishing co-operative work or with students highly motivated to learn on their own. But motivation to learn may not be the panacea educators think it is. The data we have been presenting on the student culture of the medical school suggests that while motivation may be related to high levels of effort, students seriously committed to their work and eager to learn may, under certain conditions, direct their efforts in ways the faculty does not approve.

We are not suggesting, of course, a close analogy between mischievous grade school children and medical school freshmen, for the similarity is structural: neither group accepts the dyadic model. Medical students are like children only in that both groups have a perspective on how students ought to behave. But where children, at some point in their school careers, seem to their teachers to share a perspective that studying is the least proper behavior for students, medical students want to learn medicine and want help from the faculty. Indeed, many of them try to learn exactly what the faculty wants.

We need not go back over the students' determination to work hard enough to learn everything as expressed in the initial perspective. In many of the excerpts from the field notes in this chapter, students say they want help from the faculty in deciding what is important. They want the faculty to give specific reading assignments and tell them how deeply to go into a subject. When they define lab experiments, dissection of deep and peripheral areas, reading on material not in lectures, and lectures on research and theory as a waste of time, they are saying, in effect, that the faculty ought to help them with the tremendous amount there is to learn by stripping away what students consider inessential. The difficulty here is not that the faculty does not want to help but that students and faculty disagree on what would be helpful.

At this juncture, we must not jump to the conclusion that the actual

model of faculty-student interaction is the one commonly associated
with industry of two groups unequal in power and divergent in interests. It is true that the faculty power to pass or flunk is like that of
management to promote or fire; and students, like workers, gain certain advantages from a united front (teachers are not likely to succeed in keeping a class over the hour or persist in setting examinations
students consider unfair), but in medical school the analogy ends
there. Although each group sometimes phrases the relationship this
way in irritation with each other, the two do not engage in a tug of
war, with the faculty trying to get more work out of students and students trying to avoid it. While this may fit the situation in grade
schools and even in some colleges, in medical school the amount
students work is not in question. Nevertheless, there are serious differences between the two groups.

We will not go into the faculty's teaching philosophies in detail,
for our interviews show divergencies within as well as between departments. But, as we suggested in the beginning of this chapter, different teaching styles in gross and microanatomy point to differences
of philosophy. In gross there are large amounts of detail in dissection
and in texts, and it is in this course that students develop the provisional perspective of the necessity of selection. They spend less time
deciding what is important in microanatomy because the manual in
the course organizes the reading and lab work for them. The style
of teaching in first-semester physiology is different again. In this
course students have to think out how to do experiments and what
they mean. No manual is provided.

Gross anatomy exemplifies one philosophy of preclinical teaching.
It leaves organization of the material to the student with the intent
of teaching him to think. From the point of view of faculty members
who favor this style of teaching, microanatomy "spoon-feeds" the student by giving him only what he is expected to know. The style of
the physiology course demands thinking of the student, but the thinking is about theory and research rather than organizing a large body
of subject matter.

There is undoubtedly a relationship, although not a necessary one,
between style of teaching in these courses and advances in science.
Gross anatomy is a morphological study, and the morphology of the
body has been known for many years. Teachers of the subject are
somewhat in the position of Latin teachers in high school. Theirs is
an old discipline with many teaching traditions, among them a fear

of spoon-feeding and a conviction that training a student to think is more important than the soon-forgotten material he learns. Physiology and microanatomy are rapidly advancing fields; outmoded knowledge must be constantly replaced by the results of research and new knowledge integrated with old. The problem of what to teach freshmen is particularly acute because these sciences must provide students with enough knowledge to understand not only present medical practice but also that of the future based on scientific advances not yet made. Teachers of microanatomy and physiology must select from the many developments in their field what is important for medical students. In many cases, the selection is little more than a guess about what will be medically important in ten or fifteen years. As if this were not difficult enough, teachers are hampered by lack of experience with clinical practice and, in this particular school, by lack of regular contact with physicians at the medical center. Thus teachers of microanatomy and physiology share with students the problem of selecting what is or will be important. Some instructors solve it by limiting the amount of subject matter in their courses: in micro by presenting material in highly organized ways, in physiology by emphasizing theory and research.

As we have seen in this chapter, the limitation of subject matter in the two courses has an effect probably not intended by the faculty. It makes microanatomy and physiology less important in student eyes than gross anatomy, where students do the selecting themselves. (We have no explanation for this, but it occurs in many schools: the most difficult subject has the most prestige and, where there is choice, attracts the best students. Medical students, of course, have other reasons for thinking gross anatomy important, notably its obvious usefulness to physicians and the fact that more semester hours are devoted to it.) Furthermore, we have seen that many students solve the overload problem in gross by relying on textbooks and lectures as the quickest and most authoritative way to learn. They carry this method over into their other courses and earn themselves a reputation of being too pragmatic and uninterested in theory and research. Such differences of perspective further separate students and faculty. Students appear uninterested in courses that emphasize research and theory: they demand facts. Perversely, from the faculty point of view, in the course in gross anatomy designed to teach them how to organize facts, they ask which ones are important. Thus, by creating an area of uncertainty between faculty and students, which the latter fill with their own decisions, the diversity of teaching styles and philosophies contributes to the development of student perspectives frequently unsatisfactory to the faculty.

We do not mean that a lack of a uniform teaching philosophy in a faculty necessarily leads to the formation of student culture. As we have already seen, the isolation of the freshmen from advanced students and the magnitude of the overload problem in the eyes of the freshmen are necessary conditions of such a culture; the third condition, consensus, we discuss in the next chapter. Nevertheless, the lack of consistent philosophy among the faculty turns the students back upon themselves for a solution to their problem of how to reduce their work to manageable proportions and influences the nature of student culture to the extent that it makes it less likely for student perspectives either to mirror or directly oppose faculty views.

Chapter 9   # Interaction and Consensus
The Provisional and Final Perspectives

The Provisional Perspective

Thus far, we have seen that the freshmen, relatively isolated from other groups and beset by what they regard as serious
problems, develop situational perspectives; they have a culture of
their own. Another way to say this is that the group reaches consensus
on how to deal with much of what is problematical in its environment.

We have seen that in the initial perspective they agree on the need
for long hours of work; in the provisional perspective they agree on
the existence of an overload and the necessity of selecting the important things to study. They do not agree, however, on the proper
criterion to use in deciding what is important. Some students use a
criterion of importance for medical practice; others give up the idealistic notion that everything taught them in medical school will be
relevant to practice and begin to study "what the faculty wants us
to know," that is, what may appear on examinations.

If we classify the items of the provisional perspective according to
the criterion students use to decide what is important (Table XVI)
we find that although the "faculty-wants" criterion is most frequent
(54%), the practice criterion accounts for almost a quarter of the
items (22%).

Items tabulated under "None" are incidents in which students
make choices as to what is important, but do not specify a criterion
beyond saying that they are taking a short cut to save time, or that a
given course or activity is "a waste of time." Since students thus eco-

TABLE XVI

DATA OF THE PROVISIONAL PERSPECTIVE CLASSIFIED ACCORDING
TO CRITERION USED TO DECIDE WHAT TO STUDY
(September 27–October 12, 1956)

CRITERION	NUMBER	PER CENT
Practice	12	22.2
What faculty wants..........	29	53.7
None	13	24.1
Total	54	100.0

nomical of time are apt to have examinations in mind, we might well have classified these items as "what the faculty wants."

How can we account for this difference in criterion? If we turn to the students' situation itself for an explanation, we ask first if it could derive from differences in contact with outside groups. But because of the isolation of the freshmen, we know they are not likely to get help; and in examples of the provisional perspective, we saw that faculty members are apt to answer questions about what to study with the phrase "Do what you can," thus throwing the problem of selection back on the students. Indeed, as we suggested earlier, instructors are often hard put to it to answer in any other way; there are as many problems in selecting what to teach as there are in what to study.

Are the two criteria perhaps an artifact of our analytic procedure? The time period we assign the provisional perspective may catch freshmen in the middle of the consensual process. The many discussions students have with each other about how to select what is important show they are exchanging ideas on the problem, and such interaction might lead to consensus. Aware of the overload problem, the class may not have had time to work out a solution understood by everyone. According to this hypothesis, students using the practice criterion are a minority who will eventually adopt the criterion of the majority. The fact that the class has already reached consensus in the initial perspective and on most points of the provisional perspective suggests this may be the case.

Whatever the precedent, it is an equally reasonable hypothesis that the class is not working toward consensus. In this case, the time period we assign to the provisional perspective captures a continuing disagreement in the class. The students may be becoming increasingly divided or they may remain as they are. This possibility raises a question we have not as yet met: When there is disagreement among the members of a group on how to solve an immediate problem, what conditions lead to continuing disagreement, what to consensus, about the solution?

Although we do not expect it to apply to our data exactly, there is an analytical distinction we can make here to help us in answering this question. We distinguish the consensus members of a group work out together as they deal with a problem from the consensus that develops when group members have had similar experience in the past from which they can select behavior appropriate to the new situation. Consensus of the first type cannot be achieved without extensive interaction among group members. A group that achieves consensus by selectively transferring previously learned solutions to the present need not interact as extensively.

With this distinction in mind, we can approach an understanding of the disagreement among the freshmen by inquiring into the nature of their interaction and the homogeneity, or lack of it, of the student population. Our inquiry should provide information on whether the disagreement is likely to be a temporary or lasting phenomenon, and the nature of the consensual process itself.

Throughout this section of the book at the end of each quotation from our field notes, we have been indicating whether students are fraternity members or independents. Why call attention to this particular aspect of student life?

We first became interested in fraternity men and independents because they were different. It was the most obvious difference in the freshman class. On the first day of Orientation Week we noticed that while most students stood around after a lecture alone or in conversation with one or two others, there were larger groups of students who came up and introduced themselves to us as members of one of two medical fraternities.

There was a difference between these fraternity men and independents in dress and manners as well as gregariousness. We realized that where our relationship to one group was straightforward and serious, with the other we joked and kidded.[1]

In daily life, in the instant of meeting someone, and even before he speaks, we compile so many cues from his clothing, posture, and

[1] We use the word "group" loosely in this chapter. Here it means simply: people seen together, people we can distinguish from others. In one sense, the chapter is an effort to define "group" in relation to consensus.

facial expression to prepare our own instant response, that we know what quality of voice he will use and the sort of thing he will say before he opens his mouth. We go astray occasionally and hear a gruff voice when we expect a sweet one; less frequently, an angry note instead of kindness. But mistakes are so rare we are startled or shaken with ill-timed laughter when they happen. In fact, we are all so good at picking up cues from first impressions that the play of social intercourse is often best with no rehearsal.

Our first impression of a difference between fraternity men and independents proved good enough to use as shorthand for the clusters of differences we observed that might relate to interaction and the development of consensus. Quite early in the field work we noticed that fraternity men and independents have differing patterns of interaction in class. Later we found the living arrangements of the two groups differently structured, affording differential opportunity for interaction. Fraternity men and independents also differed in latent identity. The amount of interaction of the two groups with their own members and other groups differed. Although not large enough to prevent the class from ultimately reaching consensus, the differences between fraternity men and independents during the period of the provisional perspective were systematic enough to suggest that these groups could be identified with the two criteria in the class for deciding what to study. We tested this hypothesis by means of chi-square.

We now consider the differences in roughly the same order as they appear in the field work, beginning with students' behavior in class. Daily observation of students at times when they are free to interact provides a simple way of getting firsthand knowledge of patterns of interaction. But first let us make clear what we mean by "free to interact."

Freshmen engage in two types of interaction, different in structure and in relation to the process of achieving consensus. In the first type they interact from personal choice; they are companions. In the second type, they have been assigned by the faculty to perform certain activities together, usually in lab, and we call them associates. While associates need see each other only in lab, companions may interact in school, in living-groups, and recreation.[2] We discuss the interaction

---

[2] We consider friendship a special category of companionship, one that influences which students see most of each other within a group of companions. Students who are friends before coming to medical school undoubtedly cross group lines to continue

of companions first as it seems more likely to influence student perspectives at the beginning of the school year than that of associates.

We first noticed the interaction of companions while attending
classes with the students. The observer, who made it a practice to
sit with different students at each lecture, noted that they did not
choose seats at random but followed consistent patterns. At every
lecture members of Alpha fraternity occupied the last rows of seats.[3]
The front rows, with the exception of the very first, were occupied
by Gammas. In order to secure these seats, the Gammas sent someone ahead with notebooks to reserve them.

Members of the third medical fraternity, the Betas, did not sit
together. Since the other two fraternities had pre-empted the front
and back of the room, Betas sat in the middle on both sides of the
aisle. They did not reserve seats but simply came into the room with
several fraternity brothers and took the places available. Independents, who constituted about half the class at the beginning of the
freshman year and 85 per cent of the married men, behaved like
Betas, sitting in the middle of the room in small groups of four or
five students. There were also a few pairs of students who nearly
always sat together. These were apt to be unmarried independents
who also shared a room.

These seating arrangements were so stable that the observer soon
took them for granted and only commented on them in the field notes
when the pattern was disturbed. It remained consistent throughout
the freshman year and held over through the move from Lawrence to
the medical center at the beginning of the sophomore year, although
there are no fraternity houses in Kansas City.

Figure 3, made at a lecture in September of the sophomore year,
shows the seating pattern as substantially the same as that recorded

seeing each other. Our impression from the field work is that only a few students knew
each other well before medical school, and of these still fewer continued to see much
of each other as school went on. We checked into this after leaving the field by estimating possible pairs of friends in our random sample of 62 students and found:

$$\frac{7}{15}$$ (average number of possible pairs of friends per class)

(average number of students per class in the sample.)

That is, in a class of 100 students, about 47 went to the same college in adjacent
classes. (This seemed a better measure than childhood friends.) But from our present
study of undergraduates, we know that in large colleges the chances of making close
friends of the same sex are relatively small unless students live in the same dormitory
or fraternity house. All students in the sample who were possible friends went to large
colleges, but none of the 1956 freshmen in the sample who were K.U. graduates lived
in the same house.

[3] We named the three houses: Alpha, Beta, and Gamma.

for the freshmen with the exception that Alphas now seem to confine themselves to the left side of the room, and Gammas, while still on the right, have not entirely captured the front rows.

Alphas and Gammas also showed a capacity for concerted action when students chose desks in the microanatomy lab on the first day

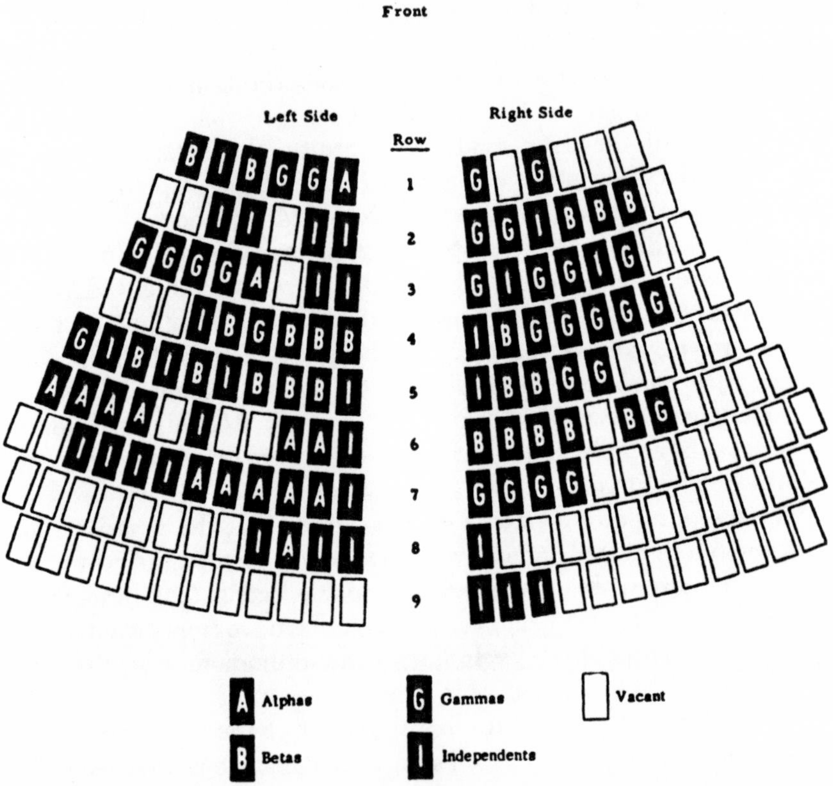

Fig. 3 – CLASS SEATING PLAN – SECOND LECTURE (September 5, 1957)

of classes in the fall. Students were permitted to sit where they wished, but choice was constrained by the fact that the class did not come into the lab at the same time, but four at once, each student with the three dissecting partners assigned him in the preceding anatomy lab. Even under these conditions, by saving seats for fraternity brothers Alphas and Gammas managed to pre-empt most of the right-hand side of the room so that the rest of the class sat on the left.

At a conservative estimate, students spent twenty-three hours a week in class and in the microanatomy lab. Those who sat together exchanged a certain amount of information in lab and had opportunities to talk freely during the ten-minute break from lectures. But the interaction of companions was not confined to these periods. Companions often went back and forth together between their homes and the medical school, and shared living arrangements or residence areas.

On noting this pattern of interaction in the class, we wondered if students would develop situational perspectives within subgroups. The cohesive behavior pattern of Alphas and Gammas suggested that each might develop its own way of solving the overload problem. The scattered pattern of the Betas and independents suggested that these groups were less likely to agree on a solution among themselves.

The Betas were difficult to understand. On the face of it, fraternity living provides maximum opportunities for interaction. We assumed that it was because Alphas had been able to get to know each other well that they were cohesive, and that this was also true of Gammas. Presumably Betas had the same opportunities as the other fraternities, yet they did not sit together. Evidently opportunity for interaction is not necessarily related to cohesiveness as we observed it, and this made us less confident that cohesiveness might foreshadow development of group perspectives.

Since in the course of our observations we were able to attend fraternity meetings and talk to the officers about the way the houses were organized, we turned to the structure of the groups themselves for more information about differences among subgroups in the class. Because Alphas and Gammas were organized in essentially the same way, we use Gammas as an example of both.

About twenty students, all unmarried, lived in the fraternity house and took their meals there. They held meetings and elected officers, initiated members, and ran their affairs very much as they wished. There was minimal supervision by a graduate student who lived in the house, but in the absence of upperclassmen (all at the medical center), freshmen had almost complete autonomy. Election to the fraternity came in the spring before the freshman year. Premedical students from the University of Kansas and nearby colleges, known to the members or interested in joining, were invited to smokers at the house and pledged if they met with approval. Gamma officers obtained names of prospective students from more distant colleges from their faculty adviser.

In October the Gammas pledged nonresident members, most of

them married. These new members might have lunch at the house and a few of them did, particularly the single students, but on the whole the formal contact of nonresidents with the fraternity came only at Wednesday night guest dinners when wives were also invited. Although a student could put in a bid himself, names of prospective nonresident members were usually suggested to the house by one of its officers. In every case known to the observer the officer recommended a student who worked with him at the same anatomy tank.

The organization of the Betas was similar to that of the Alphas and Gammas. They differed from the other fraternities, however, in recruitment of new members. In the year the observer was there, there were a number of vacant rooms in the house when medical school opened in the fall, and the head of the house and some other students who had been elected the previous spring went about openly among the students suggesting that they join. There was an embarrassing incident in which several students simply moved into the house without having joined the fraternity or asked anyone for permission. The officers accepted this as a *fait accompli* and invited the newcomers to join.

Whereas all fraternity men except the few who did not live in the house were single, two-thirds of the independents were married. Independents had no formal organization, officers, or meetings. Some of them studied together in the evening in small groups. Married independents lived in apartments or trailer camps off campus, and either went home for lunch or ate at the Student Union. Single students followed a similar pattern but usually ate at the Union, frequently with a roommate.

Thus far, our examination of the four groups in the class has shown that two of the three groups with highly organized living-structures, the Alphas and Gammas, displayed a cohesive seating pattern in class. The unstructured independents, with their limited opportunities for interaction with each other outside of class, had a scattered seating pattern. We could predicate a relationship between the amount of interaction afforded by the structure of a group and its cohesiveness in class (and go on to seek a relationship between these characteristics and perspective) were it not for the Betas, highly structured but not cohesive.

Betas differed from other fraternities, however, in recruitment, and this suggests we need to know something about the members of a group, in addition to its organization, before we can relate organizations to cohesiveness. In discussing the freshmen, we have been talking about student culture as the perspectives students develop in dealing with situations that arise in the school environment. Another way of looking at student culture is to consider it the *manifest*, as opposed to the *latent*, culture of the group.[4] People carry culture with them when they leave one group setting for another; they do not shed their cultural premises. Something is true of the person by virtue of the fact that he has another social identity which draws its being from another social group. Among the things true by virtue of this fact is that he holds some ideas which are part of the culture of that group.[5] In short, the members of a group may derive their understandings about things from cultures other than that of the group they are participating in at the moment. To the degree that group participants share latent social identities (related to membership in the same "outside" social groups) they will share these understandings — there will be a culture which can be called *latent*, latent in the sense that it has its origin and social support in a group other than the one in which persons are now participating.

The strength and unity of a group's latent culture will, of course, depend on the character of the recruitment to the group. To the degree that it is restricted to persons who come from a similar cultural background, latent culture will be strong and consistent; there will be no variant subcultural groups within the larger group, and everyone will share the premises of the culture associated with common latent identities. To the degree that group members have different latent identities, a latent culture will not be possible.

The concept of latent culture may help us to understand what is happening in the class; to decide whether it is an aggregate in the process of becoming a consensual group, with independents (and possibly Betas) constituting a briefly deviant minority, or whether differences of latent identity in the class are great enough to make consensus unlikely. We use what are often called "background variables," social class or ethnicity, for example, to discover what we can

[4] Several of the following paragraphs are adapted from Howard S. Becker and Blanche Geer, "Latent Culture: A Research Note," *Administrative Science Quarterly,* V (September, 1960), 304–13, in which we make use of the concept of latent and manifest identities advanced by Alvin W. Gouldner in "Cosmopolitans and Locals: Toward an Analysis of Latent Social Roles — I," *Administrative Science Quarterly,* II (December, 1957), 281–306.

[5] We do not mean to imply that latent identities are necessarily based on prior group membership, for Gouldner's example of "cosmopolitan" and "local" identities makes clear that such identities may arise out of the internal "politics" of organizations.

about group members. In doing this, we assume that background variables may be related to latent identities and latent culture, which may in turn provide a basis for the development of situational perspectives.[6]

We turn to our random sample of sixty-two students to learn about the membership of each of the four groups in the class.[7] Table XVII gives the per cent of the members of each group having certain characteristics of home and college background in common.

The particular variables used in the table were not put in the interview schedule to distinguish subgroups, but merely for general information about social class and previous schooling.[8] Variables of this sort are rather unsatisfactory to deal with because we know they are confounded. Our intention in selecting them for Table XVII was not to find the best indicators of similarity or difference, but to use as many variables as possible, thus making it as difficult as we could to obtain consistent patterns.

We use all the easily quantifiable items in the schedule on social

TABLE XVII

Per Cent of Each Companionship Group Having Certain Background Characteristics in Common
(Random Sample of 62 Students)

Group	(1) No Gaps in Schooling: High School to Medical School	(2) Father With Some College	(3) Mother With Some College	(4) Urban (10,000 +)	(5) Parental Support (50% +)	(6) Fraternity in College	(7) Graduate of K.U.	(8) Professional Father
Alphas N 12	83	75	50	66	66	100	75	58
Gammas N 21	85	57	71	52	47	47	43	47
Betas N 14	50	57	43	43	28	14	43	43
Independents N 15	46	46	40	26	13	33	20	20

[6] One point needs further clarification here. The use of the terms "manifest" and "latent" connotes nothing about whether the cultural items operate with or against the openly expressed aims of the organization. It might be thought that manifest culture, for instance, would not operate at cross purposes with stated organizational aims, but it well may. In medical school, the student culture has as one of its functions the support of organized deviance from the goals of the administration and faculty. Yet we refer to this as manifest culture because it is tied to the students' identities *as students* and grows up around problems of the student identity. Similarly, latent culture may support stated organizational aims.

[7] We feel free to use students from all years in school since the background variables antedate medical school. The use of the entire sample also permitted us to see if the 1956 freshmen differed, at least in these variables, from upperclassmen. We made separate tables for the whole group and the freshmen (not given here), and found little difference between them.

[8] The entire schedule appears in the appendix to this volume.

class and school experience, omitting those which did not distinguish the groups. Virtually all students in the sample are Protestant Midwesterners. Those who are married have wives with some college education; siblings have some college education and are engaged in professional work.[9]

Items relating to home background (columns 2, 3, 4, 5, and 8 in the table) are parents' education, size of home town, amount of parental support in college, and father's occupation.[10] In each case we dichotomize the variable, entering in the table the per cent of group members sharing the characteristic indicative of higher social standing. For example, for the father's education variable we enter the per cent of group members having fathers with at least one year of college (the most educated category of any size), as opposed to those without college.

The variables related to previous school experience (columns 1, 6, and 7 in the table) are also related to social class, perhaps more meaningfully than home variables, since they indicate current status.[11] Students who have gone straight through from high school to college to medical school (column 1) are more likely to have financially able families. Membership in a college fraternity indicates higher social standing in college than being an independent. For those students (the vast majority) who come from Kansas, to be a graduate of the University of Kansas carries more social prestige than to have gone to other colleges in the state.

More important for our purposes in estimating similarities in latent identity, those who have gone straight through in a fraternity share many experiences, academic and social. This is strikingly so, if we compare them with those students who have been in military service or held jobs, who have not been exposed to the highly organized social life of a fraternity but have been on their own in college or attended one of the many small colleges of the region.[12] Thus, on the college variables, a high figure indicates a large amount of shared experience; a low figure indicates not only that few members of the group have gone to the University of Kansas, for example, but also that those who

[9] Questions 133, 16, 12, 23, and 22 in the interview schedule.
[10] Questions 20, 21, 16, 7, and 18.
[11] Questions 24, 39, and 29.
[12] We feel reasonably sure of these statements since we are presently investigating these and other matters in the course of a study of University of Kansas undergraduates. Our understanding of social class in the region was enhanced by Richard Coleman's "Social Class in Kansas City" (unpublished Ph.D. dissertation, Committee on Human Development, University of Chicago, 1959).

did not attended many different colleges and have not shared anything but the fact of having gone to a college.

Our analysis of Table XVII will not be exhaustive as we are not interested in particular characteristics of each group but in relating these data to what we already know of the structure and cohesiveness of the groups. We ask two questions of the table: 1. How similar in latent identity as measured by these variables are the members of a given group? and 2. Are any of the groups similar to each other in latent identity?

Answers to these questions should give us more information on whether the class is in process of working out a common perspective on how to select what to study or is divided into subgroups, each possessed of its own criterion derived from previous experience.

Although this is a small sample, and each of the groups includes students from the four medical school classes, Table XVII shows that there are indeed differences among the groups in the number of members with similar latent identity. We have shaded the cells which show that 50 per cent or more of the group members have a characteristic in common. By this rough measure, Alphas have more members who are homogeneous in background than any other group; they exceed 50 per cent on every variable. Gammas hover about the halfway mark on most variables and exceed it in four. Betas reach the mark twice; independents not at all. Thus, the groups form a hierarchy in which each group has a larger percentage of members sharing a characteristic than the group below. (The larger percentage of Gammas with college-educated mothers is an exception.[13]) Since the figures indicate the per cent of members in the upper range of each dichotomized variable, the table also ranks the groups in social class.

We have no way of telling, of course, where to draw the line and declare a group too varied in background to share latent culture. Homogeneity diminishes gradually from one group to the next. The data does tell us that Alphas are quite different from independents in latent identity and that the latter are much more varied in background. Where Alphas have a large proportion of members who have gone straight through from high school to college to medical school, belonged to college fraternities and graduated from the University of

[13] The reversal in mother's and father's education for Alphas and Gammas suggests there is less difference between the two groups than might appear on the basis of father's education alone. Coleman, *op. cit.*, p. 261, believes the wife's education is more predictive of social status than the husband's in Kansas City.

Kansas, more than half the independents have had their schooling interrupted by jobs or military service. This means that many independents are older than the typical Alpha and that they have had greater experience of the world. Included in the independent group are students who have gone to large state colleges, small denominational colleges, municipal colleges, teachers' colleges. By living at home, in apartments, or in dormitories, two-thirds have not experienced the highly structured social existence of a college fraternity.

On the home variables, where Alphas have a relatively high proportion of members raised in cities, whose parents contribute more than half their support, and who have professional fathers, independents are rural, self-supporting, and most of their fathers are engaged in one of the many nonprofessional occupations. Of the groups, one would surely nominate the Alphas as most likely to have a latent culture based on similar latent identities and independents as least likely.

What can we say of the two middle groups, the Gammas and Betas? Except in the matter of parental support, much lower for Betas, the two are alike on home variables, but on college variables, to which it seems reasonable to give more weight because they are more recent, Gammas are like Alphas, Betas like independents.

Our picture of the freshman class has now become more detailed. The class consists of four subgroups. Alphas and Gammas are highly structured, cohesive, and similar in latent identity. They are slightly higher in social origin than the less cohesive, less homogeneous Betas and independents whom we may consider (despite the organized living-structure of the Betas) residual groups, less likely to possess a latent culture consistent enough to affect the formation of the manifest culture of the class.

Having come thus far, what can we now say of the relationship of these groups to the criteria students use to select what is important to study? While it is tempting to speculate, before we fit the four groups to the two criteria, we need information in still another dimension: the amount of interaction in the class.

We have been discussing the groups as if they were static and nothing about them changed. While it is true that each group continues to follow the same seating pattern in class throughout the freshman year, and neither the structure of its living arrangements nor its latent identities change, we commonly expect interaction patterns to be fluid. When a number of people come together at the start of an undertaking, differences in latent identity and living arrangements may present barriers to interaction, particularly to the interaction of companions. Thus, at the beginning of the school year we expect students to interact more frequently with members of their own group than with members of other groups, but as the year goes on and they associate with each other in school, we expect this pattern to change, at least to some extent. With our knowledge of latent identity in the groups we can go further than this common sense approach and look for a pattern of interaction related to these identities that would help to explain the difference of perspective in the class. We approach this problem in the next table.

Table XVIII shows what per cent of the recorded interaction of each group is with its own members and what per cent with members of other groups. Data for this table were secured by going back through the field notes for the period between September 5 and October 12, the last day of the first examinations, and counting the number of times each student was observed interacting with another student or students. This includes mention of students observed sitting with each other in the classroom, talking to each other during breaks, walking back and forth to the medical school, or eating together. It does not include laboratory situations where students were working associates but not companions.

The data are limited by the inability of the observer to be in more than one place at a given time, and we wonder if the observer spent more time with one group of students than others, even though a conscious attempt was made to observe all groups. As a check on this possibility, the number of students in each group can be compared with the number of observations, and it will be seen that the proportions are about the same, except for the girls.

We separate the girls from the rest of the independents; they are such a visible minority in the class that they evidently turn to each other for company.

Table XVIII shows that from the beginning of the year until the time of the first examinations members of each group in the freshman class interact much more frequently within their own group than with members of other groups.

If we compare Table XVIII with Table XVII, we find that the differences in amount of interaction among subgroups, although slight, are in the direction suggested by our findings on latent identity. For instance, both Alphas and Gammas are more exclusive than either of the two other groups in that not more than 16 per cent of their

TABLE XVIII

Per Cent of Recorded Interaction of Group Members With Own Group and Other Groups
(September 5–October 12, 1956)

Group	N	Alphas N	Alphas %	Gammas N	Gammas %	Betas N	Betas %	Independents N	Independents %	Girls N	Girls %
Alphas	18	96	60.8	31	11.8	4	2.6	26	12.2	8	8.0
Gammas	23	31	16.4	170	63.6	15	7.2	34	16.7	9	9.0
Betas	18	4	2.5	15	5.0	92	58.2	46	22.6	3	3.0
Independents	36	28	15.9	34	15.5	46	30.0	94	46.1	6	5.0
Girls	6	8	4.4	9	4.1	3	2.0	6	2.4	80	75.0
Total	101*	165	100.0	259	100.0	160	100.0	206	100.0	106	100.0

* Two non-fraternity boys are not included; they were identical twins, and the observer could not distinguish between them at this date. One student left school during this period.

interaction is with an outside group. This fits the cohesive behavior of Alphas and Gammas in class, their selective recruitment, and relatively homogeneous home and college backgrounds.

Interaction with another group runs as high as 30 per cent for the Betas; 22 per cent for independents. The lack of cohesiveness of both these groups in class and their heterogeneous backgrounds fit this tendency to interact with others.

Our several sources of data suggest that Alphas and Gammas are likely to be able to achieve consensus about the problems they face in school, but Betas and independents are not. We know that the interaction of Alphas and Gammas in class is patterned in the same way. In Table XVIII the two fraternities show an almost identical pattern in amount of interaction: a relatively large amount of interaction with each other (16% and 12%, respectively), frequent interaction with independents, but little with Betas. If we combine this information with that of Table XVII, which indicates that Gammas approach the homogeneity of the Alphas in home and college background more closely than other groups do, we conclude that Alphas and Gammas may be sufficiently alike in latent identity to share a previously learned solution to the overload problem.

Outside their own group, Betas see little of anyone but independents. Their failure to interact with other fraternity men is understandable if we remember from Table XVII that only 14 per cent of them were Greeks (fraternity men) in college, and that many of them differ from men in the other two houses in that they are older, have had experience in the army or jobs, and are supporting themselves. At the same time, half the Betas have been in school continuously and 43 per cent are from the University of Kansas; there are differences inside the group that make it unlikely that Betas share a latent culture.

Independents are the most catholic of the groups in interaction. They see less of their own and correspondingly more of other groups than fraternity men do. At first glance this is surprising, although we might argue that married independents who were Greeks in college might continue to find fraternity men congenial. But Table XVII, since it describes the whole student body, provides a poor estimate of the number of undergraduate Greeks who are independents at the beginning of the freshman year in medical school. The medical fraternities pledged nonresident members in October of 1956, and the interaction of these men with fraternity men probably raises the amount of interaction between the groups. These considerations, of course, do not apply to all independents but indicate it is a divided group unlikely to solve the overload problem on the basis of shared latent culture.

Our examination of subgroups and their interaction helps us to understand the failure of the freshmen to work out a collective solution to the overload problem at the beginning of the year. The relatively high degree of homogeneity of Alphas and Gammas and the similarity of their latent identities suggest that these two groups may share a latent culture from which they can transfer previously learned solutions to academic problems to their present situation as medical students.[14] Independents and Betas appear less homogeneous in latent identity and less given to interacting within their own group. Their social origins and college experiences are not only more varied than those of Alphas and Gammas, they are also indicative of lower status and prestige. We do not expect them to have a latent culture capable of providing common solutions to current problems or to share the solution of the more unified and influential groups. It therefore seems probable that if we classify the data given in Table XVI by the group membership of students using each criterion, the fraternity men will be more apt to use the majority criterion, "what the faculty wants us to know," in deciding what to study; independents, the minority or "practice" criterion. Table XIX tests this hypothesis.

Although the numbers in Table XIX are small, the preference of fraternity men for the criterion of "what the faculty wants us to know," and the indecision of the independents is clear.[15] (There are too few Betas represented to say much about them, although this very absence of data on what criterion they use is suggestive of their differences from other groups since they are not underrepresented in the field notes.) We conclude that companionship groups in the class

[14] It is important to see that latent identities will not affect either individual behavior within the group or the collective behavior of the group unless they are in some way mobilized and brought into play in the daily interaction of group members. In other words, these latent identities must be taken account of and people must orient their behavior toward latent as well as manifest identities for understandings which are part of latent culture to have any influence on behavior in the group. The fact of being an "old-timer" in the organization or of being a member of some particular ethnic group will not affect behavior unless these distinctions are made use of in daily interaction in groups which support and maintain the culture associated with these "extraneous" identities. Latent culture is thus only a potential, and it needs to be developed in the new situation in the sense that it has to be brought into play and applied to the new problems arising for group members. It does not influence group behavior simply because there are persons present who have similar latent identities.

[15] χ^2: 9.3, df 2, P < .01.

TABLE XIX

DATA OF THE PROVISIONAL PERSPECTIVE CLASSIFIED ACCORDING TO CRITERION USED
TO DECIDE WHAT TO STUDY BY FRATERNITY MEN AND INDEPENDENTS
(September 27–October 12, 1956)

CRITERION	FRATERNITY MEN[*]	INDEPENDENTS	TOTAL OBSERVATIONS
Practice	6 (16%)	6 (37.5%)	12
What the faculty wants........	25 (66%)	4 (25.0%)	29
None	7 (18%)	6 (37.5%)	13
Total	38 (100%)	16 (100%)	54

[*] Betas: Practice, 0; Faculty, 1; None, 1.

affect the development of student perspectives at the beginning of
the freshman year.

The Final Perspective

By analysis of the companionship groups in the class and their interaction, we have sought further understanding of the fact that freshmen use two criteria for deciding what to study in the provisional perspective. In the second part of the first semester the provisional
perspective is succeeded by a final perspective on academic work
which students use throughout the remainder of the freshman year.
Like the others, the final perspective is an outgrowth of previous perspectives closely related to the immediate medical school environment. We now expect it to be related to two other features of the
students' situation — the pattern of interaction in the class and the
latent culture of companionship groups. We discuss the perspective
itself and the medical school environment in the next chapter; interaction and latent culture in this one.

Table XX gives a second compilation of the recorded interaction
of group members with members of their own and other groups. The
accounting begins after the first major examinations and includes
data from the latter part of continuous observation and short periods
(one or two days) of observation through March of the second
semester.

Comparison of Table XX with Table XVIII shows that interaction
of group members with members of their own group has gone down
an average of 28 per cent. Interaction with own group is in some cases
less than that observed with other groups.

It may be, of course, that the observer's attention was more directed

TABLE XX

Per Cent of Recorded Interaction of Group Members With Own Group and Other Groups
(October 16, 1956–March 18, 1957)

	N	ALPHAS		GAMMAS		BETAS		INDEPENDENTS		GIRLS	
		N	%	N	%	N	%	N	%	N	%
Alphas	20	13	17.6	23	12.0	8	7.3	30	17.7	0	0
Gammas	30	23	31.0	82	42.6	38	34.9	49	28.8	0	0
Betas	17	8	10.8	38	19.8	23	21.1	35	20.6	5	21.0
Independents	23	30	40.6	49	25.6	35	32.1	49	28.8	7	29.0
Girls	6	0	0	0	0	5	4.6	7	4.1	12	50.0
Total	96*	74	100.0	192	100.0	109	100.0	170	100.0	24	100.0

* Two non-fraternity boys are not included as they are identical twins and the observer still could not distinguish them at this date.
Five students who had either left school or flunked out by the end of the first semester are omitted.

toward cross-group interaction at this period of the field work or so accustomed to in-group interaction that records of it were not made, but although bias of this kind is likely and little trust can be put in any single figure of either Table XVIII or Table XX, the gross difference between the two tables is clear. Students do not hesitate to cross group lines after the first block. In fact, since in two of the five groups interaction with other group members is as great or greater than with own-group members, we conclude that the original divisions in the class are no longer meaningful.

This is a dramatic change; it calls for more explanation than merely the passage of time. Initial barriers to communication have broken down and the class is now capable of working out a solution to the overload problem together. How has this come about?

We have already mentioned one of the things that lower barriers to interaction in the class: the election of married independents to fraternities. Another is the close association of students in laboratory work. At the beginning of this chapter we distinguished two types of interaction, that of companions and working associates, and we now describe the latter.

When classes begin in the fall, each student is assigned an anatomy partner by the faculty. Anatomy lab is held twice a week. A two or three hour lab follows morning lectures and another, usually three hours' long, occupies the afternoon. At these times the student works continuously with his partner dissecting half the cadaver and is closely associated with the two students dissecting the other half. This enforced association lasts throughout the first semester. Although it is possible for a student to change his working associate by applying to the faculty member in charge, it is made clear to the students that they are expected to get along with their partners and few changes are made. The fact that the student himself has to find another student willing to change with him makes a change difficult. We observed only one case.

In the second-semester biochemistry lab, students are assigned table space alphabetically. In physiology the class is assigned to four laboratories according to anatomy tank numbers, that is, students from the front section of the large anatomy lab go to one physiology lab, students from the second section to another physiology lab, and so on. They choose partners from students in the room. Many students remain with their anatomy partner; a few have the opportunity to join class companions. Thus, every student spends at least ten hours a week with three working associates, and some spend all their lab time (about twenty-seven hours a week) with them.

When faced with serious problems about what to study and how, a student exposed by his working associates to the perspective of a group other than his own may well carry the views of his working associates back to his companions. At the same time, working together in lab provides associates with many opportunities to influence each other as to what and how to study. For instance, some lab partners decide to omit the dissection of peripheral nerves and vessels, as they can get the knowledge more easily and quickly from the text.

Although the continued interaction of working associates as the school year goes on provides opportunities for discussion, and the isolation of the freshmen together with the tremendous amount they think they must learn suggests they will discuss the overload problem with associates as well as companions in the effort to solve it, we do not know what solution they will choose.

One possibility is that groups with prestige or power will dominate manifest culture. If differentials in prestige or power between subgroups are not great enough for one of them to win out, we expect the eventual solution to be a compromise. There is also the possibility that there may be one subgroup which shares a common latent identity and culture while the remainder of the larger group is relatively diverse in latent identity. Members of the culturally similar group will be more able to influence manifest culture than their unorganized mates. Communication between them will proceed more easily because of shared premises, they will have operating agreements almost before others are aware that there is any problem calling for solution. Once established, good communication implies organization which suggests the general proposition that the development of latent culture will depend on the relative strength of organization in people of differing latent identity. One subgroup may have such strength and others not.

The freshmen have several kinds of (latent) social class identities, and they belong to groups which differ in degree of organization. Alphas and Gammas are upper middle class, while Betas and independents are lower in social status. The three fraternities are highly organized; independents are not. We note that formal organization should not be taken as an infallible index of the existence of latent culture, for such an organization may in fact recruit haphazardly, as the Betas did, and end with a membership of diverse latent identities, thus weakening the organization. Furthermore, when people sort themselves out into groups, as the students did when they joined fraternities, many "mistakes" may be made so that people who are not of the "proper" class end up in the organizations.

Such situations warn us to keep other variables in mind. For instance, two groups defined by common latent identities may be present, yet the cultural background of one may make it less likely that its members will effectively combine. It may be that upper middle class culture provides more experience in "combining," so that when this group competes with members of a lower social class the situation parallels that in which one group competes with a diverse aggregate. Even where the background culture did not provide this dividend of combining power, it might be that persons with certain kinds of latent social identities and cultures are more visible to one another than other persons sharing a different latent identity, thus making it easier for them to combine (as, for example, Jews as contrasted with Protestants, drug addicts in many settings, homosexuals, and so on).

Where there are two groups distinguished by common latent identities and a third which is an aggregate of diverse identities, the group with less power to maintain exclusiveness may find itself further weakened by the fact that it becomes, in effect, a residual group: everyone who does not belong to the more exclusive groups finds his place in the less exclusive group, which then has even less strength to achieve latent cultural consensus and contribute to the manifest culture.

In cases where one group's latent culture furnishes the material for the manifest culture, the process can be aided or hindered depending on whether the group more nearly fits the general public's cultural image of what members of the organization or group should be like. Although membership in an organization does not legitimately raise questions about characteristics of the member other than those clearly relevant to the stated operations of the organization, Everett Hughes has noted that auxiliary status traits are attached in the public mind to many statuses and that dilemmas and contradictions of status can arise when a person possesses the key or master status trait but is deficient in the auxiliary status traits.[10] Thus, all one needs to be a doctor is a license, yet it is typically assumed that an

[10] Everett C. Hughes, "Dilemmas and Contradictions of Status," *American Journal of Sociology*, L (March 1945), 353–59.

M.D. will be male, white, and upper middle class. A group which most nearly fits the auxiliary status specifications attached to the manifest identity (i.e., has the proper associated latent identities) may be seen as having more authoritative information or more legitimate right to suggest solutions for the manifest culture.

Thus, our knowledge of the increased interaction in the class after the first block tells us the freshmen are capable of resolving their disagreement about what criterion to use in deciding what to study. The cohesive, highly structured, and socially homogeneous nature of the leading fraternity groups, together with their closer approximation to the popular image of a physician, lead us to expect the class will adopt the fraternity solution to the overload problem in its final perspective on academic work. In the next chapter we see that there are also situational factors that convince independents they should abandon the effort to learn what is important for practice, and confirm both independents and fraternity men in studying "what the faculty wants."

Chapter 10 # The Final Perspective

"What They Want Us to Know"

W<small>E</small> have seen that during the period of the provisional perspectives students in the two major subgroups in the class (fraternity men and independents) make different decisions about how to select what to study. The increased interaction in the class after the provisional period and the pre-eminence of the fraternity group suggested to us that the whole class might, in time, adopt the fraternity criterion. We must be cautious about this prediction, however, since clearly the latent culture of a group will provide solutions to current problems only if it is relevant, and no solution will continue in use if it is not successful.

Our present study of undergraduates has shown that such students, particularly members of college fraternities, have elaborate techniques for pleasing the faculty and passing examinations. Undergraduates coach each other and make use of files of old tests to maintain the house average. Alphas and Gammas, most of whom belonged to college fraternities, bring this knowledge to medical school as part of their latent culture. At the very beginning of school, during the period of the initial perspective, they do not use it, idealistically preferring to try to learn everything; but when they find they cannot learn everything in the time available, they revert to the undergraduate practice of learning the things that will appear on examinations or, as they phrase it, "what the faculty wants us to know."

Independents, isolated from fraternity groups until the time of the first block, do not accept this solution to the overload problem as readily. They do not share a latent culture based on college fraternity

158

norms; they cling to the notion of studying not for examinations but for themselves. When they decide there is too much to learn, they choose to study things that will be most useful when they get into practice.

As they develop the final perspective on their academic work which we present in this chapter, both independents and fraternity men decide on the relevance and success of their method of selecting what is important.

The decision they make is not, of course, a conscious one for most students. They are, after all, engaged in a series of trials, reacting to the demands and constraints of their environment and estimating their success from cues given by grades, test questions, faculty perspectives, and the various events, scheduled and unscheduled, of the school year. Thus, although our examination of the groups in the class suggests the freshmen are likely to reach consensus and that they will choose the solution of the fraternities to the overload problem, we can confirm this only within the context of situation and event.

The students' situation — the given, repetitive detail of their lives as medical students — continues much as before, although it is marked, with the beginning of the second semester, by a less demanding style of teaching. We have already discussed the effects of this teaching style. Students have more time off (one or two afternoons a week), although this time is made up in Saturday classes. They have more frequent tests. Since there is less demand that they organize the material for themselves than in gross anatomy, in the eyes of some of the faculty they are more "spoon-fed." For students, the changes make it relatively easier to find out from tests and lectures what the faculty wants.

Although they are less apt to be "clutched" as they become accustomed to them, the examinations at the end of each block of work continue to be the "traumatic" proving ground of student perspectimes. This is so, not only because the penalty of failure is severe (repeating a course or possibly leaving medical school with poor prospects of getting into another), but because test questions reveal to the students whether they are studying the "right" things, and discussion of tests in class or papers returned with comments indicate whether they are answering in the "right" way. The fact that fraternity men appear to do better on the examinations and their system

for finding out what the faculty wants more accurately predicts the
questions are still other factors in the adoption of the fraternity criterion by independents.

The progress of the class toward consensus is also influenced by
out-of-the-ordinary events. These are unusual happenings which
require student discussion because, unlike the routine situations defined in perspectives, such events have no commonly accepted meanings. Thus, many of the statements of the final perspective in our field
notes occur in the context of unusual happenings. Figure 4 lists the
scheduled and unscheduled events of the period of the final perspective.

October 24 — Grades abolished.

October 25 — Exodus from the anatomy lab.

November 27 — Examinations in gross anatomy.

January 15 — Examinations in gross anatomy.

January 24 — Correlation clinic at Kansas City (neurology and psychiatry).

January 25 — Correlation clinic at Topeka (neurology).

Final practical examinations in microanatomy and neurology.

January 28 — Final written examinations in all subjects.

February 4 — Beginning of the second semester.

February 23 — Examination in biochemistry.*

May 20 — Beginning of final examinations.

* We were not at the medical school on any further examination dates, but there
were probably tests at the end of each block as listed on p. 86.

Fig. 4 — EVENTS OF THE PERIOD OF THE FINAL PERSPECTIVE (October 16, 1956, to
September 5, 1957)

Two chief events of the year were the announcement, after the first
block, that grades were abolished, and a trip in January to the medical
center to see neurology patients. A similar correlation clinic was held
in Topeka.

In abolishing grades, the administration inaugurated a policy already in force for students of the three upper classes at the medical
center. The dean, in making the announcement, spoke against competition for grades among students and the fraternity house practice
of keeping files of old examinations. Henceforth, students would not
have examination papers returned to them with numerical or letter
grades and would not be ranked in the class. They would be notified
if their work was not satisfactory. The change reduced tensions in

some students and increased them in others. It had the general effect of drawing the class closer together.

The visit to the medical center, which came after the freshmen completed the study of neuroanatomy, provided them with an opportunity to test their knowledge and compare first-year teaching with the clinical approach. It was particularly meaningful to those students still in process of adopting the final perspective.

At the end of October something happened which we can classify as neither situation nor event: the symbolic ending of the students' "rebellion" against the faculty. In the excerpts from the field notes presented in the provisional perspective, students often expressed resentment of the faculty. They did not complain in general of the teaching, but of specific things: a particular examination question that was unfair because it was "not in the book" or "would not happen in practice"; a misleading "tip" on what to study. As we have seen, it was situations like these in which students felt the faculty had gone back on the universal bargain between teacher and taught to put "important" things on examinations, that provoked resentment.

Although it bewildered some of them because it was a new experience, getting a "pink slip" for failure seldom made students resentful of the faculty. They knew that everyone in the class had done well in college, and recognized that medical school put greater premium on ability and preparation. But the faculty was uneasy. After the first block but before final grades were given out, a graduate assistant spoke to us dramatically of the "coming crisis" between faculty and students. An instructor lecturing late Friday afternoon of the second day of the first block when students had been taking examinations for a day and a half, felt the need to "crack down." He startled the class by taking sharp disciplinary action; something the students had not yet met in medical school:

Dr. S. put some diagrams on the board and then said suddenly, "I rather feel that I am talking to a group that is used up. I suggest that you take a fifteen-minute break. Then if you are ready to come back and take it like a man or woman, you can come back." The classroom had been quiet although there was some restless shifting around in the seats. As we went out of the room, a student said to me, "Hey, did you get that? Did you get that? Put that in your book." He stuck out his tongue in the direction of Dr. S. As we got outside they exploded into such comments as, "I wasn't doing anything, I didn't see anybody doing anything." We stayed outside for less than the usual break of ten minutes.

(October 12, 1956. Single independent.)

But such incidents were rare. It may be that the faculty of state universities must always keep the possibility of student rebellion in mind, since instances of complaints to the state legislature have been known to occur.

We observed the students daily during this period but saw only one instance of overt rebellion. It took the form of exaggerating an undergraduate custom: lining up on the sidewalk to watch the girls go by. The incident is best understood with reference to the anatomy lab regulations. Students were told at the beginning of the year: "There will be no breaks; you are expected to be there [in the lab] all the time."[1] Although many students regularly took short breaks from lab in groups or two or three, this time:

> While we were talking at tank nineteen Shep and I looked up. Great numbers of boys were leaving the lab in a rather self-conscious way. Tom said, "I didn't think they would go out." Shep looked at his watch and said to me significantly, "It's time." I knew he referred to the fact that there is a girl with a very large bust who goes by the building at ten minutes of eleven every day. Last week about one third of the boys went out to see this phenomenon. Jay Downing, the fourth man at this tank, said, "I guess everybody is going out this time." We went too and by the time I left the lab there were only about a dozen boys left in the big room. Outside they were all lined up on the very edge of the sidewalk. Some of them were standing on the stone seats so they could see better and they were watching students as they came along, laughing and joking somewhat loudly together. One of the graduate assistants came out behind me and looked around in an amused way. Sitting down on a bench was Judy Noyes and I kidded her about coming out. She said, "Well, we always take our break at the same time at our tank and besides I have to have my coffee." Her partner Dean Campbell, had a large thermos of coffee and he was passing it around. The business of looking for the girl went on until a little bit after eleven but she did not come, and we all went back into the lab rather sheepishly.

(October 25, 1956.)

Thereafter the rebellious spirit in the class died down; it never became prominent in the students' final perspective.

We may think of rebellion as a possible, if dangerous, solution to the overload problem. Students might have demanded that the faculty lighten their work load instead of deciding to do it themselves by one process of selection or another. This is not to say that com-

[1] See p. 90.

plaints about specific matters ceased, but only that the freshmen did not unite in further direct action against the faculty. Instead, in the daily activities of the final perspective, the class unites in a common endeavor to get information about what the faculty wants; continuing, as they had throughout their shifts of perspective, to define the academic situation for themselves and set their own level and direction of effort.

The final perspective predominates in the second half of the first semester and thereafter throughout the freshman year. Students carry over parts of their earlier situational perspectives: hard work from the initial perspective, the necessity of selection and the most economical ways of learning from the provisional perspective. They add to this behavior the use of the fraternity criterion of selecting what is important according to whether it is "what the faculty wants us to know" and develop techniques to discover what this is.

The many instances of the final perspective in our field notes may be summarized as follows:

1. We select the important things to study by finding out what the faculty wants us to know. This is the way to pass examinations and get through school.

2. We continue to study hard and in the most economical and efficient ways.

3. We try to find out, in every way we can short of cheating, what questions will be on the examinations and how they should be answered and share this information with other members of the class.

In developing the perspective, students find not only a solution to the overload problem that reduces strain and tension for the rest of the year, but also a co-operative way of behaving that draws the class together in the effort to predict and fulfil faculty wants. The level of effort remains high. Most students feel that in directing their effort toward learning what the faculty wants they are also learning medicine, but they are not without resentment and a feeling that they have somehow been forced to give up the ideal of learning for themselves in order to pass the examinations.

In presenting incidents from our field notes as illustrations of the perspective, we argue that each incident expresses one or more points of the final perspective outlined above. There are four types of incidents. We begin with the transitional phase: statements showing students in process of change from the practice criterion to "what the faculty wants." Next come incidents showing that students continue to work hard and study in the most economical and efficient ways. After this, we present statements on how to find out what the faculty wants and the relation of this endeavor to grades and competition between students. Finally, we allow a student a retrospective look at the freshman year.

We have already noted the increased interaction in the class and the stimulus of certain events of the school year on the rapid formation of consensus about the proper solution of the overload problem. While we do not have enough data to document it thoroughly, what we have suggests that the shift from the practice criterion to the criterion of what the faculty wants is easier and quicker for students who interact frequently with fraternity men, that such students are hardly aware of the change. The student in the example below, a married man who belongs to a fraternity but does not live there, explained to us at some length in October how he had studied things "important for practice" for the first block:[2]

This was right after the mid-term examination, and happening to get into a conversation with Eddie Cawley I remembered that I had talked to him right after the first examination and wondered whether he had any different thoughts. I asked him how things had been going since then, and he said, "Gee, everything has gone along just right for me since that first exam. It is hard to believe that it really has." I said, "Have you been having trouble figuring out what is important?" He said, "No, not since that first time. Of course I may be just lucky in guessing." An uncomfortable look came over his face then, although he had looked very pleased with himself when he fire told me that he was a good guesser. He went on, "You just have to try to figure out what they want you to have, and then it makes it easy. I guess I just hit it every single time. You see, there's so much work to do you can't do it all. It's just the way they tell you in the beginning of the year, so you have to do the important things. I don't mean just to beat the test, and yet that's about it. You have to figure out what's important, and it is pretty easy to do. You can tell from what they say."

(February 4, 1957. Married fraternity man.)

This student's change of criterion is not entirely a matter of interaction with his fraternity brothers, of course. He did poorly on the first block; he was not prepared for questions on the scapula and wrist which he considered unimportant in practice. But the fact that he now uses the criterion of what the faculty wants, and not some other criterion of his own devising, has been made more likely by

[2] See p. 123.

the agreement among his fraternity brothers on the faculty criterion and his exposure to it.

In the next excerpt from the field notes, a student who has recently joined a fraternity communicates part of his perspective to a friend who has remained an independent. Another independent is also present:

I sat next to Bob Simpson and Ken Thomas, during an intermission from a class in which the professor had been discussing the results of an anatomy examination with the class. Ben Black was also there. Bob said to Ken, "Now you see, I was right. The way to study for this is to pick out the important things and learn them. There's no point in trying to get too many details that are not important. That was what you did for the first exam and I'll bet you did much better on this one." Ken agreed to this statement and said to me that on the first quiz he had tried to memorize everything in a given region and had not done very well. I said to Ken, "How do you decide when a thing is important?" He blustered at this a bit and finally said, "For instance, you know that some little muscle which raises your palate is less important than one that has to do with swallowing. A guy can get along without that little muscle in the palate, but he can't get along without the things about swallowing."

(November 27, 1956. Married fraternity man, married independent, single independent.)

Like the first excerpt, this conversation demonstrates how situation and interaction combine in the consensual process. Whether or not the fraternity student interprets what the instructor says about the examination correctly according to the instructor's view is irrelevant. The student clearly feels that he knows how to study for examinations and that the instructor's remarks confirm this. He does not hesitate to try to persuade his friend. The independent is only partly convinced. He still thinks he can pick out the important things by his knowledge of medical practice. But he is exposed to the fraternity perspective (the reader will have to take our word that these two students were often together) and may adopt it if his own proves unsatisfactory on subsequent tests.

As independents get to know fraternity men working together in lab and the barriers between groups in the class begin to break down, students discuss with each other the common problem of the overload and how to select the important things to study.

The following incident in which an independent discusses what is important with a fraternity man is the first instance of serious cross-group discussion we noted. It takes place here with the observer as catalyst:

I sat next to Dick Porter during lecture, and asked him how things had been going during November. He said, "Things are really about the same as they were. I think this is still a kind of orientation time. They are still trying to show us how little we know and how much there is to learn. They are still trying to scare us. This is just an introduction and we have still the same problem of trying to figure out how much we should know or what is important to learn. I think it will get better later on." Al Jones joined us and listened to what Dick was saying. Dick continued, "I went to see Dr. N. and I asked him what was important, and he said, 'Everything we do here is important,' but I don't think he was speaking for the whole place up here. I think he was just speaking for anatomy." Al said, "Hell no, it's not important. Take all this stuff we had in the lecture this afternoon. That's not important. It wouldn't be important to you unless you wanted to be an ophthalmologist. I've been talking to some of the guys down at the Center, and I know. I think most of this stuff they give us here will only be useful for one specialty, and I think that's a waste of time." I said, "Well, what do you think they should give you; what is important?" Al said, "I think they ought to give us basic understanding of these things. For instance, about the retina, and vision. I think that's important, but heck, I don't know. I really don't know what to think now."

(November 26, 1956. Single fraternity man, married independent.)

Both the fraternity man and the independent in this incident have a certain amount of resentment of the faculty. The fraternity man consults his instructor about what is important but disbelieves the answer. He thinks the faculty creates the overload deliberately to make students set their own level and direction of effort.

The independent is bewildered. According to the practice criterion, little of what he is being taught seems important. Where the fraternity man accepts the necessity of deciding things for himself and incorporates it into his perspective, the independent is no longer sure that he knows what to think or do.

The realization that it is often difficult to decide what is important on the basis of usefulness in practice also comes to students in a way that touches them very closely — examination questions. Some faculty members believe that students resent the fact that there is so little clinical medicine in the first year and try to interest them, or please them, by including clinical material in lectures and tests. This good will on the part of an instructor sometimes angers students rather than pleases them. The next excerpt, which takes place the day after the one just quoted, illustrates this point. "Al" in the incident is the same student as in the previous example:

As he and his partners worked at dissection, Al said, "Well, there was one question that N gave us that made me mad. It was that one about abscesses." Joanne said, "Yeah, what is an abscess?" Al said, "That's exactly right. We haven't heard of these things. They're not in the book. He just assumes that we know these kinds of things, but we're not doctors. We're not practicing medicine. How does he expect us to know things like that?"

I said, "Yes, I remember on the first test about that embolus." Al said, "Yes, I knew about that one because I had worked in a hospital." Joanne said, "Well, I didn't. I never heard of an embolus before."

(November 27, 1956. One married independent, one girl independent.)

In this case the instructor's attempt to please students misfires; they think he is unfair. What the instructor probably considered common occurrences in clinical practice are things the students have not heard of. In his bitterness, Al puts the dilemma of all students trying to decide what to study by the practice criterion into one ironic phrase: "We're not doctors." The criterion is beginning to seem unworkable.

His phrase "They're not in the book" is further evidence the independent is adopting the criterion of the fraternity men. He has adopted their defense and rallying cry. Where independents condemn test questions by saying, "That never happens, you'd never see *that* in practice," fraternity men use books as weapons against the faculty. When they think a question unfair, they appeal to the textbook as an authority higher than the instructor, and the latter is not likely to improve his case by saying the text is out of date or inaccurate. Thus, in changing from the practice criterion to the criterion of "what the faculty wants," a student does not give up his independence. If he gives up the demand that he be taught what he will later use and asks instead that he be examined on what is in the book, he acquires a powerful defensive weapon against the faculty that has the advantage of being close at hand.

The limitations of the practice criterion in choosing what to study were highlighted when the class visited the medical center. The excited student in the following example, a Beta, had been using the practice criterion up to this point:

On the day that we went to the Medical Center the lecturer, a clinical professor, asked one of the freshmen a question which he couldn't answer.

It was about nerve roots, which he said were very important. Later, as I was coming out of the lecture with Shep Boas and Dennis Young, Shep said, "Things have been going much better. I've been sleeping and all that, really it's O.K. now. We don't have to worry about these examinations coming up; they will be easy." I asked some questions about the amount of work and Dennis said, "No, it is not too much any more. It is just about right." Shep said that he thought so too, but then as he stopped to think he got excited and said loudly, "These goddam Ph.D.'s don't teach us the right things, they never gave us anything about the nerve root." I said, "Why do you think that is?" Shep said, "They expect us to figure out what's important. As if we could do that! Hell, we don't know anything, how do they expect us to do that?" Dennis nodded in agreement. Shep said, "I wish they had brought us down here earlier, then we would have known what to study. It doesn't do us any good now; we have finished with this stuff."

(January 25, 1957. Two single fraternity men.)

The realization that their knowledge of medical practice was not extensive enough to help them decide what to study bewildered many students and led them to seek another solution to the overload problem. Low grades on the first block frightened many of them and provided an additional situational stimulus to change. As their interaction with fraternity men increased, independents learned from them how to find out what the faculty wanted and adopted this method of deciding what to study as the more workable criterion.

The final perspective of the freshman year continues to include parts of earlier perspectives. Since we were not at the medical school long enough to see for ourselves how many hours the students worked, we asked them about it:

At the end of the day I was talking to Scott Dawson who said, "I don't think I'm going to do well [on the test] because I don't seem to have been studying as hard. I don't know why, I really can't explain why." I said, "Well, how much time have you been putting in?" He said, "Four or five hours a night I guess. But it doesn't seem to hang together as well. There has been so much detail to this stuff, so much to learn."

(November 26, 1956. Married independent.)

The hours of work this student mentions are the same as the norms of the initial perspective. In the second semester, lab hours are slightly reduced, and students feel they have been "goofing off":

During physiology lab Jay Downing asked me, "Have you noticed any changes in us since the beginning of the year?" I said, "Oh, yes, a great many changes. Don't you think there have been?" Jay looked doubtful and then said, "Yeah, I guess you're right. We are more used to it now and we don't get so clutched up for examinations." I said, "Seriously, Jay, how about the amount of time you spend studying? Is it more or less or what?" Jay said, "Well, I've been goofing off a lot this semester. You know the first week we had two afternoons off in one week. I think I've only been working two or three hours a night and maybe once a week I don't do anything. Spring is coming, you know, and it is a lot harder to make yourself study. But then other times I work four or five hours a night. I still work over the weekends, maybe five hours or so, but it is not nearly as much as I used to."

I said, "Do you think that is pretty general in the class?" Jay said, "Yeah, I think so. We are all more relaxed than we used to be."

(March 16, 1957. Single fraternity man.)

This "relaxation" amounts to approximately sixty study hours a week, rather than the seventy-seven hour schedule generally followed in the first semester.

Students continue to study, when they can, in the most efficient and economical way. Although they do the lab work because it is required, they consider it a waste of time:

At tank seventeen the students were discussing dissection. Pete Tyler said, "I don't see why we have to do all this. I think a lot of these tank-hoppers do better than we do." Max Bender said, "You have to do your dissection. They flunked out two guys last year for not doing it." (The term "tank-hopper" is applied to students who go around during lab, looking at other dissections. It has an overtone of not attending to your own business.) Pete said, "I don't know why it makes any difference whether we do this or not, though. We are not learning anything." Joanne Bond said, "I don't see why they should care whether we do it or not. You could really get it all from the book."

(October 18, 1956. Two fraternity men, a girl independent.)

In an earlier example, a student protested bitterly over an examination question about something that was "not in the book." He was using the text as a standard with which to judge the faculty. Here the textbook presents the easiest and quickest way to study; faculty reasons for requiring other work are not understood. In the next excerpt a student discusses this point more fully:

In physiology lab I said to Bob Simpson, "How about these dog experiments, Bob? Do you think you get a lot out of them?" Bob said, "Well, I don't like to work with dogs very much. I think they're a waste of time. This is all in the book, and we don't really get anything out of doing it.

I suppose you could say that you could remember it better when you see it, but it doesn't seem worth it to me to spend so much time on it. Then a lot of experiments don't come out." I said, "What do you mean?" Bob said, "Well, we've been pretty lucky and all of ours have come out and we've gotten good records [of the experiment], but lots of times they don't. It isn't anybody's fault. Maybe the dog dies on you; each one is different and you can't figure out how he works. Maybe that's part of what they're trying to teach us, though, that each one is different."

(March 18, 1957. Married fraternity man.)

This student also looks at the textbook as a final authority and the most efficient source of knowledge. He appreciates that the faculty may want him to learn how animals differ, but he implies that he knows this and need not learn it so repetitiously.

Students did not have this perspective on the live animal experiments in physiology at the beginning of the semester. Many of them were excited by being able to operate, even if without asepsis, and at getting the chance to apply their knowledge of anatomy. But the enthusiasm had worn off for most students within a month. There is still an overload: so much medicine to learn that methods of learning that "waste time" seem wrong. The final perspective retains the emphasis of the provisional perspective upon economy and efficiency in the learning process.

In the effort to save time, we have seen that many students take short cuts in lab by omitting dissection that can be gotten more easily from the text or making out lab reports the way they come out in the book rather than in the experiment. They do not regard this as cheating either themselves or the instructor but as a reasonable way to save time. If they know what results they should get, they feel they have done what is important. Their perspective is pragmatic: they regard books, lectures, and experiments as means to knowledge. The fact that they are not examined on lab techniques undoubtedly re-enforces this belief.

The line between practices of this kind and what students consider cheating is a fine one. In the example below a student has found a way to save time in lab and thinks other students do the same thing:

In biochemistry lab the students were making a test involving Benedict's solution. They filled test tubes with it and boiled them in a flask over a Bunsen burner. All but one of the solutions turned red. This one remained a greenish color. Chuck Dodge said to his neighbor, Keith Shelby, "Did yours all turn red?" Keith said, "Yeah." I said, "But what about that greenish one, how do you know they are all supposed to be red?" Keith pointed to his lab manual where it was written in red ink: *red*. Keith said, "You know you have to do this kind of thing to get through, all K.U. students do it. You have to do it." I understood that the reason they knew how the test was supposed to work out was from having a lab manual from the previous year. The rest of the day I checked up on whether other students were doing this but did not see any lab manuals which had marking in them beyond the point where the assignment went.

(February 4, 1957. One married independent, one married fraternity man.)

Using a lab manual marked by a former student is evidently not something students do. This man is an exception, although he does not know it. At first glance it is difficult to see why using a marked manual is cheating when writing up experimental results by remembering how they came out in the text is not. Perhaps the distinction lies in the fact that in the former case the student uses another student's work, in the latter he uses his own.

That this distinction is not always important to students, but depends upon their definition of the situation, comes out in the next example:

During my conversation with Cowper, Bob Prentis came up and said, "You know that assistant in the upstairs lab, you know what he did to me? On those notebooks we had to hand in, and it counted 10 per cent, he gave me 'D.' Boy, I hadn't done anything, the way I look at it. What it was was that I just didn't put down the answers to two or three things in there because he set up the experiment so late in the afternoon that we all didn't get a chance to look at it. So I went and asked him about this 'D.' He said he didn't grade the notebook on whether they were correct or not, he just marked them on whether all the questions were there. Boy, that burned me up." Al said, "Yeah, I should think so. That was 10 per cent of the grade." I said, "What can you do when something like that happens?" Bob said, "There ain't," and then he corrected himself, "there isn't much you can do about it. I went in and showed it to G [his instructor] but he wasn't going to do anything about it. He didn't say anything. They're not going to change anything like that around here. That guy is not a good lab instructor. He doesn't know what he is doing.

"The thing that really griped me was that three guys copied from my notebook and one of them was in another lab and nothing was said about his at all." Al said, "I know how it is. George O'Day was really chewed out by G for not handing in that graph. It wasn't important. But G said to him that it was his responsibility to do all of these things and he'd better see that he did them. I don't see what there was to get so excited about that about."

C never looks at the notebooks. He just takes what the lab assistant says about them." Bob continued to look very belligerent about his difficulty with the lab assistant, but he ended on a milder note. "He is too conscientious," he said.

(March 18, 1957. The chief speaker is a married independent, the other a married fraternity man.)

Conversations like this one will probably be familiar to anyone who has to hand in papers in school. Most students are concerned about the correctness of their work as evidence of learning and want to be graded on this. They are disturbed to find that the faculty cares only that a complete paper is handed in as evidence that the work or some semblance of it has been done. It is probable that under these conditions students do not hesitate to copy, since they know it is the form of things, the "motions," and not learning that is rewarded. Thus, when the faculty wants a complete paper, they may get a copied one from students who extend the final perspective to cover this case, thinking such behavior an economy since it frees time for studying the important things.

We are not saying here that many freshmen cheat in this way, but pointing out that cheating is situational: dependent upon faculty perspectives and regulations as students understand them.

Student emphasis upon economical ways of learning in the final perspective extends to their judgments of teaching. They reserve their praise for instructors who do not waste time:

Jim Hampton said to me, "You know who the realistic guy about things around here is, that's Johnson. He really gives it to you straight. He knows you have to work hard."

(October 18, 1956. Single fraternity man.)

Another student puts it even more strongly:

I talked to Shep Boas after psychiatry conference. He was very tense. He said, "I don't like this kind of thing at all. I don't like these conferences where people [students] ask questions. I can't think of anything to say. And besides I think it really wastes your time; even in class I don't like it when they [instructors] ask questions because we are here to learn and take it from them. . . . It is up to them to give it to us. It is not something to be argued about."

(February 7, 1957. Single fraternity man.)

Thus, teaching methods that do not approach the concrete finality of a textbook seem wasteful to the students. They think of medicine as a tremendous body of well-established facts that they must learn. Their efforts are so directed toward entering the examination room knowing these facts, the things the faculty wants them to know, that they do many things along the way that the faculty does not like. They slight assignments and, in a situation that calls for completed rather than knowledgeable work, some of them cheat or condone cheating.

The phrase "give it to us straight," favorably used in an earlier example, is the student counterpart of the derogatory word "spoon-feeding," used by the faculty. In our interviews with faculty members, those who oppose spoon-feeding the students or do it unwilling-ly* often complain that students are too pragmatic, impatient of everything imprecise; they want only hard facts. Some professors associate this impatience with variation and anything uncertain with students' dislike of research and experiment. They deplore the tendency to accept the textbook as final arbiter and point out that texts often contradict each other and rapidly become out of date. Faculty members with this perspective want students to master a subject sufficiently to be critical of experts in the field and the field itself. They worry about what kind of physicians students will become if they accept only facts as material for learning and are uncritical of these facts in a rapidly changing discipline. They ask the perennial question of elders: Why aren't they more like us?

While it is probably true that many freshmen find the tentative, scientific approach of some of their teachers as disturbing to the learning process as exceptions to spelling rules, it is not true that freshmen are uncritical. They show the critical spirit (in a way teachers seldom appreciate) by appealing to the authority of the textbook over the heads of the faculty. The challenge is often more than a show of independence, however. It can be deliberately instrumental, for the discussion which follows may bring out an instructor's perspective on his subject and help students to anticipate what questions he will put on the test and how he likes them answered:

During the class in which he was discussing the test results, N went through some of the things he thought should have been used in answer to a question. Harvey Stone asked him about additional material, arguing that it would have been important and that Morris said it was. N listened

* The faculty perspective here is either that the large amount of material medical students must be taught necessitates spoon-feeding or (less flatteringly) that students are not good enough for greater self-direction.

carefully to Harvey's point, but before Harvey had finished his sentence N interrupted and started explaining that this material really had nothing to do with the question. They went back and forth two or three times on this. N explained that there were both major and minor structures involved. I heard Bob Simpson say to the guy on his left, "Major and minor crap."
(November 27, 1956. Two married fraternity men.)

Here the student appeals to the authority of the text over the head of the instructor, but does not get far. He does, quite aside from the question of his grade, get information on the kind of thing the instructor thinks relevant answers on his examinations.

The co-operative technique for finding out what the faculty wants of which the faculty is most aware is the use of files of old examinations kept in the fraternity houses. The most useful papers include answers and instructor's comments. They are corrected papers returned to a student after the examination which he has donated to the house files.

The use of such files, although often condemned, has been handled in a variety of ways by school faculties. In some schools or departments within a school, the faculty maintains files for the students or posts old examinations before a test. This may be done in approval of the practice, as in prep school cram sessions for college boards, or with resignation in the belief that students will get copies anyway. (Tales of students who have memorized entire examinations and written them out for the benefit of their fellows are usually a part of faculty culture.) In other schools, every effort is made to prevent students from getting copies of old examinations on grounds that they use them to memorize answers rather than do their own studying, or take unfair advantage of students without access to files.

When the administration condemned the practice in late October and announced that grades would not be given out or examination papers returned, students recognized that it would be several years before the files became too out-of-date to be used:

I found a group of students discussing the announcement and joined them. They were all Gammas. The president of the fraternity went by as we were standing there and Larry Horton said, "Boy, that's a guy I wouldn't like to be now." I said, "Why is that?" Terry Smith said, "All this fraternity business, you know. Of course we have always had the tests to study with, although I didn't think they did much good. I didn't use them very much." Larry said, "Well, if they go on like this and never give them back, in ten years we will have to study medicine!" At the word "medicine" his voice went up into a shriek and everyone laughed uneasily.

(October 24, 1956. Two single fraternity men.)

The irony of the words "we will have to study medicine" is clear in the light of the students' expressed desire to do so in the long-range and initial perspectives.

Public condemnation of the files did not, however, discourage their use. As interaction among the groups in the class increased, the files were no longer the exclusive property of the fraternities, but spread throughout the class:

Scott Dawson was telling me about the dissection of the head and neck, which I had missed. I asked him whether he had tried to learn all the details. He replied, "Well, you can't really. You have to try to figure out which ones are the most important." I said, "How do you do this?" Scotty said, "I don't really know. Of course you get some of it in lectures, and then there are the old examinations. I try to figure out what seems to be important and think about what the faculty wants us to know." I said, "Where did you get this copy of last year's examination?" He said, "Oh, I got it from a fellow. He isn't a fraternity member. They're pretty general now; most everybody has them. There isn't any trouble getting one."

(November 26, 1956. Married independent.)

Old examinations are not as useful in finding out what the faculty wants, however, as papers returned with corrections:

Hap Garrett said, "Well, I found one thing that is good from looking at those last year's exams with the answers on them; they [the faculty] take any reasonable answer. I think that's good. I hope they tell us what is wrong with our exams and be specific, because I really don't know what they want now and I don't know whether I gave them enough or too much or what." Bob Warren said, "They will say that when they hand back the tests to us."

(October 16, 1956. Two married independents.)

Analysis of corrected papers helps students study for the next block. It does not help, of course, on the first test an instructor gives. In this situation, students may resort to graduate assistants and a bit of sociological analysis of departmental history and structure:

Eric Post was explaining to Duane Norris some dope about the coming exam he got when he went to see one of the physiology assistants. After Eric had finished explaining this to Duane and to Bill Boynton, who was leaning over his shoulder, Duane said, "Do you think we will have this on the test?" Eric said, "Well, there's a lot of these questions on last year's." Duane said, "Yeah, that's right, but these are Baker's questions, and the guy you talked to used to work with him. I don't think we will have that kind of questions on this test, because Jones [the present instructor] isn't that way." Eric said, "I know, it will probably be about philosophy, like his lectures. I'm going to study the lectures very carefully." I said, "Gee, that makes it hard to find out, doesn't it, when a guy isn't here?" Bill said, "That's funny, isn't it. It's a good example of two professors looking at the same thing in different ways." Eric said, "Yeah, Baker always has these diagrams and figures. He had a lot of physics and engineering, but Jones is more on the philosophical side."

(October 17, 1956. Three single fraternity men.)

In deciding that the assistant's advice is not likely to be helpful because he worked with a former instructor in the subject, the students conclude that the lectures of the present men are the best source of information about what will be on the examination. No one suggests asking the man himself; there is kind of unspoken understanding among students against pressing the teacher too closely about the examination just before it is given. Immediately after the test the teacher is fair game again:

I saw Terry Smith and asked him the question about what had been happening since Thanksgiving. Terry said, "Well, between Christmas and last week they were really giving it to us. Boy, they gave us so many exams everybody got real tense. You know before that histology final, I went out and drank a quart of beer, and that usually puts me to sleep. I took a couple of aspirins, and I still couldn't sleep. That never happened to me before in my life. Boy, that exam was the worst damn thing I ever heard. You know I'm sure all the questions were given to us by R. It was just ridiculous. . . . I just couldn't do it at all. Maybe I got 20 per cent of it. Of course, I know I didn't fail it, but it was just something to laugh at. That guy, R, I don't know what was in his mind. It was nothing but minutiae. Those things weren't in his lectures and they weren't in the book; they weren't anywhere. I went up to him and I said, 'How do you expect us to study for a thing like that?' It was ridiculous; when they passed out the papers there was one whole page I didn't know."

(February 4, 1957. Single fraternity man.)

The student does not say what, if anything, he learned about the instructor's point of view in this exchange. He does make it very clear that according to the final perspective a faculty member should play ball with the students and ask questions only on material in the lectures or text. The instructor should teach and examine in such a way that students, with proper effort, can determine what the teacher thinks important and study these things. Students look upon this as a bargain between them and the faculty; breaking it brands an instructor as incompetent. In thus defining the academic situation, students forget the faculty is not a party to this "bargain" except in the students' perspective.

Although they provide less information than an instructor's verbal or written comments, students also use grades to help them determine what the faculty wants. The following conversation took place immediately after the announcement that grades were to be abolished. The mixture of students, independents and fraternity men not seen together before, suggests how an important event helped to draw the class together:

Outside the lab I saw Joe Jensen, Al Cowper, Sandy Dobby, Jerry Hartwell, and Curt Hughes talking together. Al said, "Well, I'm glad about the new grading system. I think it's a good idea to cut down on the competition." Curt spoke for some while on the fact that he would like to have his papers corrected and handed back to him. He said, "I don't care whether it has a grade on it or not." Jerry said, "Well, the thing that gets me is how can you tell whether you are doing what they want, or not? I get so clutched on those tests that I can't remember what answer I gave. They [the faculty] said they would discuss the tests with us in class; but I don't think that would do me any good because I couldn't remember what I said on it." Sandy said, "I think it's a good idea, I really do, as long as they let us know how we are doing and don't let us go on without knowing, the way it was with that guy a couple of years ago." I said, "Well, couldn't you go and ask your counselor?" Sandy said, "Yes, I guess you could, but I wouldn't feel like doing that, I don't think. I think I'll just wait, the way they say, until someone tells me I'm not doing all right." Joe said, "It's not as simple as that, though. What if you got thirty or twenty on the first test, and you went in to your counselor [after the second] and he said you were doing better; maybe you would be doing thirty or forty, but that wouldn't be good enough and you wouldn't know. I think it's possible to misunderstand a question, or give them an answer that they don't want and you wouldn't realize that you had done so."
(October 24, 1956. Two single fraternity men, two single independents, and one married independent.)

After giving lip service to the evils (unspecified) of competition, these students immediately get down to the problem of information. Corrected test papers provide the best means of information; they allow a student to decide for himself whether he has understood the questions and given acceptable answers. Counselors may not be helpful; they may not give exact enough information for students to know how to improve.

Implicit in the discussion is the students' feeling that the perspective of the examiner himself is important to them. They think examination questions may be interpreted and answers written in a number of ways, that they cannot know which ways are most acceptable to an examiner unless he tells them. They are confident that if they can only find out what he wants, they can do it.

We are not saying that all or even many students reacted to not getting grades in this way, for most of them accepted the change as relatively unimportant. They were more concerned about whether they would get examination papers back. What we want to emphasize is the difference between the student perspective and that of the faculty.

The students' premise in the final perspective is that there are many things to learn and many ways of demonstrating learning on examinations. They believe that each instructor or department[*] has its own ideas about what should be learned and how this learning should be expressed. Quite aside from the question of their own abilities, they believe they must make every effort to find out what an instructor wants in order to study intelligently for an examination and do themselves justice in taking it. They see it as part of their job as students to understand a teacher's perspective on his subject, and they direct their efforts toward this end.[5]

Teachers are apt to forget that they themselves are an object of student learning. In faculty culture, a poor examination paper means a dull student, or one who does not know how to "organize his time." Allowances are also made for students with personal problems or illness on the day of the test. This is a perspective focused on individual students.

When teachers think of the relationships among students, they seldom consider collective phenomena of the kind we have been concerned with here in which students take co-operative action to get at faculty perspectives, for it is a commonplace of the academic world

[*] Examinations are often made up jointly by members of the department. We speak of one teacher for simplicity; since students can identify each man's question, little violence is done to the facts.

[5] Studies of teachers' grading has shown that the same mathematics paper may be graded anywhere from zero to one hundred by different teachers.

(which students themselves subscribe to) that students do not co-operate; they compete with each other for grades. When the administration abolished grades in October, competition was given as one of the chief reasons.

Perhaps we can clarify the confusion on the relations of students to each other by reference to an informative paper extending game theory to the various forms of competition by Jessie Bernard.[6] The paper distinguishes two kinds of competition: autonomic and decisive. In autonomic competition, entities are ordered or winners determined by the process itself. The particular type of competition that students are said to engage in is called Richardson, an autonomic type in which competitors try to out-achieve each other and the maximum of one becomes the minimum of the other. The relationship among competitors is one of stimulation and reaction. But the competition of students is actually not of this type; it is the decisive type in which winners are decided not by self-selection but by a judge or decision-maker.

Dr. Bernard notes that in the decisive type of competition one "has to learn how to win the judge or decision-maker rather than how to win the game. . . . The variable that is being maximized tends to become ability to please the decision-maker."[7] In speaking of the freshmen we prefer the word "satisfy," for "please" is a word with overtones of apple-polishing. It suggests that flattery may be more effective than good work in influencing a teacher, a notion foreign to the freshmen. Nevertheless, our knowledge of the students' final perspective, their efforts to find out what the faculty wants, leaves little doubt that the competition they engage in is of the decisive type.

Student interest is primarily focused on the faculty, from whom they try to get information on what and how to study, rather than on competing with each other. This explains why students did not mind having grades abolished. It deprived them of their least specific source of information about faculty wishes. Since very few, if any, freshmen were using grades to measure themselves against other students in an effort to out-achieve them, not knowing how others were doing was unimportant.

Decisive competition engaged in co-operatively takes on several aspects of a game. The relationship between faculty and students in

[6] Jessie Bernard, "Autonomic and Decisive Forms of Competition," *Sociological Quarterly*, I (January, 1960), 25–35.
[7] *Ibid.*, p. 33.

the final freshman perspective is similar to that of opposing teams. The faculty protects its position while students attack. In many instances, the stars of the student team (those who get the most information) are fraternity men. With their greater social ease, they do not hesitate to argue in class with a professor or complain to him about examination questions, and the class learns more about an instructor's perspective on his subject.

The social distance between faculty and students becomes more understandable from the vantage point of the game analogy. If students are a team sharing their knowledge of the decision-maker, an individual who appears too intimate with him may be cheating on his team, getting information which he is not sharing; hence the common phenomenon of dislike of "teacher's pet," and isolation for the able student who studies independently.

The hesitation freshmen show in seeking help from their counselors may be related to this aspect of the final perspective. Students are unwilling to take action that may mark them as not participating fully in the information-sharing team.

We remarked earlier on the tendency of educators to define the ideal relationship of teacher and student as dyadic. Many teachers think of themselves as contending with each student in the class individually. When the dyadic condition is approached, as in schools where pupils are given much individual help by the teacher, decisive competition may be maximized. The student has no fellows to support him if his definition of a proper level and direction of effort differs from that of his teacher. He must make every effort to please.

Boarding schools where teachers go to great lengths in supervising study halls to make sure their pupils' work is done independently approach the dyadic idea. These schools frequently put much emphasis on grades and encourage students to compete with each other for them. But we rather believe that there have been few instances where teachers entirely succeed in getting students to ignore the teacher's role as decision-maker and compete only with each other. When they are out of earshot kids exchange the vital information about what old so-and-so is like and the kinds of things he will ask on the test. Note the kinds of things, for on the whole, this is what students want to know, not the question itself, for this would break the rules of the game.

Before we present evidence supporting our contention that the final perspective is the customary way students deal with their academic problems after the first months of the freshman year, we let one of the students sum up his successive perspectives during the year in his own words. He is an independent who came unwillingly and late to the use of the criterion of what the faculty wants:

Late in the afternoon I found Al Jones in the physiology lab. I asked him how things had been going. Al said, "Well, before Christmas was all right. They threw a lot of stuff at us toward the end of that. You know we had more in those last weeks of anatomy than we had in the first two months. After Christmas there were a lot of tests. My God, the tests we had, about six I think, coming about every two weeks. You know that got me awfully upset, a lot of those tests. My stomach is still bad. I went home and I just lay there for a whole week. That was good for me; that was what I needed. But it makes you stop to think about yourself. It's not very mature to get so upset about things like that. Sometimes I wonder about this anyway, you know. After Christmas I looked in the mirror and I thought: am I a medical student? And I didn't look like one and I still don't feel like one. I don't know why that is."

We were interrupted by Terry Smith who wanted to talk about some students who had flunked out. After he left Al went on: "You know it scares me the way we go through these courses. I think that anatomy ought to be at least a year long. I don't really feel as if I knew anything. Oh, I know a few things. I know more than I did before, but it worries you. I suppose there will be review later on and there'll be lots of repetition. But I don't know. I don't think medical education is so good really. I think they do the best they can and they do a good job here but it is all over the country. I think they've got to make it longer. I think they've got to make it six years.

"You know how I feel about this. I think medicine is terribly important. I know one thing. I don't want to go out and practice by myself right after I get out of medical school in one of these little towns like out my way. There's a couple of guys fresh out of medical school out there now in a town near me and they just don't know what they are doing. They are always carting people off to the hospital because they don't know how to deal with them. . . . I certainly wouldn't want to be on my own. I don't think you know enough."

I said, "What do you think of your courses now that you have finished them?" Al said, "Well, of course anatomy is the important one. Histology — that's not important. Using a microscope is something we don't have to do as doctors and looking at all those slides doesn't do any good except maybe to be able to identify tissues. But when you get to pathology you really need anatomy. . . . They haven't mailed me anything. [Al is referring to the practice of sending the boys a pink slip if they have not done well in exams.] That wasn't unusual though. A lot of guys, if they knew they passed the first one they didn't worry about the third one. But I'm not that way, I worry about all of them.

"But you know the thing is that when we first came here, we came here to learn. We just wanted to learn things for ourselves. It's too bad that it has be this way in medical school. It's just like any other school and after a while you get going and you just do it and you don't think about it at all. You just don't think that you are a medical student."

(February 5, 1957. Married independent.)

This student expresses a rather profound disillusion. He is ashamed of himself for continuing to "clutch" about examinations. It is unworthy of a medical student. But by working back through his original idealism about medicine, which he maintains, and his initial perspective on school — to learn for himself what he will need in practice — he explains his own trouble. He cannot study the things he thinks he will need for practice; he must study for examinations. He wanted the operating word in the term medical student to be "medical," but it has turned out to be "student."

In conclusion we present evidence that the final perspective is in frequent, widespread, and legitimate use among the freshmen from mid-October through the end of the year. Table XXI shows that there are fifty-nine instances of the final perspective in our field notes; six negative cases are not shown. The number of instances is about what we can expect for the ten days or so in the field represented.[9] Table XXI also classifies the statements of the final perspective according to whether they are volunteered or directed, made to the observer only or to other students in everyday conversation. Since all the statements are volunteered and a substantial proportion (65%) made to others, we conclude that, under our definition, the final perspective is considered legitimate behavior by the freshmen.

TABLE XXI

STATEMENTS EXPRESSING THE FINAL PERSPECTIVE CLASSIFIED
BY THOSE PRESENT AND WHETHER VOLUNTEERED OR DIRECTED
(October 16, 1956–September 5, 1957)

STATEMENTS	VOLUNTEERED	DIRECTED	TOTAL
To observer alone.........	21 (35%)	0	21
To others...............	38 (65%)	0	38
Total	59 (100%)	0	59[*]

[*] There are six negative cases in which students continue to use the practice criterion.

[9] See p. 99 and p. 125.

Table XXII shows the distribution of the final perspective among student companionship groups. We note that it is widespread. (The proportion of Betas represented, four out of seventeen, remains as low as it has in previous perspectives.)

TABLE XXII

DISTRIBUTION OF OBSERVED INSTANCES OF USE OF THE FINAL
PERSPECTIVE BY STUDENTS IN DIFFERENT GROUPS
(October 16, 1956–September 5, 1957)

STUDENT GROUP	NUMBER		PER CENT
Fraternity men:	35		59.3
Alphas		7	
Betas		4	
Gammas		24	
Independents:	24		40.7
Married men...........		14	
Single men...........		4	
Girls		6	
	59*		100.0

* Six negative cases are distributed as follows: Betas, 1; Gammas, 3; married men, 2.

We conclude that the final perspective is the customary behavior of the freshmen from mid-October through the rest of the year.

Table XXIII reclassifies the same items according to the criterion used by the speaker in deciding what to study and whether a fraternity man or independent makes it. Eight statements express the final perspective but do not specify a criterion; we include these in the table so that it may be compared with Table XXI.

The six statements of the practice criterion are, of course, negative to the final perspective and do not appear in Table XXI or XXII.

TABLE XXIII

DATA OF THE FINAL PERSPECTIVE CLASSIFIED ACCORDING TO CRITERION USED TO
DECIDE WHAT TO STUDY BY FRATERNITY MEN AND INDEPENDENTS
(October 16, 1956–September 5, 1957)

CRITERION	FRATERNITY MEN*		INDEPENDENTS		TOTAL OB-SERVATIONS
Practice	4	(10.3%)	2	(7.7%)	6
What the faculty wants........	28	(71.8%)	23	(88.5%)	51
None	7	(17.9%)	1	(3.8%)	8
Total	39	(100.0%)	26	(100.0)	65

* Betas: Practice, 2; Faculty, 4; None, 0.

If we compare Table XXIII, with Table XIX, the same breakdown for the data gathered before October 16,[9] we find that fraternity men maintain about the same proportion of use of the practice and faculty-wants criteria in the two tables (6 :: 25 and 4 :: 28), but independents have changed. Where they formerly favored the practice criterion slightly (6 :: 4), they now overwhelmingly favor the faculty-wants criterion (2 :: 23). The class has reached consensus on how to decide what to study.

We conclude with a last bit of evidence that the final perspective remained in force through the freshman year and dominated students' retrospective views. In the fall of 1957 we observed the '56-'57 freshmen as they began their sophomore year at the medical center. One morning during a break from lecture, the new freshman class arrived for a tour of the center. We were present as two sophomores gave advice:

Paul Inkles and Bob Warren were talking to a new freshman whose name I did not get. Paul had just asked him whether he had bought his books yet up at Lawrence and the boy said that he had not, but he thought he would get Morris. Paul said to him, "Well, if you want my advice, don't get more than one book for each course. That's what they [the faculty] told us to do last year and I think they were right. You just can't get through more than one book. In fact, there is so much more in them than you have time to learn that you can't really get it. You can't really get all there is in one." Bob nodded agreement to this and the freshman looked bewildered.

At this point the freshmen were called to continue their tour. Paul turned to me and said, "You know, you can't give them very much advice. I wouldn't have listened to any myself last year. . . ." Bob said, "I think it's going to be very different this year. I have an entirely different feeling about it. Last year we were working for examinations, but this year I have the feeling that when I go out and see a patient with diphtheria, I'm going to learn all about that for myself."

(September 5, 1957. Two married independents.)

[9] See p. 152.

A NOTE ON THE
SOPHOMORE YEAR

W<small>E</small> did not do much field work among the sophomores, but we observed enough to come to the decision that we need not make a thorough analysis of students' experience in the second year. We made this judgment very early in our work and have not systematically attempted to demonstrate it. In many ways, this was an error, for it is the major lacuna in our analysis. All we can do here is suggest the reasons for our judgment; later research may subject these impressions to more systematic testing.

We do not think the second year unimportant. It clearly is a year in which students learn a very great deal. They bring from the first year their knowledge of the basic medical sciences — anatomy, physiology, and biochemistry — and apply these to subjects which are much closer to the drama of medical practice. In pathology, the course to which most time is devoted, they study in detail the range of diseases to which the human organism is subject. They learn the etiology of diseases, the diagnostic signs by which they may be recognized, the characteristic pathological lesions (both gross and microscopic), and the appropriate methods of treatment. They participate in autopsies, examine diseased organs preserved for their study, study slides of diseased tissue microscopically, and perform experiments.

In microbiology students learn the characteristics of bacterial, viral, and other organisms which produce disease. They learn to identify these by microscopy, by making cultures, and by observing the diseases they produce. In pharmacology, they acquire a knowledge of the drugs physicians use to treat various diseases, the dangers associated with use of those drugs, and the methods by which new drugs are discovered and tested.

In these courses, the "Big Three" of the sophomore year, students learn most of the basic medical knowledge they will need in order to get the most out of the time they spend in the hospital wards and clinics in the last two years. Seniors, looking back on their four years of training, often told us that they considered the second year the most important of the four, that they wished they had studied even harder than they did because the material was so important.

In a fourth very important course, physical diagnosis, students have their first direct contact with patients and learn to examine and diagnose them. This course means a great deal to students, for it is their first actual participation in the core drama of medicine, the treatment of diseased human beings. (Students, of course, have still other courses during their sophomore year: lecture courses in obstetrics, public health, biostatistics, and so on.)

In spite of the fact that the work of the second year is so important, both objectively and in the eyes of the students, we have chosen not to deal at length with it. Why? The answer lies in the fact that we are not, after all, attempting to study medical education in its entirety. Rather, we have confined ourselves to studying one aspect of medical education: the way students collectively formulate and act on perspectives which influence the level and direction of their academic effort. However important the second year might be from the point of view of pedagogy, in our judgment it is a year in which the styles of student effort are not unique. That is, much of what the students do is a continuation of the perspectives formed during the freshman year; what is not represents the beginnings of perspectives which will become dominant during the clinical years.

Several students, when queried about the sophomore year, made the paradoxical statement that the work was much harder than the first year but that they had not been panicked and had been able to take it in stride. This seemed to us to indicate that, from the students' point of view, the problem of what and how to study remains in the second year and that, while it is harder in the sense that there is more of it, they have already devised ways of dealing with this problem so that it does not upset them as it once did. Observation of the second year showed us that the problems it presents to students are not, in fact, very different from those presented by the first year. Lectures and laboratory sessions, combined with very substantial amounts of reading, still constitute the basic mode of pedagogy. Students must still choose what to learn from the great amounts of fact they face. The faculty still gives examinations which constitute one of the important ways, as students see it, that they are likely to be judged. Students still know so little of the problems of medical practice that, even though the relevance of their work to medicine is now much clearer, they have no good way of choosing what to learn on the basis of what will stand them in best stead when they begin to practice.

Our brief observations seemed to show that sophomores, insofar as they are faced with the same problems as freshmen, deal with them in similar ways. They study what they think the faculty wants them to know, assessing the faculty's desires just as they did earlier: by careful examination of current and old examinations, by careful analysis of hints dropped in class, and so on. They are somewhat more convinced as sophomores that what they are learning will be of use later on even if, just as before, they have no particular basis for making this judgment.

In their work in physical diagnosis, however, the problems students face differ markedly from those of freshmen and the same solutions do not apply. Since the succeeding seven chapters deal with these problems and the solutions to them developed by students, we will not bother to summarize that material here. Suffice it to say that the new perspectives students begin developing in their work in physical diagnosis foreshadow those which become dominant in later years, when the work is largely clinical in character.

For these reasons, then, we ignore the sophomore year in this volume. We do this in the belief that we have not thereby missed anything of major importance to the main theme of our study.

Part Three:
STUDENT CULTURE IN THE CLINICAL YEARS

Chapter 11 # The Work of the Clinical Years

T<small>HE</small> student now enters the clinical years of school. For the first time the major part of his work consists of direct participation in the care and treatment of medical patients. He works in an institution which is only partly devoted to educational activities — a university medical center in which the care of patients is paramount and in which research also plays a prominent role. What happens to the level and direction of student effort in this setting?

In this section of the book we document in detail the proposition that the students' level and direction of effort in the clinical years are a function of the immediate, situationally-based perspectives they develop in order to deal with the problems they face as students. Although they now work in a medical setting, they remain students, and the characteristics and limitations of the student role decisively shape the problems they face and their solutions of them. Working in the medical center, they become involved in medical culture and might be expected to begin to internalize it; but we shall show that while medical culture influences student culture (and indeed furnishes much of the material from which it is constructed), it operates only within the limits permitted by the students' immediate situation.

Medical culture consists of the shared understandings and perspectives of the medical profession as well as of the technology of diagnosis and treatment of human illness. Although it probably possesses a core accepted by almost all physicians, it varies greatly among functional, regional, and other subgroups in the profession. Students come into contact primarily with the version of medical culture held by the professional subgroup represented by their faculty but also meet other versions in their contacts with visiting physicians, staffs of other hospitals affiliated with the school, and other doctors with whom they have contact outside the school.

Students absorb medical culture in a selective fashion as it helps meet the problems posed by their school environment. Thus, what they use of medical culture is by no means the same as, or simply a junior version of, the culture of the practicing physician. Rather it contains characteristic distortions and omissions which, as we shall see, account for many of the disagreements, both overt and implicit, between students and faculty.

Student versions of medical culture differ from those of the practicing physician because the position of the student in medical school differs radically from the physician's. Although the distinctive characteristics of the student position are obvious, they are so necessary to analysis of student behavior that they must be pointed out. The student is someone who is learning to be but is not yet a doctor. He cannot become a doctor without completing his training in school. This training is supposed to provide him with some necessary minimum of knowledge and skill so that he can be certified as fit to practice medicine. Until such time as he has completed his training he cannot be allowed to carry on the full range of activities or exercise the full range of prerogatives associated with the physician's role. His training consists in great part of carrying on some of these activities under supervision, with a greater range being allowed him as he progresses through the years of school.

Students enter this environment with two goals: 1. to be allowed to complete the training (not to flunk out of school) and 2. to learn what they will need to know in order to carry on medical practice successfully after graduation. In attempting to achieve these goals in the school environment and within the confines of the student position, students face a number of problems. In particular, they must decide how hard they are going to work and on what things they will work hardest.

This section of the book describes the students' collective solutions to the problems of setting a level and direction of effort. These collective solutions are the student culture of the clinical years, the perspectives students share about proper behavior in the student role. Student culture, so conceived, is not, to repeat, merely a junior version of the culture of medicine. It does show, inevitably, a close family resemblance to the professional culture, for it is constructed in some part out of the aspects of professional culture the students are directly exposed to in school. But it is constructed as a set of answers to the problems of students, and these are not the same as the problems of practicing physicians (although, again, the two have some family resemblance). Student culture thus consists of a set of answers to student problems which draw, where possible, on what the students know of medical culture; but only those aspects of medical culture relevant to student problems become involved in the student culture, and they are given a characteristically "student" phrasing.

To the degree that student culture is drawn from medical culture, it furnishes students with the rudiments of the professional culture they will participate in after graduation. In Part IV we consider some of the ways students make use of these rudiments of medical culture in thinking about what they will do when they leave school. But we consider here those aspects of student culture more directly tied to problems of being in school. The chapters to follow in this section deal with the development of student culture in the clinical years.

Chapter 11 describes the curriculum of the clinical years, in the form it took while this study was made: courses, teaching methods, and the activities students are required to engage in. It provides much of the necessary ethnographic background for what follows and also specifies some important conditions for the development of student culture.

In Chapter 12 we analyze one of the basic problems students face: what to study out of the mass of material they are presented with. We show further that the faculty and the organization of the school suggest a solution to this problem in the form of two criteria which appear to be important parts of medical culture: clinical experience and medical responsibility. Chapter 13 describes the perspective students develop on the problem of what to study.

Chapter 14 turns to the question of student relations with faculty where the faculty function as examiners who have the power to prevent students graduating and describes the perspective students develop on problems arising for them in this area. The problems arising out of the relations between students in work situations and the perspective which develops in consequence are considered in Chapter 15. Chapter 16 shows the influence of student culture on one very important area of student activity: student relations with patients in the teaching hospital. Finally, Chapter 17 discusses the question of student autonomy in the clinical years, asking to what extent students are free to set their own level and direction of effort.

Beginning in a small way in the second year of school, and thereafter completely, the student does clinical rather than academic work. That is, he gets his training primarily by working with patients rather than through lectures and laboratory work (though, of course, these continue through the last two years of school). Though he remains in many senses a student, he becomes much more of an apprentice, imitating full-fledged practitioners at their work and learning what he will need to know to be one of them by practicing it under their supervision. That he now becomes, in a sense, a functionary of the hospital is symbolized by the uniform he dons at the beginning of the third year: the white shirt, trousers, and jacket he will wear through the remainder of his undergraduate and postgraduate medical training. He now works in a hospital surrounded by hospital personnel; the work itself is in large part that demanded by hospital routine.

The bulk of the student's work consists of "working-up" patients who come to the clinics or are admitted to the wards and then assigned to him and of performing minor diagnostic and therapeutic procedures on them. Working-up a patient, an elaborate exercise in discovering and interpreting the signs and symptoms of disease, is made up of three distinct parts: taking a medical history, performing a physical examination, and making a differential diagnosis. This is the same routine a physician goes through in dealing with a patient. In taking a history, the student attempts to elicit from the patient, through a relatively set list of questions, all the information the patient can contribute about his own illness. The student asks when the present illness began, what it was like, and how it has progressed. He inquires about past illnesses, how they began, progressed, and came to an end, with or without treatment. He queries the patient about possible symptoms, whose importance the patient may not have been aware of prior to questioning, in all the major physiological systems of the body — neurological, digestive, cardiovascular, and so on. He may ask about the patient's family situation, job, or other social matters which might have a bearing on the patient's difficulties.

He then performs a physical examination. The faculty has urged him to follow a set routine in doing this. He no longer relies on the patient's descriptions but instead looks, listens, and feels in an effort to make an objective appraisal of the physical signs, as contrasted with the subjective symptoms which patients report, of disease that may be present. He takes the patient's pulse and blood pressure and listens, through a stethoscope, to his heart and lungs. He inspects, with appropriate instruments, the patient's eyes, ears, nose, and throat. He palpates the patient's abdomen, looking for enlarged organs or anomalous masses. He inspects and palpates the patient's extremities. He does a rectal examination. He may make various specialized examinations, such as a complete examination of the patient's nervous system, if the situation seems to warrant it. In each of these procedures, the student is looking for those deviations from the normal he has read or been told about that may signal various disease states he has studied.

In addition to this direct examination of the patient's body, the student performs certain routine laboratory tests: a blood count and a urinalysis. He draws a sample of the patient's blood and gets a specimen of urine, which he examines in the laboratory. He also has available to him the X rays taken of the patient and the results of such other laboratory tests as have been made.

On the basis of the information gathered from the history, examination, laboratory work, and X rays, the student attempts to make a differential diagnosis of the patient's condition. The differential diagnosis is an exercise in deductive reasoning in which the student takes all the facts he has gathered and tries to determine which disease or combination of diseases would best account for what he knows about the patient. Typically, the student takes the major symptoms and signs which the patient exhibits and runs through all the known conditions which might produce them, attempting to narrow the field of suspects down to the culprit or culprits responsible by ruling out most of them. For example, he might suspect that a patient with stomach pain had a gastric ulcer but rule out this possibility on the ground that the pain occurs directly after eating, as the pain of ulcer rarely does. By considering all the known possibilities and ruling out most of them on the basis of contrary evidence, he reaches a decision about the cause of the patient's difficulty. Having done so, he decides on a plan of treatment.

All the information from the history and physical, the differential diagnosis, and the plan of treatment are written down in a standard form suggested by the faculty, and this document is placed in the patient's hospital chart, alongside similar documents prepared by other hospital personnel. The patient's chart contains, in addition to these documents, all results of tests and therapeutic procedures. If the patient is hospitalized (instead of being treated as an outpatient), the chart is kept on his floor, and the student and others add to it information gathered by daily contact with the patient, further questioning and examination, and possibly by further diagnostic procedures (such as spinal taps). The chart, while not a public record, is available to all authorized hospital personnel. After the patient's treatment is completed, the chart is filed with the hospital's medical records. Consequently the student's work-up can be seen by a great many people.

In various departments of the hospital students help out with therapeutic procedures. They may attend to minor injuries in the emergency room, be given a place in the surgical team in the operating room, or assist or even officiate at the delivery of babies.

The student's social world, while he is engaged in school work during the clinical years, is made up largely of other students, patients, and other hospital personnel. Since students are assigned to their courses by the administration and have very little choice of what they will take or when they will take it, the students they associate with at work are those who have been assigned to the same hospital ward or clinic. They do have some opportunity during free time to meet with other students, but hospital routines and the common interests aroused by being in the same situation conspire to keep student associations within the bounds of these work groups except for lunch periods and coffee breaks. This means, of course, that they associate almost entirely with students in their own year of school.

The student meets patients either when they are hospitalized or when they come to a clinic for outpatient treatment. Although hospital personnel classify patients informally in many ways, administratively they are either "private patients" or "clinic patients." The private patients have come by referral to be treated by a particular doctor; they pay their own way, either directly or through some form of insurance. Clinic patients may be paid for in whole or in part by the state or various agencies; they may also pay part of the cost of their care themselves, in accordance with their circumstances.

The other hospital personnel the student has contact with can be divided into medical personnel and nurses and auxiliary personnel. He has some contact with the nurses, aides, and housekeeping personnel found everywhere in the hospital, as well as with the laboratory and X-ray technicians. Of these people, the nurses probably play the biggest part in the student's activities, assisting him in examining patients and performing such procedures as drawing blood. However, aside from the occasional unmarried student who would like to become more friendly with an attractive nurse or student nurse, there is little informal contact.

Laymen tend to think that nurses play a more important part in the students' training than they actually do. There is a great deal of lore about how nurses who know more about medicine than medical students use their superior knowledge to help, influence, or correct the inexperienced students. During all the time we spent in the hospital wards and clinics, we did not observe one instance of nurses acting in any of these ways; it is not difficult to understand why. Though the school and hospital occupy the same physical space and encompass many of the same categories of people, they consist of two quite separate chains of command and authority. The nurse operates in the hospital hierarchy but has no place in the line of authority of the medical school. This makes it illegitimate for her to attempt to interfere in the student's training. Of course, such formal obstacles are often ignored in the routine interaction of organizational personnel. However, the fact that the nurse has no place in the formal structure of authority in the school also means that the medical student is not disposed to pay much attention to her, just on that account. We suspect that nurses know this and do not attempt to have any influence on medical students. The idea of the nurse's importance in the medical student's experience may possibly derive from the very much larger role she plays in the work lives of interns and residents. Both the nurses and the young doctors of the house staff are part of the hospital hierarchy and under the orders of the same superiors. They have a common stake in many of the hospital's activities, and the nurse has more influence on the residents and interns with whom she comes in contact.

Of all the people the student has to do with in the hospital, the most important to him are the doctors, of whom there are many kinds. The most basic distinction is that between the faculty of the school (who are also the practicing staff of the hospital) and the house staff, who are the interns and residents taking postgraduate training in medicine. (From now on, we refer to the first group as staff members or faculty, to the second as house staff, interns, or residents.) The faculty have all completed their graduate medical training, almost always in some specialty, and usually (although not necessarily) carry on the practice of that specialty in the university hospital or elsewhere. They have primary responsibility for teaching, examining, and passing or failing students. The faculty may work full-time at the medical center, having their offices and seeing and treating all their patients there; or they may be members of the visiting staff, physicians who have their practices elsewhere in the city, serve on the staffs of other hospitals, and come to the medical center occasionally to help out with the teaching.

The house staff consists of those who have graduated from medical school and are either serving a mandatory one-year internship before entering practice or, having completed that, are taking further training as a resident in some specialty. Members of the house staff do not have private patients of their own, though some clinic patients are assigned to them to handle. Much of their work consists of working up patients in the wards and in the clinics and in this way resembles the work of the students. But members of the house staff are licensed physicians and, as such, can be and are left in charge of medical affairs and decisions when their superiors, the faculty, are not present (although always available). Residents and interns also have some responsibility, which varies in parts of the hospital, for teaching and overseeing the work of the students.

Though the student spends some time during the clinical years in academic lecture halls and classrooms, the bulk of his work is carried on in the hospital's wards and clinics. A ward is a unit of the hospital, some part of a floor and under the authority of some one department, such as Medicine or Surgery. It consists of a number of rooms for patients, a nurses' station, one or more treatment rooms, and usually a small laboratory in which students do blood counts and urinalyses. In addition to the patients hospitalized there, a ward is peopled by a number of nurses and auxiliary personnel, an intern and one or more residents, and one or more staff members (typically, a senior staff member, who holds high academic rank and his associate who, holding lower rank, may be called a junior staff member).

The time these people spend on the ward and the kind of contact the student has with each category of person vary. The student himself is expected to be on the ward most of the time when he is not in classes; he may, of course, spend some time in the cafeteria or library. Patients are in their rooms and available to the students for examining and history-taking at all times except when they have been taken elsewhere in the hospital for special diagnostic or therapeutic procedures. Nurses are on the floor most of the time for the student to consult if he wishes. The student interacts with both patients and nurses when he chooses, insofar as they are available.

The student, on the other hand, interacts with faculty and house staff when they choose. Since the faculty and house staff have other activities, they are not always around, and the student sees them either at administratively appointed times when classes or other educational activities are scheduled, when they want him for some special activity, or when he is able to catch them. It is easier to catch the house staff than it is to catch faculty, as their work keeps them on the ward a good deal of the time.

It must be remembered that the medical faculty have several responsibilities, of which teaching is only one. They have patients to attend to in the hospital, patients to be seen in their offices, residents and interns to train, and research to do. Consequently, in contrast to some other kinds of teachers, there is no expectation on anyone's part that they will be available to the students all or most of the time. It seems understandable and justifiable to the students that this should be the case.

The student spends the bulk of his time, in fact, with the other students assigned to the same location. He not only attends such formal activities as classes in their company but shares his spare time with them as well. They are all at the beck and call of the same staff member, residents, and intern, and must necessarily be on the same ward most of the day. The student laboratory furnishes a natural meeting place, where students study, loaf, do lab work, talk over events of the day, and discuss patients they have seen. Some of our most interesting field materials come from "bull sessions" in these student laboratories.

The clinic, unlike the ward, does not operate twenty-four hours a day. It is open on specified days for a specified number of hours, and patients come to it for outpatient treatment. In most clinics, particularly those in which the students do the bulk of the work, charity patients are a considerable proportion of the total.

Clinics are held in a suitably appointed part of a hospital floor, containing a hall (with chairs for waiting patients), a reception desk to which patients report, many small offices in which patients are seen, and a few rooms in which students may consult with others about the patients they are examining.

In addition to patients, the clinic is peopled by several other kinds of persons. Nurses sit at the reception desk and take patients' names as they come in. They turn the names over to the resident or intern in charge of the clinic, who assigns each new patient to a student and sees that returning patients are seen by the student who saw them last. The house staff collaborates with the faculty (which ordinarily includes several of the visiting staff) in hearing students present the findings of their examinations and their diagnoses. Nurses occasionally assist the student in his examination.

The student works-up his new patient (or checks over the old patient) and then presents the case to one of the clinic staff, describing the positive findings in the history and examination, giving his tentative diagnosis, and suggesting either further diagnostic procedures, therapeutic measures, or both. The staff member may accept the student's findings and discuss the case with him on that basis, agreeing on some plan of therapy; or he may decide to have a look at the patient himself, in which case he may demonstrate important kinds of findings to the student during his own examination. In either case, the student ends up with a supervised diagnosis and plan of treatment. He then sends the patient to get whatever additional diagnostic procedures are necessary and gives him instructions on how to take care of his illness and prescriptions for necessary medication. All orders for diagnostic procedures and drugs must be signed by one of the staff, although the students ordinarily make out these forms and usually suggest what drugs to use. Occasionally, a staff member helps the student discuss the case with the patient, pointing out to the patient the necessity of following the prescribed treatment. The staff member, with greater experience and greater authority in the patient's eyes, has an easier time convincing him that he should follow directions than do the students.

Patients are usually required to return to the clinic at frequent intervals to have their progress checked. On these occasions they are seen by the same student who saw them originally; this gives the student an opportunity to follow the case from start to finish and get experience in handling patients over a long period. On these return visits, too, the student makes use of the findings produced by the diagnostic procedures prescribed earlier. He again has to check the case with a staff member, just as with a new patient.

Although, as we noted earlier, most of the student's work is built into hospital routine in the ways we have just described, he still has some more academic responsibilities and activities. The responsibilities take the form of examinations and other procedures in which the faculty test the amount of knowledge the student has acquired. These include written examinations of both the multiple-choice and essay type; oral examinations in which several faculty members quiz a few students at a time on material mentioned in lectures or reading or suggested by the patients the students have had assigned to them; and ward rounds, during which the staff member in charge of a ward accompanies the students on a tour of the patients on the ward, the students present their findings and diagnoses on the patients assigned to them, and the staff member quizzes them on their presentations.

The student's academic activities consist of lectures, laboratories, and small discussion classes (often referred to in the hospital as conferences). During lectures, members of the faculty present material of various kinds: rough overviews of their specialties, selected details on the diagnosis and treatment of particular diseases, presentations of patients who display pathological conditions, and so on. Students listen and sometimes take notes. Much of the teaching is done to small groups of students assigned to a particular part of the hospital, and here lectures are less frequent. Instead, these conferences are most often handled with some form of the discussion method. The teacher, who may be a member of the faculty or an intern or resident assigned to the same service as the students, quizzes and talks with the students about topics relevant to the patients they are seeing or the specialty they are studying. Students have some laboratory work while they are in surgery, consisting of the examination by the methods of pathology of tissue removed from patients at surgery.

All of these academic activities require the student to do some reading. Students buy texts for some of their courses and in addition make use of the collection of medical and scientific books contained in the school's library.

Student assignments to various parts of the hospital, as we have said, are made by the administration. Students are assigned to a "service," i.e., that part of a ward handled by one staff member or one team of staff members, or to a series of clinics under the direction of one department. Each student takes the same group of courses as his classmates in the same year, but all students do not take the same course at the same time, instead rotating through the various services and departmental clinics. The students do not move individually through this sequence but as one of a group of five or six students who are assigned together to each service or course.

We now describe briefly the courses students take in their last two years. It must be remembered that the school is in transition. The curriculum we describe here no longer exists in this form; many changes have taken place and more will follow. What we describe is what the students we observed went through. It is the environment in which the perspectives students developed in the clinical years, their student culture, grew.

The Third Year

The third year is divided into three quarters, each of about eleven and one-half weeks. The student body is likewise divided into three groups, and there are three main courses during the year, each group being assigned to one of these fields each quarter. The groups rotate through these fields, so that by the end of the year each group has each of the subjects: medicine, surgery, and pediatrics. Keeping in mind that each group has these three subjects in a different order, we will discuss each one separately, describing what a quarter's work in each consists of.

Not all of the training is carried out at the medical center. In the quarters devoted to medicine and surgery, affiliations with both a large private hospital and the local Veterans' Administration hospital are made use of. At any one time, half the group assigned to medicine, for example, will be located at the medical center; the other half will be divided between these two local hospitals. At the halfway point in the quarter, these groups exchange places, so that everyone will have spent some time both at the medical center and at one of the two affiliated hospitals. The course in surgery is split between the university and the Veterans' Administration hospital. Pediatrics also makes use of an affiliation with a local pediatric hospital. This program is run somewhat differently. Half of the group assigned to pediatrics spends the entire quarter at K.U., while the other half spends its entire quarter outside. So, for medicine and surgery, each group has about the same experience, while for pediatrics the experiences may be quite different, depending on the hospital to which one is assigned.

Finally, each student spends one week with a psychiatric unit during his third year, either at the medical center or at the VA hospital. This assignment may come at any time of the year and, consequently, will take one week out of the student's time in one of the other three courses.

Medicine. The student taking his five and one-half weeks of medicine at the medical center will be assigned to one of three services, as a member of a group of five or six students. Two of these services are permanently headed by senior staff members working in conjunction with a junior staff member. Each of these two services is also manned by two residents and an intern. The third service to which students may be assigned was formerly devoted to Negro patients; various members of the permanent and visiting staff of the department of medicine are assigned there in rotation, but the patients do not "belong" to them. A permanent staff member supervises students for a period of each day throughout their five and a half weeks on this service. When the student group changes, the staff member changes too. Another period of supervision is provided by a different staff member each day. A resident and an intern are also assigned to this service.

The services headed by the senior men each have a sizable number of beds on the general medicine ward of the hospital, both those for private patients of the doctors involved and those for clinic patients. We will describe the experience of the student by going through his typical daily schedule, as we saw it operate on the services headed by the senior staff.

The student's day begins at eight in the morning, when he must arrive in order to get around and see all his patients and check on their status before ward rounds begin at nine o'clock. Approximately once a week — this job is rotated among the five or six students on the service — he must get in at seven-thirty in order to draw all the samples of blood that are needed from different patients on the service. Since many samples are likely to be required, and the student is likely not to be skilled, this is a long and tedious job. The major teaching exercise of the day, ward rounds, takes place each weekday morning from nine until eleven. The students, residents, and intern go around with one of the physicians in charge of the service to see each of the patients under their care. Each patient has been assigned to a student, who is responsible for presenting that case on the first day it is seen and for continuing to be ready to present further information on it when requested.

The remainder of the day is devoted to lectures in a number of medical specialties, to informal conferences with residents, and to "ward work": seeing one's patients, performing laboratory work, and performing special medical procedures under the supervision of a resident or intern. The conferences with residents and the perform-ance of medical procedures take quite different forms, depending on the resident in charge of the service. Some residents involve students in most of the procedures that occur on the service; others do not. Some residents take great pains with the conferences, turning them into highly organized series of lectures and discussions; others treat them as informal discussions.

Students are usually free over the weekend (Saturday afternoon and Sunday). However, those men next in line to receive a new pa-tient are considered to be "on call." They are required to be available so that if a patient should come in they can be notified and complete their work-up in time for rounds on the following Monday. Evenings are free, except for students on call, who may be called in at any hour of the night to work-up a new patient.

The medical services at the private and the Veterans' Administra-tion hospitals offer the student experiences essentially like those he has at the medical center. Students make rounds with attending phy-sicians, discuss cases with them, work-up patients, draw blood, and perform other minor procedures. Since these hospitals are not uni-versity medical centers, the services are somewhat less demanding of the student.

Both the private hospital and the VA have the care of patients as their primary purpose and teaching must, in the nature of things, assume lower priority. Thus it happens that teaching rounds and lec-tures may be interfered with at the private hospital when the attend-ing physician is forced to leave on a house call. The routines of these hospitals are not set up to take account of students, who thus find themselves more frequently unattended. Similarly, there are fewer residents at these hospitals (and no interns at all at the VA hospital) so that the house staff is not so readily available to the students. In practice, this means that the amount of time the students get is very much up to the individual resident; in fact, some residents may spend more time with the students than do their opposite numbers at K.U. The number of formally assigned lectures and conferences is about the same, although different subject matter may be covered at the different hospitals.

Two other factors differentiate the three hospitals: the amount of freedom to perform minor procedures given students and the degree to which they are allowed to play important roles in the treatment of patients. Since the patients at the private hospital are private patients of staff physicians, there is some tendency for the students to be more purely students: onlookers and learners rather than doers. At the VA, since all patients are being treated by salaried physicians, and since there are no interns to share the work load, students are apt to be given somewhat more responsibility.

Surgery. Two-thirds of the students assigned to surgery are, at any one time, at the medical center, while the others are at the VA. The surgical services at the medical center are split up in much the same way as the medical services. The student can expect to be assigned to one of three services. Two of these are private services, under the charge of senior staff members. Each has an intern and resident assigned to it, as well as the two surgeons in charge. They differ from their counterparts in medicine in that they have few clinic patients under their care. The third is the Ward Surgical Service, to which are assigned all patients who have entered the hospital for surgery by way of the outpatient clinics. Some are indigent patients from Kansas, referred by various agencies; a considerable portion are Negroes, many of whom turn up on the hospital's doorstep from the state of Missouri. The Ward Surgical Service is under the charge of the senior residents. As in medicine, the student in the junior surgery program is assigned patients as they come into the hospital, the assignments rotating in order through the group of five or six of which he is a part, and he is required to do an initial work-up on them. He is also responsible, as in medicine, for initial laboratory work and for further routine laboratory work as needed.

In other ways the student's schedule in surgery differs greatly from that in medicine. It starts at seven, when the students meet with the resident to make rounds on patients who have already been operated on. The surgeons begin operating at eight o'clock, and those students whose patients are scheduled for surgery that day are required to scrub in for the operation. A second student is assigned to each patient, to assist with the anesthesia. Those students not due in the operating room have a lecture at eight.

Most operations we witnessed were handled by a team of four: the operating surgeon (a staff member), resident, intern, and student. Ordinarily, the student's main job is to hold retractors, in order to help expose the operative field; occasionally, he may be allowed to cut sutures and to sew up incisions. Anesthesia is ordinarily given by a member of the senior staff or by a resident in anesthesiology. Students assisting the anesthesiologist check the patient's pulse and blood pressure and help set up and administer various anesthetics.

An operation may last anywhere from a half hour to four or five hours, or even more. Ordinarily, several operations are scheduled each morning for each service; each staff member on each service alternates days in operating. The operating schedule of a service may be completed by eleven or twelve, or it may run well into the afternoon, depending on the kind of cases on the schedule. The hours from nine to twelve are left open on the student's schedule, for operating room work for those whose patients are so scheduled and for work on the wards, either in working-up new patients or making progress notes on old ones, for the others. Several hours of lectures and conferences are scheduled each week, and three hours a week are spent in the surgical pathology laboratory, where students dissect and make a microscopic examination of tissue removed at surgery.

The student is required to spend four or five nights in the hospital on call. On these nights he may be awakened to work-up a newly admitted patient, or to perform minor procedures, such as starting an intravenous setup. Two students are on call each night and must stay in the hospital from six in the evening until eight the following morning. On Saturdays students are on call from noon until eight the following morning, and on Sundays for a full twenty-four hour shift starting at eight in the morning. The student on call sometimes participates in an emergency operation in the early hours of the morning.

An important difference in the three surgical services is that the students on the service headed by the department chairman go to surgery clinic with him two mornings a week. The six students in his group are assigned patients as they come into the clinic and work them up, taking a history and doing a physical examination. Then the staff member brings the other students in and discusses the case with them, speaking particularly about possible surgical treatment. The other groups do not have this experience in the clinic.

Surgery at the Veterans' Administration hospital offers students much the same kind of experience. As in medicine, there are no interns, so that students are given somewhat greater responsibilities; since residents do much of the operating, the student is apt to find himself nearer the center of activity. Students see somewhat less of the senior staff than they do at the medical center. Finally, the schedule is looser, and students who desire more operating room experience need not wait for one of their own patients to go to surgery but can assist in whatever operations happen to be going on.

Pediatrics. The group which has this training at the university is made up of about sixteen or seventeen students, divided into three groups. Each of these groups spends equal amounts of time, in rotation, on each of the three floors in the pediatrics building. Each floor is devoted to a somewhat different set of patients: one floor largely to infectious diseases, one to other medical and surgical cases, and the third to infants. Each floor is manned by a different set of residents and a different intern.

Each of these smaller student groups is again divided in two, and these subgroups alternate between the hospital floors and the clinic. The student's duties on the pediatrics ward are essentially the same as those on the other third-year services. He must complete a full medical work-up — history, physical examination, and laboratory work — on each new patient assigned to him. He must also see his patients each day and enter progress notes in their chart.

Pediatrics differs from surgery and medicine in some respects. In the first place, the student must deal with the parents of his patients as well as with the patients themselves. In most pediatric cases, what medical history there is has to be taken from the parents rather than from the child. This introduces certain difficulties into the student's work, because the person from whom the history must be taken is not always present when the student would like to take it, as is the case with adult medical and surgical patients.

In pediatrics the teaching is somewhat more informal and relaxed than in the other services, but there are daily lectures and conferences. In the conferences the students are expected to ask questions to generate discussion. The lectures often take on the form of discussion in which the students may be quizzed on reading which has been assigned.

Staff members make rounds daily, at various times; in addition to students assigned to the floor in question, others may turn up and go along with them. The students are not required to attend these rounds, but note is taken of consistent absence. They are not asked questions about the cases. The rounds seem to be oriented more toward the residents and interns and to be concerned with the management of particular cases. But the students may ask questions; if they do, they are answered, sometimes at great length. So there is always an element of teaching in the seemingly informal procedure. The residents also do a great deal of informal teaching. They are on the floors most of the day; the students, who occasionally find time on their hands between admissions or other duties, engage them in discussions and question-and-answer sessions.

The student also attends general and specialty pediatric clinics and the "well baby" clinic. In the specialty clinics, he does not ordinarily work-up patients. Typically, the man who is teaching the specialty will demonstrate a patient and discuss the case and the general principle involved in it. In the pediatric psychiatry clinic, however, each student is assigned to either a disturbed child or the mother of that child and sees these patients each week. The students take turns interviewing their patients in the "goldfish bowl," a room with a one-way mirror and microphones in which they can be observed by the staff and other students and their technique criticized.

In afternoon clinics the student sees a variety of pediatric cases. In the well baby clinic he takes care of newborn infants, checking their growth and giving directions on feeding and other problems to the mother. When he has seen the patient, he goes to one of the residents or junior staff members and presents his findings and recommendations and has them checked. In the routine pediatric clinic, he does a complete examination on each patient, makes a diagnosis, and thinks about possible treatment. Then he consults with a resident or staff member and gets his opinion and directions as to what to do. Frequently, the person who is checking the student will go with him to see the patient, repeat parts of the examination, demonstrate important findings to the student, and discuss what ought to be done for the patient with the parent.

The work at the affiliated pediatric hospital is similar to that at the medical center. The students are again divided into three groups, spending their time in turn on each of three services: 1. isolation ward, including afternoon clinic; 2. a ward containing children with chronic disease, usually polio or some orthopedic problem, and morning clinic; and 3. boys' and girls' ward and baby wards, catchall wards to which all children are sent who do not belong in either of the other two wards. Ward work is similar to that at the medical center, although there are some minor differences in routine. Children are admitted through the clinic, and the student takes the history and does his physical (including the laboratory work) in the clinic; he then follows the child through its hospital stay, making daily examinations and reporting his findings. The routine in the clinic is essentially the same as at the medical center: patients are examined, the case is discussed with one of the attending staff, and treatment recommended. Students periodically spend an evening on call and help the residents and interns with night clinic, seeing the many children who are brought into a hospital in the early evening.

The teaching schedule is less crowded than at the university. There are fewer classes and formal conferences. There are, however, many informal conferences with residents, just as at the medical center. It is probably true that the student has more free time to spend at tasks of his own choosing in pediatrics than in the other third-year services. It is also true that they see less of the older staff members in pediatrics than in any of the other third-year services.

Psychiatry. Each student takes a week off from his regularly assigned service sometime during his junior year in order to spend a week on psychiatry, either at the VA Hospital or the medical center. Only the work at the medical center was observed.

Students have very few formal responsibilities. The faculty attitude appears to be that the students should take advantage of the week to acquaint themselves, at their own convenience, with various kinds of psychiatric disease and the hospital procedures used in treating them. Each student is assigned one or possibly two new patients for work-up while he is on the service. A work-up consists of the ordinary physical examination, the taking of a psychiatric history (which often proved very difficult with extremely disturbed patients), and a mental status examination. This latter is designed to reveal the patient's level of mental functioning and is new to the student; one purpose of his week in psychiatry is that he learn to make this examination. In addition to seeing a new patient, the student is encouraged to become acquainted with a few other patients exemplifying typical psychiatric disease states. He is briefed on these patients by the resident. Students spend a good deal of time hanging around the locked ward observing and talking with patients. They also see insulin and electroconvulsive therapy given each morning.

On their first day, they attend an orientation talk by a staff member and have a long conference with a staff member later in the week as well. They also attend the Tuesday morning staff conference at which all patients are discussed by the medical and nursing staffs and auxiliary workers.

We have been told that student responsibilities at the VA Hospital are quite similar, although there is some variation due to differences in the patient population and hospital policy. Almost all VA patients are male. Such procedures as group therapy are used at the VA Hospital, and students sit in on these sessions.

The Fourth Year

The fourth year program is divided into four quarters of approximately nine weeks. These quarters are devoted to four major courses of study: medicine and psychiatry, obstetrics and gynecology, surgical specialties, and a preceptorship.

Medicine and Psychiatry. The students in senior medicine are divided into two groups of approximately fifteen. The schedules of the two groups differ in some respects; halfway through the course, groups exchange schedules, so that each group gets all the kinds of teaching given during the quarter.

The major activity for students is work in either the general medicine clinic or in the neurology or psychiatry clinics. No matter which schedule the students are on, about half of their time in school is spent in clinics. They spend the remainder of their time attending conferences and lectures.

The students find the general medicine clinic the most important of their activities. In the clinic each student has a small office, containing a desk, chairs, and an examining table, where he sees patients who are assigned to him. The student ordinarily sees somewhere between three and six patients in each four-hour clinic session. Some of these are "new" patients, who have not been to the clinic before for their current difficulty; others are "old" patients, whom he has seen before and is now treating for the ailment diagnosed earlier. Seeing a new patient takes longer than seeing an old one, and some effort is made to make sure that students all get their fair share of new and old patients. Aside from this, no effort is made to insure that a student gets any particular variety or range of cases. He gets what is assigned to him in rotation. The student works-up his new patients, checks over his old ones, and talks over his findings, diagnoses, and proposed plans of treatment with members of the staff.

The routine of work in the neurology clinic is essentially the same as in the medicine clinic. These patients are typically referred from the medicine clinic, and the same student who has seen them there ordinarily sees them in the neurology clinic. The only difference lies in the fact that the staff members he consults with are neurologists.

The psychiatry clinic meets two afternoons a week. It has three major activities. First, students have diagnostic cases, on which they work in pairs, one student interviewing the patient and the other interviewing a friend or relative of the patient. They ordinarily see these patients twice, once for a diagnostic session and a second time to make disposition of the case. Some of the patients become part of the second activity of the clinic; psychotherapy is recommended for them, and they are assigned to the student as a "treatment case." He sees these patients every week for an hour-long therapeutic session.

Supervisory hours with the faculty constitute the third major activity. This consists both of group discussion of cases and problems encountered in dealing with them, and of supervisory hours, in which two students meet with a practicing psychiatrist for a detailed discussion of how to handle the cases they have under treatment.

The student sees a wide variety of kinds of disease in these clinics. In the medicine clinic, he sees anything from cases requiring immediate surgery to cases in which there is no pathology at all. Similarly, his psychiatric patients (those there for diagnostic purposes) range from people suspected of mild neurosis to persons who are quickly disposed of by commitment to one of the state mental hospitals.

The student devotes the rest of his time in senior medicine to attending conferences, lectures, and discussions, dealing with a great range of special subjects. These classes meet for an hour or two weekly for one-half the quarter; the differences in schedule between the two groups of students lie in the particular classes they have. The following are among the subjects discussed in these short four-week courses: clinical biochemistry, metabolic diseases, allergy, dermatology, prescription writing and practical problems of drug therapy, cardiology and the interpretation of electrocardiograms, clinical physiology, neurology, gastrointestinal disease, and psychiatry. In addition, the students participate in ward rounds on the chest and hematology services for two hours each week for one-half of the quarter. They also have a conference on medical pathology for half of the quarter; here they work in pairs, one student giving the clinical history of a patient who died in the hospital and the other discussing the pathological findings.

For half the quarter students have a weekly conference in which problems of medical judgment are discussed with a senior staff member. This is connected with the clinical pathological conference (C.P.C.), one of the high points of the year for the students. This hour-long conference is held each Saturday at noon throughout the year and is attended by all students on the Kansas City campus of the medical school, by interns and residents, and by members of the hospital staff.

Obstetrics and Gynecology. The student works harder, perhaps, on obstetrics and gynecology than any other service in the hospital. This is due probably not so much to a difference in teaching philosophy on the part of the staff as to the nature of their cases. Two activities take up almost all of the students' time. One of these is clinic; the other, the care of women who have entered the hospital to have babies.

Obstetrics clinic is held every morning. Here the student sees pregnant women, both when the diagnosis of pregnancy is first made and later for routine prenatal check ups. When a woman comes to the clinic for the first time, thinking that she is pregnant, the student takes a complete obstetrical history and does a physical examination, including measuring her pelvis in order to make sure that it is of sufficient size to allow a normal birth. On subsequent visits to the clinic, up until six weeks before delivery, the woman will be seen for a very short time, just long enough to have her blood pressure checked and be asked a series of questions relating to possible complications of pregnancy. Starting six weeks before her expected date of confinement, the woman will have an abdominal examination in which the student seeks to determine the position and general state of the fetus. This goes on until she is admitted to the hospital for delivery. Residents and staff members are present in the clinic, but the student only needs to have those patients checked who are being seen for the first time, and those he feels present some complications.

Gynecology clinic is held every afternoon. The patients present a wide range of symptoms, and the student is required to take a history, perform a physical examination, and arrive at a diagnosis and plan of treatment, after consultation with a member of the staff. The importance of GYN clinic for the students lies in the fact that it is here that they get experience in doing pelvic examinations.

The morning clinic runs for about two and a half or three hours, the afternoon clinic for about two. The morning clinic is preceded by a lecture, and the afternoon clinic is followed by one. These lectures are given by members of the hospital staff and the visiting staff who happen to be in the clinic that day. The schedule of lectures is informally arranged and flexible; lectures are not always held when scheduled.

The more dramatic part of the students' experience on this service comes with the delivering of babies. Two students are on call at all times, and as each one gets a patient he is replaced by another student. When a patient comes into the hospital for delivery, a student and a resident examine her and decide about when she is likely to deliver and whether there are any complications. She is then moved to a labor room, and the student assigned to her case stays with her, timing her pains and doing rectal examinations to determine the downward progress of the baby, until she actually delivers. The differences in the length of time various women spend in labor produce great disparities in the amount of time students are required to spend attending them. One patient may deliver thirty minutes after she enters the hospital; another may not deliver for thirty hours.

When the indications show that the patient is about to deliver, she is taken to a delivery room. The students and a resident scrub for the delivery. The student himself delivers patients of certain kinds; he assists the residents and staff members in delivery of others. He does not deliver women who are having their first child or those expected to have a difficult time. Those women who are private patients of members of the staff are examined and delivered by their own doctors.

The student has certain other responsibilities in connection with any delivery. He ties off the umbilical cord, puts silver nitrate in the baby's eyes, and weighs, measures, and examines the placenta. He also fills out a form giving details of the delivery, to be inserted in the patient's chart along with a similar form filled out by the resident. Finally, he does such laboratory work (blood count and urinalysis) as is required while the patient is in the hospital.

The obstetrics department, as the nature of its work requires, runs on a twenty-four-hour basis. Students on call may have to wait until the middle of the night before patients come in; the student who is next up may be called out in the middle of the night to come over to the hospital to wait for the next patient to come in. A room furnished with double-deck beds is provided for students who must stay in the hospital overnight. Students frequently are awakened an hour or two after they have gone to sleep to examine a new patient, and they are frequently called from home at the same hour. (Work with patients on the OB floor takes precedence over work in the clinic.)

After a woman has delivered, the student visits her daily to see how she is coming along and writes progress notes in her chart. Occasionally a student will see a patient several times in the clinic, and then deliver her and watch her postnatally as well.

The student must also work-up all patients who come into the hospital for treatment of gynecological diseases; that is, he must take a complete history and do a physical examination and laboratory work on each one, make a tentative diagnosis, and suggest a plan of treatment. These cases do not play an important part in the department's training program. Rounds are not made frequently on the GYN service, and students often do not accompany the patients to surgery. GYN patients are assigned to the students on a rotating schedule during the day. At night the man who is on second call has as his responsibility the working-up of all GYN patients admitted.

The students see staff physicians for lectures, occasionally during clinic, and when private patients are having their babies. Otherwise, they spend most of their time among themselves and with the residents and interns on the service. The relations between students and residents are perhaps more intimate, whether in a hostile or friendly direction, here than on any other service in the hospital.

Only half of the group assigned to OB during any quarter has its training at the medical center. The other students go to Kansas City General Hospital, the charity hospital in Kansas City, Missouri, where they have a very similar experience. Clinic, classes, and delivery room work are the same as at the university. Students see somewhat less of the senior staff, though this difference is not marked. There are no private patients, so students are not denied access to patients on that basis. However, at the time this study was made students were not allowed to deliver white patients in the then-segregated hospital; their practical experience came from the delivery of Negro women.

Surgical Specialties. The students spend ten days in each of five surgical specialties. The specialties included varied during the two years we were conducting our observations. During 1955–56 the course was made up of otorhinolaryngology, neurosurgery, urology, orthopedics, and plastic surgery. During 1956–57 anesthesiology was substituted for plastic surgery. Groups of five or six students rotated from one service to another during the quarter.

In many ways, student experience is similar on all of the services. With the exception of anesthesiology, students on each service are assigned patients as they enter the hospital for an ordinary admission work-up (although they frequently do not have to do admission laboratory work). They follow patients during the time they are assigned to the service, conduct daily examinations, and make progress notes in the charts. They are not expected to spend as much time in surgery as during their junior year. The specialty services do not have as many patients as general surgery and ordinarily do not operate every morning. Furthermore, the operations are either so long and complicated that the student cannot learn much from them, or quite repetitious since most patients on the service have similar diseases; students are usually expected to attend one or two operations during their time on a service or to step in for a few moments in order to see the pathology when it has been surgically exposed.

On all services except anesthesiology, students attend clinic for a varying number of half-days a week, usually as frequently as clinic is held. They see patients, take a history, and do a physical, then call in a resident or a staff member who suggests treatment or arranges for hospital admission. Typical disposition of cases varies greatly between services, according to the nature of the diseases they deal with; on some services students perform a great many minor therapeutic procedures.

General lectures in surgery and its specialties are scheduled each day for all the students; in addition, each specialty has its own schedule of ward rounds, lectures, conferences, and informal discussions. The teaching in each specialty, since time is so short, tends to concentrate on one or two important things the faculty thinks students should know or be able to do. Typically, instructors try to teach students to do the kind of examinations characteristic of the specialty: the ear, nose, and throat examination of otorhinolaryngology, the neurological examination of neurosurgery, and so on.

Students on anesthesiology spend every morning from seven-thirty on in the operating room, working at the side of a resident who is giving anesthesia. They move from one operating room to another so that they may have experience with all the major kinds of anesthetics given. They are ordinarily given a chance to administer and become familiar with most of these anesthetics. A good deal of informal teaching goes on before, after, and during surgery. Patients are followed up postoperatively in the recovery room. Conferences are held with a staff member or resident each afternoon, in which cases done during the morning are discussed and the general principles illustrated in each brought out. Occasionally, therapeutic anesthetic procedures, such as nerve blocks, are demonstrated.

Students spend four or five days of their time on anesthesia in the emergency room. During this period they have no responsibilities to anesthesiology but are on twenty-four-hour call in the emergency room. They spend this time with the intern on call, and their work varies at his discretion. They sleep in the hospital during this time. Typically, they help the intern work-up patients coming into the emergency room and get some training in handling minor injuries and sewing up lacerations.

Preceptorship. The preceptorship is divided into two four-and-one-half-week periods. During one of these the student lives with a general practitioner in a small town in the state of Kansas, doing whatever work the preceptor assigns him. The preceptors are carefully chosen by the faculty. The aim of the program is to give students an intimate understanding of the nature of a rural general practice. We did not observe any preceptor-student pairs in the field, and our knowledge of the preceptorship is based on what students and faculty told us about it.

In general, it appears that the program works about as it was intended to. Students accompany the preceptor on his house calls and work with him in his office. They do not do any laboratory or similar routine work; instead, they participate in the diagnosis and treatment of patients in about the same way they do in the hospital. The primary differences are that here they see the kinds of patients typical of a rural general practice, instead of the more selected patients who come to the medical center, and the work of a private and general, as opposed to an academic and specialized, practitioner.

During the other half of the preceptorship, students work in one of the state mental institutions. Again, we did not observe any of these situations. Conditions vary greatly between the various hospitals to which students are assigned. In some the students handle the general medical problems of the inmates much as they handle clinic patients at the medical center; occasionally, the institution is so shorthanded that the student becomes a *de facto* intern, with most of the responsibilities of that position. In other institutions, their work is more psychiatrically oriented.

Conditions for the Development
of Student Culture

Several features of the work in the clinical years create the conditions necessary for the existence of a strong and effective student culture in the clinical years, a culture which constrains important areas of student behavior and thus has important consequences for the operation of the medical school. This culture consists of a set of perspectives held collectively, perspectives embodying agreements on the level and direction of effort students should put forth in their work as students.

Though features of the immediate situation forcefully constrain student behavior, we should keep in mind that these constraints are effective, in part, because of certain basic assumptions students make about why they are in medical school. Let us recall, first of all, that these students intend to go into the private practice of medicine. Though a few may conceive of alternatives, students ordinarily take it for granted that sometime after graduation they will be installed in a doctor's office, seeing and treating patients. They do not expect to go into research or into administration. They therefore look on school work, even when its details appear irrelevant to the actual practice of medicine, as a means of becoming a medical practitioner.

Let us further recall that these men have no very specific notions about what kind of medicine they will practice, no notions that specify the areas in which they must be especially competent. Many of them intend to become general practitioners. Those who intend to become specialists seldom settle on any particular specialty before graduation, so that they also have no clear directives as to special areas in which they should become competent. Lacking career plans which might give direction to their school work, they assume that anything taught them may be of value in practice.

The first condition for the development of student culture in the school, given these assumptions by students, is that the school presents students with a set of common problems. Though we discuss the problems related to particular student perspectives in more detail in later chapters, we can characterize them briefly as follows: Students all have the problem of what to study and learn from among the mass of facts they find in books, lectures, conferences, and clinical work. They all have the problem of how to deal with a faculty which examines and grades them and has the power to fail them and thus halt their progress toward the goal of practicing medicine. They all have the problem of dealing with their fellow students so as to prevent any one student from increasing the workload all must bear.

A second condition for the development of student culture is a pattern of extensive and intensive interaction among the students who share these problems. The school provides this by organizing most activities by groups and by occupying most of the student's time with school activities. The reader will have noted that the student in the clinical years, like the freshman, devotes most of his time to school. The student spends a minimum of five full days of most weeks in the hospital. These days ordinarily begin at eight in the morning (or earlier) and do not end until four-thirty or five in the afternoon. He spends Saturdays, from eight till one, in lectures and classes. Other activities oblige him to spend still more time on the premises. Various services require him to take occasional night call, which means that he does not leave the hospital for more than twenty-four hours. Many other services require him to return to the hospital to work-up patients assigned him at whatever time they are admitted to the hospital; this cuts into many of his evenings and nights. Of course, the student must find time in this crowded schedule for study and review. When we have accounted for the interaction of students with the medical staff, other students, and patients, we have exhausted the list of significant activities and contacts that students experience.

Besides these two major conditions for the development of student culture, certain other features of the school environment influence the nature of that culture. Student culture in the clinical years consists of a set of very general agreements on goals and means rather than specific agreements on how to deal with particular concrete problems, yet there is not much variation among students in the solutions they devise to their problems.

The lack of variation among student work groups in the character of student culture probably is related to the fact that certain patterns of enforced association characterize student interaction. Though, as we have seen, the student does not have much choice of his working associates during the preclinical years, what little choice he has is drastically reduced when he begins to spend all of his time in the teaching hospital. Students are assigned to the many different services in the hospital in small groups of from five to fifteen at the discretion of the school administration, and have no choice at all about who will be in their group. (It is, presumably, possible for a student who finds a group unbearable to request a change, but this is not an ordinary event. We witnessed no such request during our field work.) When the composition of these work groups changes, it is because of administrative necessity. Little or no attention is paid to the students' preferences. The consequence is that students do not work with close friends but must be prepared to work with whatever associates administrative routine assigns to them. The necessity of working with casual acquaintances suggests that students will operate, in their work activities, on the basis of those beliefs and norms which permeate the entire class rather than on the basis of ideas peculiar to a small group of intimates.

This does not mean that the small student groups assigned to various services do not vary widely, as the faculty often insists, in ability, knowledge, initiative, and other qualities. What it means is that when students work together the basic understandings in terms of which they develop their collective activity will be those common to all members of the class. Many kinds of collective activity can be developed on that basis, and very real differences can appear.

The fragmentation of the student group during the clinical years, brought about by several features of the organization of the curriculum, creates a condition in which it is likely that student culture will consist of very general agreements requiring specific adaptation to particular situations. The splintering of the entire class among many different clinical services, each with its distinctive demands, means that the students do not face the same problem at the same time. They all eventually face much the same problems by the time they complete their training, if we assume that the demands made by the services are relatively unchanging. But at any given moment each small group has a different set of clinical problems to study, a different set of medical superiors to deal with, and so on. This means that collective agreements among them cannot be as specific and detailed as they would be if the entire class faced the same problems at the same time. Each group of students finds itself examined by different people on different materials at different times, and no collective agreement on just how to deal with this specific problem is possible.

To the extent that the services remain stable and the problems they present to students do not vary, there can be some transfer of knowledge about how to deal with the problems they present. But residents and interns move from service to service in much the same way students do (though the cycle is longer for residents and in many cases shorter for interns) so that the situation on a given service may differ radically from time to time. It is not likely, in other words, that there will be much transfer of specific information on how to deal with the problems of a given service.

The collective agreements that make up student culture, we may therefore expect, will be quite general in character and require specific adaptation to the situations in which the small groups of working associates find themselves.

To summarize, the students' environment in the clinical years creates the conditions for the development of a student culture held by almost the entire class, without significant minority cultures, and quite general in character.

Chapter 12   The Responsibility and
Experience Perspectives

The Problem and its Setting

Students moving through the sequence of clinical courses we have just described continue to face the problem, familiar to them from their preclinical work, of how to organize and direct the effort they put into their schoolwork. They must still decide what is important and worth remembering, which activities should get the bulk of their attention, and what general criteria are most useful in answering these questions.

Some of their work in the clinical years continues to be essentially academic in character. They are still presented with bulky texts and fact-filled lectures and must decide which of the multitude of facts they might learn they should try to incorporate into what the faculty refers to as their "fund of information." Some of the faculty still give examinations designed to ascertain the extent of that fund. In general, the perspective developed on similar situations during the preclinical years — that one must learn what the faculty will ask about on examinations — persists in the clinical years, although it must be adapted to the different circumstances of clinical teaching. (We discuss the students' perspective on the academic portions of their clinical work in a later chapter.)

But much of the students' work now has quite a different character and is much nearer the work of the practicing physician they expect

221

to become. They now become, in essence, apprentices who learn not by studying material from books and lectures but by doing under the supervision of those who are already doctors the things they will later do as doctors. For instance, the major activity of students in the clinical years, clearly apprentice-like in this sense, is "working-up" the patients assigned to them in the clinic or on the hospital wards. The student goes through the same actions as do the intern, resident, and staff physician in working-up a patient.

Many other activities of the students are of this apprentice-like character. They perform, under supervision, a number of diagnostic and therapeutic procedures they will perform on their own as practicing physicians. They deliver babies and assist in surgery. They perform a variety of diagnostic procedures ranging from those as simple and routine as drawing blood to those more difficult such as spinal taps. They perform such therapeutic procedures as the surgical repair of simple lacerations.

The shift in emphasis of the students' work, from the academic exercises of study, lecture, and class discussion to the apprentice activities of working-up patients and performing medical procedures, is not complete, but it is enough of a change to bring back into play the long-range perspective students had entered with as freshmen but had given up because it was irrelevant in the exclusively academic setting of the freshman year. They can now look again on their schoolwork as training for medical practice, instead of a series of academic hurdles they must clear before they are allowed to practice.

The change in the students' point of view that follows from the shift in the character of their work does not solve their problem of deciding what to study and where to put their effort. If their work will now be training for future practice, the solutions to this problem developed in the freshman year and carried over into the sophomore year are not relevant. There is no sense in studying simply to pass examinations if examinations no longer have as great a potential effect on one's school career, especially if one feels the urgent need to prepare himself to practice medicine. But to say that one's training must be used to prepare for practice is not specific enough to give clear directives about how to proceed in school. Most students know little more about medical practice than they did as freshmen and thus have no way to select from the mass of their experiences as apprentices what is most worthwhile, what should be remembered, and what deserves to have most effort given it.

There are, of course, many possible answers to the question of where students should put their major effort in order to prepare themselves for future practice. The faculty, though they disagree in many ways about the aims of medical education, would probably agree that the student in the clinical years should devote himself to mastering the rudiments of scientific medicine and the basic skills involved in getting along with patients. That is, the student should use the opportunities his clinical training gives him to learn how to make good observations and use those observations to reason his way to the best possible diagnosis. In working-up patients, the student should view each patient as an exercise in diagnostic reasoning and devote his effort to mastering this basic mode of scientific medical thought. He should try to master the skills of dealing with patients so that he will be able to work with the patient as a whole human organism instead of a collection of disease entities. If the student held such a viewpoint, he would know what to work on and where to put his effort.

In fact, we find that students do not solve the problem of where to direct their effort in this way. Instead, making use of two ideas which we think must be strongly emphasized in medical culture and in the perspectives of practicing physicians, they create a collective perspective which tells them in what direction they should put forth effort. These two ideas are *medical responsibility* and *clinical experience*. In this and the next chapter, we argue that students faced with the problem of where to direct their effort discover, in the course of their work in the hospital, these two notions and construct out of them two of the perspectives which make up student culture in the clinical years. In this chapter, we elaborate the meaning of these two concepts and indicate that they are presented forcefully and persuasively to the students, both by the faculty themselves and by certain structural features of medical school and hospital organization. In other words, even though the faculty, in their more pedagogical moments, argue for another view of the proper direction of student effort, in their day-to-day operations they express the ideas of responsibility and experience very forcefully. In the next chapter, we describe the perspectives students develop by adapting the ideas of responsibility and experience to their own school situation and demonstrate that these perspectives are the students' customary way of dealing with the problem of where to direct their effort in the apprentice role.

Responsibility

The term "responsibility" is used in different ways in the hospital, depending on who is using it and in what situation; we will consider some of these variations later. First, we must see that basically the term refers to the archetypal feature of medical practice: the physician who holds his patient's fate in his hands and on whom the patient's life or death may depend. Medical responsibility is responsibility for the patient's well-being, and the exercise of medical responsibility is seen as the basic and key action of the practicing physician. The physician is most a physician when he exercises this responsibility.

We became aware of this particular idea of medical responsibility at the very beginning of our study, long before any specific hypotheses or questions had been formulated. Shortly after the first period of observation had begun, one of our observers was making rounds with a small group of students and a staff member; this was the basic teaching activity in the department being observed. While the staff member was quizzing a student about one of the patients in a ward room, another patient began vomiting blood and, while the students stood there, in a few minutes died of a perforated ulcer. The observer, being new to hospitals and looking at everything through the lens of a layman's conception, assumed that the students, whom he still knew only slightly, would respond with horror of some kind. He thought that the first sight of actual death (which this was for most of the students) would be profoundly upsetting and that the fact of death and how one learned to take it in stride would be the focus of the students' reaction to the event.

This was not the case, however. As soon as the death occurred, the students retreated down the hall and began to discuss it among themselves and with the observer, whose notes record the following conversation:

Jones said to Brown and myself, "Well, I don't know. I don't think that this needed to have happened." Brown said, "Well, what could you do?" Jones said, "We should have operated on him a lot earlier. It seems to me that they could have operated before this, that this didn't need to have happened at all." Brown said, "Well, I don't know. You know he was in shock before. Just came out of it."

(Junior Medicine. October, 1955.)

There was very little discussion of this case for the next few days, except with regard to technical questions: what had been found at autopsy, how big the ulcer had been, and so on. But the staff member and residents spoke to the students about the case several times, emphasizing their own responsibility for the death, even though it had been, in the circumstances, unavoidable. Here is one of the staff member's speeches:

You see, a case like this, you're damned if you do and damned if you don't. He came in here [to the hospital] bleeding badly yesterday afternoon, and we had to decide whether to transfuse him up and get his blood pressure and volume up to a point where it would be safe to operate or to go ahead and operate. So we decided that it was too much risk to operate right then, so we kept him overnight and transfused him up. That seemed like a reasonable decision at the time, but then it works out like this; you sure feel like a horse's ass. . . . I'm not trying to attach any blame to anyone, nor am I trying to say that it was anyone's fault; it's nobody's fault when anything like this happens. . . . It's easy enough to see after the fact what we should have done, and I think that you have to realize that it was a touchy situation either way. I think that if they had gone ahead and operated on him at eight, that they would not have gotten his stomach open and got to the blood vessels and clamped them off before this could have happened. I think he would have died on the table anyway. Of course, we don't know. It would have been risky either way we did it — and we took this way and lost, that's all.

In other words, the students' first reaction, reinforced by the interpretations presented by the staff, was to inquire into who was to blame. It is clear that even though the staff member insists that no one is to blame in such a situation, he has raised the question of blame and responsibility for the death in a very frank way; even had the students not been aware of this possible response to the event before his speech, they must necessarily have been after it. This incident sensitized the field workers to the existence of the idea of responsibility for the patient's well-being as an important theme in hospital culture.

In our further discussion of this matter, we will consider simultaneously three questions: 1. What are the ramifications of the idea of "responsibility"? 2. In what ways is this idea presented to the student by his teachers? and 3. In what ways does he see other participants in the life of the hospital make use of the idea?

Responsibility, in this special sense, is not characteristic of everything a doctor does but only of certain situations, although a kind of reasoning can be employed to extend the area of its applicability. Responsibility is seen in pure form in a situation like the one we have just described when a patient who has been placed in the doctor's hands dies because of something the doctor did or did not do. Less melodramatically, any physician who has a patient placed in his care is saddled with the responsibility of seeing to it that the patient gets well, or as much better as is possible; more important, he has the responsibility of seeing to it, if possible, that the patient does not get worse than he was before the doctor saw him.

Students, and others in the hospital, distinguish mistakes from those errors of judgment which arise from the incomplete state of the medical arts, but in either case see the doctor as bearing responsibility even though he is not "to blame" in the same way for an error of judgment as he is for a mistake. One student discussed this problem this way with the observer over a cup of coffee:

You know, the doctor really does have a terrific responsibility. He can make some pretty bad mistakes if he's not careful, and that's quite a responsibility to carry around — the fact that you could make a mistake and cost someone their life. Now everything isn't a mistake. In other words, few real mistakes are made. There is a difference between a mistake and an error of judgment or an error of opinion: something where what you did was reasonable, but it turned out not to be right later because of things you had no way of knowing about. Maybe things that wouldn't show up until an actual autopsy was done; but that's not a mistake.

(Junior Pediatrics. October, 1955.)

A doctor can only exercise responsibility in a situation in which his action or failure to act can produce some change in the condition of the patient. The patient should be in "danger" of some kind, even though this be quite remote. It is by showing that the ultimate consequences of some action are "dangerous" that the area of medical responsibility is extended to cover relatively routine occurrences. Where the doctor, by his actions, can fail to reduce the danger or can even increase it, he is in a position to exercise medical responsibility. The situations in which responsibility can be so exercised range from the obvious ones of the medical emergency — where the victim of an accident or heart attack will die without proper medical care — to routine physical examinations in which, it is argued to the students, the failure to perform a thorough examination may jeopardize a patient's life by leaving undiscovered a potentially remediable condition.

The student's experience in the hospital teaches him that medical responsibility is an important characteristic of the full-fledged physician in two ways: through his observation of hospital organization and through repeated mention in formal teaching and in the informal conversations he takes part in or overhears about cases coming to his attention. We expect students to take cognizance of this theme and incorporate it into their own perspectives because it is ubiquitous and because it comes to their attention in particularly forceful ways, the incident quoted earlier being a dramatic example. We heard the faculty or house staff express the idea of responsibility in every one of the services in which students worked during their clinical years. Furthermore, such expressions appear in our field notes at all stages of the research, both before and after the idea was formulated by us.

One of the first recurring phenomena we saw as a use of the idea of responsibility was a phrase we heard staff members use in both their formal and informal teaching: "Getting into trouble [with a patient]." This phrase referred to the situation in which a patient got worse while under a physician's care; the physician was "getting into trouble" when his patient showed signs of getting worse. Clearly, the connotations of this phrase depicted a situation in which the patient's welfare depended on the physician's actions. Our field notes do not contain many full-length examples of this, because the observers quickly took to characterizing a staff member's discussion as using the "getting-into-trouble gambit." The following example comes from a lecture by a staff member to a small group of seniors:

The thing is that you can really get yourself into an awful lot of trouble with a patient like this. Every once in a while one of them will turn up with a blood sugar of two hundred or so instead of twelve hundred or eight hundred, which is what you would expect. You give this guy too much insulin and he goes into hypoglycemia. Then you are really in trouble because there isn't any combination of things that is more difficult to treat than diabetic acidosis and hypoglycemia. You're really in a bad way then. Diabetics who die in coma nowdays die because they were given too much insulin and became hypoglycemic. In other words, it's the doctor's fault that they get into trouble now, so you give that glucose at the beginning just to cover yourself when you give the insulin. At least until you begin to get blood sugars on them.

(Senior Medicine. February, 1956.)

Another typical teaching device we identified as a use of the idea of responsibility was what we quickly labeled the "emergency room" or "the patient comes into your office with . . . What are you going to do?" gambit. We heard this in classes taught by the discussion method and in many casual and informal teaching situations. Here the staff member presents a hypothetical medical emergency to one or more of the students and teaches him how to handle it by correcting the wrong answers he gives. The heavy emphasis on the supposition that the patient's life hangs on the correctness of the student's decisions led us to see such teaching sessions as these, in which a staff member quizzes a group of five students whom the observer was following through their school day, as presentations of the responsibility theme:

The staffman kept giving hypothetical examples of patients, in order to start off a discussion. For example, he would say, "All right, Green. Here comes old Brown into your office and he has the following signs," and he would name off a list of symptoms and signs and then say, "All right — now what are you going to do for old Brown? Is he going to die if you don't do something pretty quick? Sure he is. Now what are you going to do?" Or he would say, "Here comes old Brown in the emergency room. He'd just gone out for a swim in his big fancy swimming pool but he forgot that the pool had been drained that day and he landed on his head, and now they've brought him in the ambulance to the emergency room. This is what he looks like — " and he would give a list of signs and symptoms. "Now what are you going to do for him?"

The student he asked the question of would start to answer and if he suggested something wrong the staff member would say, "Come on now. Old Brown is lying there bleeding to death or something. We'd better find out what it is, don't you think? After all, there he is — he's your patient. He's going to die if you don't do something pretty quick, isn't he? But he doesn't have to die. You can save his life if you want to, if you know how to. Now what are you going to do? Come on now, quick, you have to make these decisions quickly when they come in that way."

(Neurosurgery. September, 1956.)

We saw, too, that the many incidents we observed in which students were told about cases where a doctor's mistake had led to a patient getting sicker or a mistake could be made causing a patient's condition to deteriorate were also reiterations of the idea that the doctor held the ultimate responsibility for the patient's welfare. Here are two typical incidents in which students had the importance of responsibility so impressed on them:

An internist discussed a case with a group of fifteen seniors. The patient was described by a student as having undergone exploratory surgery for a liver obstruction, but none was found; after surgery he developed a small gastric ulcer, probably as a result of having a suction tube in his stomach for a long period, and died when it hemorrhaged. The internist said, "From the evidence we have it looks like he was already on the road to getting well when they operated. His death was obviously a result of them putting a suction tube into his stomach and keeping it there too long. I think it is safe to say that he probably would have recovered successfully if he had not gone to surgery. I really think he did not need to die at all—it was one of those things that happen. If the surgeons had let him alone he would have been all right."

(Senior Medicine. March, 1956.)

A urologist lectured to the entire sophomore class on the subject of catheterization. He told a story about a boy who had come to the hospital for an emergency appendectomy which had gone off perfectly well. The boy was having trouble urinating so they put a catheter into him. The next day his temperature was 99.8. The following day it was 102 and the day after 104. The boy was dead within two weeks. The urologist said the death was not a result of the appendectomy at all, but because the catheterization had not been done in a sterile fashion and bacteria had been introduced. A kidney infection had started and the boy had died in uremia. He said that while catheterization was a very useful procedure, it had to be done in a very aseptic manner to avoid things like that.

(Sophomore Physical Diagnosis. April, 1956.)

In each of these instances, the students learn that a doctor's action can be mistaken and cause great damage, even death. They learn also that relatively minor procedures such as catheterization can produce grave consequences, so that responsibility is not confined to such dramatic situations as the operating or emergency rooms.

This idea of responsibility is presented to the students even by staff members who feel that the whole matter is overemphasized. Thus, one staff member told the students to avoid overwork when they started practice: "Pretty soon you really get unbalanced and begin to think that you are really saving lives or killing people, which is a lot of nonsense, as we all know." Nevertheless, the same staff member had been observed to use the "emergency room" gambit on a number of occasions.

The idea of responsibility, finally, is seen by the student as it is embodied in the hierarchical organization of the hospital. The performance of therapeutic and diagnostic procedures is generally seen as involving some measure of medical responsibility, since an error may have untoward consequences for the patient.

A staff member took five students and the observer with him into a small treatment room in the clinic so that they could watch him sigmoido-scope a patient. [In this procedure a long tube is inserted through the anus into the lower bowel so that the physician can view the bowel di-rectly.] As he demonstrated the procedure to us he said, "You noticed that I was being extremely cautious in the way I inserted the sigmoidoscope. It is very easy in a bowel which is diseased as hers is to go right through the bowel wall with your sigmoidoscope and that is a tough thing to try to repair because it is diseased to begin with and it doesn't heal well. This is a thing which happens quite frequently and is very bad. I know of at least one case of it happening in every hospital I have been associated with."

(Junior Surgery. January, 1956.)

All kinds of procedures, from routine drawing of blood to complicated and dangerous procedures like sigmoidoscopy, are parceled out dif-ferentially to persons of different rank in the medical school hierarchy. Students are allowed to do progressively more each year, interns still more, and residents still more with each year of their training. The very organization of the hospital thus presents students with an im-portant illustration of the idea of responsibility by showing them how it is associated with rank in the organization.

This array of examples indicates the range of materials which led us to conclude that the idea of responsibility was frequently pre-sented to the medical student during his years of clinical training. The same examples show that this idea was presented to the student in such a way as to capture his attention and make a deep impression. First, there is almost always a reference to the possible death of a pa-tient at a physician's hands; since this is an experience the students can easily envision themselves having when they become physicians, and since death is such an ultimate fact, such a presentation will be forceful. Second, the idea is frequently presented by asking the stu-dent to project himself into a situation in which he will actually be exercising responsibility (as in the "emergency room" gambit), which must strengthen the impression. Finally, the idea is frequently pre-sented to the student in situations in which he is highly involved emotionally, situations in which he is being put on the spot for an im-mediate answer to a staff member's question and is thus liable to the twin sanctions of failing an informal examination and embarrassing himself before a small group of fellow students if he fails to answer correctly.

Experience

A second major idea expressed in the organization of medical practice in the hospital, and one closely related to responsibility, is "experience." This term refers to clinical experience, to actual experience in dealing with patients and disease, and a major part of its meaning lies in its implied polarity with "book learning." Clinical experience, in the view implied by this term, gives the doctor the knowledge he needs to treat patients successfully, even though that knowledge has not yet been systematized and scientifically verified. One does not acquire this knowledge through academic study but by seeing clinical phenomena and dealing with clinical problems at first hand. Clinical experience, even though it substitutes for scientifically verified knowledge, can be used to legitimate a choice of procedures for a patient's treatment and can even be used to rule out use of some procedures which have been scientifically established.

The reason clinical experience is viewed as necessary is that "book knowledge" may be deficient in a number of ways. It may simply be wrong when tested against the staff member's knowledge, gleaned from his own handling of patients. Or the book knowledge may not be available, the necessary research not having been done for important kinds of diseases for which the physician feels he must do something, with or without scientific basis. It may be an insufficient basis for learning important and necessary things; for instance, students would find it difficult to learn to recognize heart murmurs from "the book" alone, for this is one of the many things that may be learned only by use of the senses. Finally, "the book" may not take into account the practical facts of life, as when laboratory tests which are in principle useful, are discounted because of practical difficulties in their administration and interpretation. Because of all these things, it is believed that a person must learn much of what he needs to know by actual clinical experience. Whether this is true or not, it is probably an important perspective in medical practice.

The idea of experience, like that of responsibility, is presented frequently to the medical students and in ways that are likely to so impress them that they will incorporate it into their own perspectives. The students are told, at the beginning of their clinical training and often thereafter, that clinical experience is absolutely necessary for performing a physical examination and interpreting its results properly. They are told that they cannot learn to hear the things they are listening for in a chest or heart, feel the things they are supposed to feel when palpating an abdomen, or see the things they are supposed to in observing a patient without having done these things many times. Since the students have great difficulty in hearing, feeling, and seeing what they are told is there, they are happy to accept this explanation.

An internist was lecturing to a group of about twenty-five sophomores, including the group the observer was participating with, on how to examine the female genitalia. He said, "Now I know that the OB-GYN men can feel all kinds of things in the uterus. Myself, I couldn't even feel a uterus at all until I had done about five hundred [sic] examinations, so it does take you quite awhile to get the hang of how to do that."

(Sophomore Physical Diagnosis. April, 1956.)

As the students move to the hospital wards for their clinical clerkships, staff members tell them about treatments that have proved efficacious in their experience, even though no one understands their scientific basis. It is not that the faculty recommends that treatment be carried on in this way, but rather that they recognize many areas of medicine and many particular medical problems for which there is not as yet sufficient evidence for treatments to be "scientifically" chosen.

A staff member discussed a case of his with a small class. After presenting the case he had them ask questions. A number of his answers were along these lines: "What I do in such-and-such a case is so-and-so. Don't ask me why it works or why I do it, because I'm not real sure. I just know that it does work and I have a feeling that it ought to."

(Senior Medicine. February, 1956.)

We first became aware of the impact of the idea of clinical experience on students by observing its rhetorical use in discussions they had with staff members. A student who is asked a question in class answers it with a fact gleaned from a text or journal article, only to be told, in one way or another, that the staff member has never seen this occur in his own experience.

The group of five juniors I was spending my time with joined two other groups for an informal lecture-discussion by a staff member. He described a particular set of symptoms and then put his hand on John's shoulder and said, "All right, John, tell us what kinds of things might produce this." John said, "Well, let's see — I think appendicitis could do it." The staff member said, "You think appendicitis, huh?" John said, "Yes, sir." The staff member said, "Have you ever seen that happen?" John said, "No, sir." The staff member said, "Well, neither have I. What else do you think might produce it?" This got a big laugh from the other students. John said, "Well, I don't know, sir. I just know that in the book it mentioned that this was one of the things." The staff member smiled and said, "By faith alone ye shall not be saved." This got an even bigger laugh. What he meant was that it was no good to take what the book said at face value — you'd better have seen it yourself.

(Junior Surgery. January, 1956.)

The fact the student offers is worthless because in all the staff member's experience in dealing with this problem it has not occurred, no matter what the book says.

Occasionally staff members underline the importance of clinical experience in this way by allowing the students to make some mistake they have made themselves and then correcting it from their own experience.

One of the residents gave us (a dozen seniors and the observer) a lecture this morning on reading electrocardiograms (EKGs). He showed us a series of EKGs taken on a man who had come into the hospital around eight-thirty one morning, a month after Eisenhower's heart attack, complaining of vague funny feelings in his stomach. The resident said he would have sent the patient home because his first EKG showed nothing. He asked what we thought should be done with such a patient, and one of the students said, "I would just reassure him and send him home." The resident passed the first normal EKG around for us to inspect. He said that the patient seemed very nervous and upset, so after an hour he decided to have another EKG taken, figuring that two normal ones would convince the patient that he was all right. While the second EKG was being taken, the patient began to have the pain again. The resident said that the EKG girl was smart enough not to stop the machine so that the last two strips on the page showed the patient actually in the process of having an infarct. They took several more EKGs at frequent intervals so that they ended up with a series showing the progressive changes in the waves during and following a heart attack. The resident passed the rest of the strips around for us to see and said, "I don't think you ought to feel bad about your deduction because it is exactly what I would have done. I would have just figured he was upset and was the nervous type, that the publicity about Eisenhower's attack had given him something to hang it on. I can tell you that from now on I will be a lot more careful about that kind of thing. I think that is the way we really learn things in medicine, by having them happen to us, so that we know them from our own experience."

(Senior Medicine. February, 1956.)

Incidents of this kind brought us to see that the argument from experience was quite commonly used and considered unanswerable. It is in the nature of the case that it should be unanswerable, because no one can tell better than the person making the argument what his experience has been; he may be reporting his experience incorrectly or drawing incorrect inferences from it, but the person to whom he makes the argument has no way of proving it. Uttering the magic phrase, "In my experience . . ." signals the settling of many disagreements, for the only counterargument that can prevail is for the same phrase to be spoken by someone who can claim greater experience in the area discussed (having been in practice in that area for more years or having seen more cases of the type under discussion). Students had the experience of having their own disagreements with staff settled in this way and could observe faculty members ending discussions with one another summarily in the same way, as in the following case:

One student described his experience in an oral exam to the observer and a group of students waiting in a hallway for their turn to be examined. "Jones asked me questions. Brown tried to get in on the act and goof me up, but everytime he did Jones would interrupt and say something like, 'Well, Tom, in my experience it hasn't been quite that way.' And when he said that, that pretty well shut Brown up. He hasn't got much to say when it comes up against Jones and his experience."

(Senior Obstetrics. May, 1956.)

Clearly, students who had experiences such as these might well be disposed to look on the idea of experience with some respect.

Finally, we became aware, as the students do, of the obvious connection between the hierarchical organization of the hospital and the idea of experience. Experience underlies that organization, not necessarily in the sense that all gradations in rank are accompanied by differing amounts of experience, but in the sense that the major divisions — between students, interns, residents, and junior and senior staff — are legitimated with reference to the increasing clinical experience of occupants of each higher position on the ladder. The student is particularly impressed with this when, as in some of the instances above, he is subordinated and "put in his place" by references to experience.

We do not have systematic evidence on the distribution of expressions of the idea of experience in the hospital, largely because we arrived at this conceptualization early and did not bother to collect much information on it thereafter. Instead, we spent our time looking for the consequences of the idea for the student. Much of what we have to say later on these points can be thought of as substantiating the preliminary point under discussion here. In short, it seemed such an obvious point that we soon began to take it for granted and base further analyses on it. Here is how one observer disposed of the point after less than two months of field work:

One of the things that impressed me this morning during this conference [a conference in which the medical staff discussed recent cases while the students listened and occasionally asked questions] — I don't know if I have mentioned this previously or not — was the constant reiteration of this theme: "I have seen many cases where so-and-so followed such-and-such" or "I have never seen so-and-so followed by such-and-such." All of the staff members use this device of referring to their past experience and what they have and have not seen, how many cases they have seen just like this, or how many variations on this kind of thing they have seen. This is a lovely subordinating device in relation to the students and the house staff. For example, a student may ask a question which at least on the surface sounds perfectly reasonable and be answered, "I have never seen anything like that in my experience. Perhaps there is such a thing, but I have never seen it." Any older man could say this to any younger man and pretty well get away with it. Logic or reason really don't enter into it; it's just a matter of experience and naturally the older men have had a lot more of that.

(November, 1955.)

Later field notes contain occasional examples of the idea of experience, cropping up in the more or less pure forms quoted above. So, although we cannot say that we have instances of it from every department, the combination of occasional instances, elaborations of the idea in connection with other problems we shall discuss, and the obvious impression it made on the observers, is sufficient to demonstrate the presence of the idea of clinical experience in the teaching hospital, an idea which might be expected to affect students working there.

We have now presented the data that led us to conclude that students, when faced with the problem of how to direct their effort in the apprenticeship situation, would find at hand the raw materials from which to construct a perspective on this problem in the forcefully and persuasively presented ideas of medical responsibility and clinical experience. So far, we have simply argued that students might well make use of these ideas, even though the faculty might prefer them to organize their effort differently.

The proposition that the ideas of responsibility and experience are presented forcefully to the students would be weakened if our data contained negative instances. However, as these propositions are stated, it is difficult to say what constitutes a negative instance. If a staff member were to argue, or state implicitly, that the idea of responsibility should not be taken seriously by a doctor, this might be considered a negative case; we have such data for both themes. But, as in the instance cited previously of the staff member who argued that doctors do not really save lives or kill people, the people who argue this way are also observed to argue in the opposite way. Furthermore, even if it should be shown that some faculty really did not see these two ideas as important, this would not weaken the argument that these ideas are acted on in the daily life of the medical school and that the students see them frequently in a way likely to make an impression on them. To weaken confidence in the proposition, one would have to show that these ideas were seldom or never expressed for the students to observe and that the hospital organization showed no signs of being influenced by them. On this latter point, one could argue from the differential distribution of responsibility and experience in the hospital hierarchy alone that these ideas were present and capable of influencing the students. Most important, perhaps, is the argument to be made in the next chapter: that these ideas had discernible consequences in other aspects of medical school life.

Another aspect of the data presented supports the point that the ideas of responsibility and experience were forcefully presented to students. The examples cited above all show these ideas being expressed by faculty members in public situations, with the clear implication that these sentiments are legitimate to express in this public way. Were these ideas not considered legitimate by the staff, we might expect them to be communicated more secretively so that the person expressing them would not have to take the responsibility for his words; or we could expect that the ideas could not be brought forward so publicly as major values without having someone argue either that these concepts are not important at all or that they are not as important as the speakers in our examples seem to think them. In fact, no instance in which a speaker felt it necessary to communicate the ideas of responsibility or experience in a secretive way was observed. Nor did we ever observe a speaker challenged when he communicated these ideas. We deduce from this that these themes are legitimate and publicly acceptable and, therefore, likely, because of their legitimacy, to make a strong impression on the medical students.

The value of responsibility, which we have described as one that figures strongly in student perspectives, has an interest for sociologists beyond its role in medical practice and medical education. It turns our attention to a morally complicated class of values which perhaps deserves further attention.

Medical responsibility, like other values, is something that those who believe the value to be important attempt to maximize. Values can be classified according to the way one individual's maximization affects the maximization of others. One classic extreme is the zero-sum game, beloved of game theorists, in which what one wins the other necessarily loses. A poker game provides a familiar example. Each player brings so much to the game and can win only if others lose. All players cannot maximize the value around which the game is organized; my maximization affects yours adversely and necessarily so.

Other values must be maximized jointly. That is, all the participants in the enterprise can gain together. What one wins, all win. Indeed, if anyone is to win, all must win. An example might be cars maneuvering in a dangerous and uncontrolled intersection. Four cars approaching the intersection, wishing to maximize their own safety, must all achieve this jointly; otherwise, all will suffer.

Still other values can be maximized with no effect on others' efforts at maximization. Medical responsibility is a value of this kind in situations of medical practice (although it is not so in the medical school, where the intern's gain may be the student's loss). A medical practitioner, by exercising medical responsibility, costs no one else anything. Medical responsibility, however, is one of a subclass of such values which can only be maximized in certain kinds of situations, namely, in those situations where someone else has trouble. The patient's illness provides the occasion for the doctor's moment of glory.

Thus, medical responsibility, while for most people a good thing, is for the person in whose behalf it is exercised a bad thing in the sense that it could not be exercised at all if it were not for his own troubles. The doctor can be most fully a doctor only when others have trouble. Perhaps this ambiguity in the moral aura of the value has something to do with the public's ambivalence toward doctors.

Chapter 13

The Assimilation of Medical Values by Students

The Responsibility and Experience Perspectives

Sᴛᴜᴅᴇɴᴛs faced with the problems of apprenticeship described in the last chapter ask themselves, "What should I do, in this setting, to prepare myself for medical practice?" The answer to this question will solve the problem of where to put their energy and attention. But the question has many possible answers. Students might, for instance, decide that schoolwork which provides them with a maximum of verified scientific knowledge would be most valuable for future practice. They might decide that they can best prepare for a medical career by assimilating some over-all point of view within which they would find the answers to problems they might face with particular patients. Thus, they might decide that a basic understanding of physiology would serve them in this way. They might even decide that what their work in the clinical years should do is give them a good "bedside manner."

The students we studied made none of these decisions. Instead, they took the hints furnished by the faculty and the organization of the school and developed perspectives on the problem of where to put their effort in their apprentice-like activities around the concepts of clinical experience and medical responsibility. Although they used these concepts from medical culture, they neither used them as practicing physicians do nor did they mean the same things by them. They adapted the core meanings to apply to their immediate situation as students. The student perspectives built around the concepts of responsibility and experience are thus influenced by medical culture but take their shape from the pressures of the situation in which students find themselves.

When students developed and used the responsibility and experience perspectives, they were presented with further problems because their apprenticeship was served in an organization embodying these ideas. We describe these further problems presented by the environment before going on to a discussion of the responsibility and experience perspectives, because the perspectives themselves contain reference to these features of the environment.

The medical personnel in the teaching hospital is organized into a hierarchy requiring different amounts of experience and responsibility of those occupying the several ranks. The student occupies the lowest rank in this hierarchy. He has had little experience and has not exercised medical responsibility in any form when he enters his clinical training. Nor can he legally exercise medical responsibility except insofar as it is delegated to him and carried out under the supervision of a licensed physician. He may examine a patient and make a diagnosis, but a licensed physician must take the final responsibility for accepting it or requiring further checks by those higher up in the hierarchy. He cannot independently undertake any apprentice activities but must wait for staff permission to do so.

Furthermore, the staff have a great deal of leeway in how much apprentice activity they allow a student to engage in. These activities can be roughly classified as more or less difficult and as involving more or less danger to the patient. Students, obviously, are not allowed to perform more difficult and dangerous procedures until their superiors feel sure that they have mastered simpler ones. A student who appears to learn quickly and perform well is allowed to do more and more things while a student who does not do simple tasks well tends not to be allowed to go any further until he has given evidence of improvement. There is no orderly progression of tasks through which all students go, as is the case in the academic studies students engage in. How much of what the organization says is important a student gets depends a great deal on how much the staff allow him to get. A student is given only what the faculty think him capable of handling and thus his education depends on their judgment of him.

The organization of the hospital is such that students may also be denied opportunities to exercise responsibility because they are low men in the hierarchy. As a medical training center, the school trains not only students but also interns and residents in the various specialties. This creates what is in some respects an economic problem. Responsibility can only be exercised on patients. Further, responsibility is indivisible and can only be exercised by one person on any one patient in a given situation. Responsibility may be delegated to another, but only one person can actually exercise it. This means that opportunities to exercise responsibility are strictly limited by the number of patients in situations of danger or potential danger. The supply of this commodity never equals the demand. If, for example, we consider the minor responsibility of closing a surgical incision, it is obvious that there are only as many opportunities to do this as there are patients on whom an incision has been made and, further, that each incision can only be closed once. The supply of incisions does not meet the demand of the many people who would like to have experience in closing them. The students' demand is the last to be satisfied, for the residents and interns who make up such a sizable segment of the population of the teaching hospital have prior call on this material, by virtue of their superior training and experience.

Since the student, by definition, is the lowest man in this system and has the least of those things which are the equipment of the practicing physician, he is also by definition unable to tell what kinds of training he should be getting. As the system is organized, he has no legitimate grounds for expressing discontent with his situation, since that situation is defined by men more experienced and more capable of exercising responsibility than he. If a resident tells a student that this baby will be too difficult for him to deliver and the resident will have to do it, the student has no acceptable grounds for disagreement available to him. This stands in marked contrast to his position as academic student, where he is defined as an independent thinking being to whom propositions must be demonstrated logically and empirically before he need accept them.

These characteristics of the student's apprenticeship give greater specificity to the problem of what he should study in order to prepare himself for practice. The organization in which he plays his apprentice role suggests that he seek opportunities to get clinical experience and exercise medical responsibility. But that same organization may make it difficult for him to get those opportunities. Since the students organize their perspectives on apprenticeship around these ideas, they automatically face the problem of how to handle these difficulties. In short, adopting a perspective solves some problems, but creates others.

We now consider the perspectives students developed on the problem of how to direct their effort in the apprentice-like situations of the clinical years, elaborating the character of the responsibility and experience perspectives and then demonstrating that these perspectives were used widely and frequently and that they were held by the students collectively.

The Clinical Experience
Perspective

One of the answers students develop to the question, "How can I best make use of my apprentice training to prepare for medical practice?" is contained in a perspective built around the concept of clinical experience and summarized in the following statements:

    1. It is important for a doctor to have had clinical experience.

    2. School activities are good insofar as they give students the opportunity to acquire clinical experience or give them access to the clinical experience of their teachers; they are bad when they furnish neither of these things.

    3. A student is making real progress toward his goal of preparing for practice when he can demonstrate to himself and others that he has absorbed some lessons from clinical experience; conversely, he has cause to be worried over his own abilities when he fails to absorb such lessons.

We conclude, from an examination of our data, that students hold this perspective and organize their behavior in ways that are congruent with it.

We formed the hypothesis that students held this perspective early in the field work, when an occurrence involving one of the students in the small group we were observing in third-year medicine suggested it. The observer was accompanying the students on regular morning rounds, during which students presented their findings on patients they had worked up:

The next patient was Green's. This was an old man, who had come in with some kind of skin irritation. Green was asked to present the case. He read the history, when the disease had come on, etc. He mentioned, in the same businesslike tone, that in the course of his examination the man had begun to cough and wheeze. Actually, this was not during the course of the examination, he never got to that; this was during the taking of the history. The man had begun to cough and wheeze and seemed to get worse and worse. So Green pulled out his stethoscope, listened to the patient's chest, and could hear that he had gone into pulmonary edema. (I found out later that this is a condition where there is some kind of heart failure, blood plasma is taken into the lungs through the walls of the blood vessels, and you either choke to death or die of heart failure in fifteen or twenty minutes if something isn't done immediately.) Green said he had heard the characteristic sounds, recognized them, and called the intern, and that the two of them had then administered the proper drugs. While he was telling this story, the staff member turned to the resident and said something about "Lucky Pierre!" In fact, there was a good deal of envious eying of Green by the other students, and the staff member and resident both looked at him as though he had had some kind of really great experience.

Later in the day the observer asked Green, "What was all of this talk about you being so lucky about this man that had pulmonary edema?" He said, "Well, I was very, very lucky. We had just had a lecture on pulmonary edema a few days before and had all of the signs pointed out to us and everything. I was in there taking his history, and he started this coughing, and I put my stethoscope up to his chest, and I could hear it very clearly, just the way it had been described, and you could just hear the fluid rising in his lungs. . . . I was very lucky to see it from the beginning that way and actually hear it happen while I was there. I could just hear it gurgling in his lungs, so it was a very lucky thing to have seen that so clearly. Most fellows probably won't get a chance to. Usually it happens before the doctor is called, and you just see the end product, but you don't see how it actually happened."

At lunch, two of the students asked Green about this episode, and he told the whole story all over again. They seemed impressed by how lucky he had been to see this. References to this episode kept occurring during the next few days.

(Junior Medicine. September, 1955.)

This incident clearly indicated that students valued events that gave them something beyond the systematized knowledge they got in lectures and suggested that they might judge school activities on the basis of whether or not they furnished that something extra.

Several casual comments by students suggested that this might be a commonly applied criterion, representing a perspective of the students worth further investigation. A few days after the above incident, the observer noted:

Another thing is the kind of pressure that is on the students while they're on the medical ward. I think the basic pressure on them is to get experience, as much and as varied experience as they can, to see as many different things as they can.

We began to search for evidence to substantiate this proposition and for evidence that would require its revision and refinement. From this time forward, we made it a point to record information bearing on the topic.

Many kinds of observations can be seen as expressions of the clinical experience perspective by students. We now discuss the variety of student statements and activities we so interpret. Our discussion, to reiterate a point made earlier, serves two purposes. First, it gives detail and body to the bare statement of the perspective given and allows the reader to see how students express it in concrete situations. Second, it specifies the characteristics of the items of observation later used as evidence that students actually use this perspective in their daily activities. In the tabulations that follow this discussion, every item that is counted as evidence for the customary character of the perspective has one or more of the features we now describe.

Students expressed the clinical experience perspective most obviously when they made direct statements that the degree to which school activities furnished them with such experience was an important criterion of the worth of those activities. The following conversation between two students is typical of several such direct statements found in our field notes:

Bell said, "The advantage to this is that you get to see all of these different diseases and see what they really look like, and that's something that you won't see or get from a textbook. If you get a good look at what the thing looks like close-up, why you won't forget it." Compson said, "That's right. I had a kid in here not so long ago that had Hand-Schüller-Christian's disease. She had a bulging eyeball, a little lump on the side of her face, and all the other signs. Some local doctor had sent her in, and he didn't know what it was. I sure as hell didn't know what it was when I saw it, but Dr. Maxwell caught it. Well, I saw her case close-up, and I don't think I'll ever forget it. . . . I'll sure as hell recognize it if I ever see it again."

(Junior Pediatrics. October, 1955.)

Similarly, we often heard students pass judgment on lectures, conferences, and teachers on the basis of how much knowledge they furnished that was the fruit of clinical experience:

A staff member gave a lecture on the treatment of diabetic coma. It was intensely practical, filled with detailed instructions on just what to do, what kinds of signs to watch for, how to handle all kinds of contingencies that might arise, etc. The lecturer occasionally referred to cases he had treated in which various of these possibilities had occurred. After the lecture, one of the students said to me, "You see what I mean, Howie? His lectures are really good." I said, "Yeah, I was thinking while he was talking that this was just the kind of thing that will be awfully useful to you when you intern. You'll probably have people come in just that way, and it must be nice to have it all laid out, what to do." He said, "You're damn right it is. His lectures are really very practical. Almost all of them are. About 90 per cent of the time they're like that. Every once in awhile he gets real abstract and goes off into something that is pretty interesting to him, I guess, but as far as I'm concerned it's just way up in the wild blue yonder and just doesn't make a hell of a lot of sense. So when he gives us one like that it's really invaluable."

Several other guys commented on how good the lecture was — they all seemed to feel that this would stand them in good stead on their internship and afterward. Barnes said, "I'm sure glad I heard that. I sort of knew about diabetes, but I never really had it laid out for me, just what you would do if a person came in in coma that way. I'm sure glad I heard that — I know just what to do now."

(Senior Medicine. March, 1956.)

Not all instances of judgments based on the clinical experience criterion are so explicit. Frequently students simply speak approvingly or otherwise of a department, teacher, or particular teaching activity on the ground that these did or did not provide "information" or "pearls." These are both shorthand terms for the kind of material the lecturer in the preceding example was praised for providing — "information" is the generic term, "pearls" are particularly valuable single pieces of information.

The group of seniors I was with met another group of seniors in the clinic. This second group asked my boys how they like neurosurgery. There were no staff members or residents around. John said, "It's a very good service. Boy, they really dish out the poop [information]. . . . " The other fellow said, "Do you scrub in on operations?" Bill said, "No — we don't. . . . We mostly get stuff on diagnosis and things like that from them."

(Senior Neurosurgery. September, 1956.)

While I was sitting with the students in the big clinic office during both morning and afternoon clinics, on several occasions when one of the residents walked in one of the students would say, "How about giving us a pearl or two today?" The resident might or might not grin at this, but they never gave forth with any pearls. Crane complained to me about this. He said, "You see how these guys are? They'll never just sit around and tell you a few things out of the goodness of their heart. They could, you know. I'm really serious. After all, that's the way you pick up an awful lot of practical information—from guys like this who are a little bit ahead of you. . . . The residents we had last year would sit down and talk with you and explain things—little things they have picked up and so on. . . . These guys won't tell you a thing."

(Senior Obstetrics. May, 1956.)

Students also express the clinical experience perspective when they say that given activities are good or bad because they do or do not make it possible to see things that add to one's own clinical experience. For instance, students frequently complain about their time in surgery for these reasons:

I spent the morning with Phelps, a third-year student who was acting as third assistant on a gall bladder operation. A resident and intern served as first and second assistants. Several times during the morning Phelps said to me, "This is a hell of a way to waste the morning, if you ask me. I don't know what good it does me standing around here. I'm not learning anything. I can't see anything." Phelps is quite short and consequently can't see over anyone, even when he's standing on one of the little platforms they have around. I went and stood for awhile behind the resident and looked over his shoulder and found that, even with my height, I couldn't see anything either. All I could see was a deep opening in the patient's abdomen, but they were working far down in the opening. I said something about this to Phelps, and he said, "Yeah, a gall bladder operation is a very deep operation, and unless you're standing right over the opening you can't see a damn thing." [Since the student is almost always third assistant, and the operating surgeon and first assistant monopolize the space directly over the incision, students seldom get a good continuous view of the operative site, even though the surgeon will sometimes halt proceedings long enough for the student to have brief look.]

(Junior Surgery. January, 1956.)

In the same way, students judge a service by the kind of patients it provides for them to see. Although we will take up the question of student preferences among patients in detail in a later chapter, we can point out here that students want a service to give them experience by showing them patients with diseases whose pathological signs they can observe for themselves and by furnishing them with a variety of such pathology to observe. They praise a service that fills these specifications and complain about one that does not. In the first incident below, students tease a colleague over whether or not he has had a properly well-rounded selection of patients; in the second, a student complains that patients on one of the specialty services are too much alike for him to acquire much new clinical experience.

Michaels was set to scrub in on an anal operation, and the other students were kidding him about it. Pike said, "You're practically an expert on anal surgery and thyroidectomies, aren't you?" [That is, most of his patients had been one or the other of these categories.] Michaels said, "Well, I've seen two or three of each, but I've had some other stuff, too. A gall bladder . . ." and he named off two or three other things. "Really, it's been a pretty well-rounded selection."

(Junior Surgery. January, 1956.)

A large proportion of the patients seen in urology clinic suffer from prostate trouble of one kind or another. One of the students, looking over the chart of a patient who had been referred from medicine clinic, saw that a tentative diagnosis of benign prostatic hypertrophy had been made. When he saw this he said to me, "Another one. Boy, they're all alike up here. We see plenty of pathology all right, but it's all the same damn thing over and over again."

(Senior Urology. October, 1956.)

We also interpret as an expression of the clinical experience perspective those activities which imply a great interest in accumulating the fruits of clinical experience as these are provided by the staff. For instance, we observed certain groups of students listening to lectures by a great many different staff members; some lectures were filled with material widely regarded as containing the "practical" wisdom these men had developed out of their clinical experience; others contained little or none. We interpreted instances where the students could be seen taking elaborate notes on the "practical" lectures or few, if any, notes on the "impractical" ones as expressions of the clinical experience perspective. Similarly, we would occasionally observe students pressing staff people for information of this kind, either by asking questions during a conference or question period or by engaging them in conversation at some opportune moment, in either case asking questions designed to get "clinical experience" information.

I walked with a couple of the juniors into a room down the hall where the resident for the service was sitting. Johnson said, "Well, Dr. Carson, give me some gem of wisdom." Carson said, "Well, what do you want to know?" Johnson said, "I don't have any questions. I thought you might have some sparkling bit of information that you could give me that would be of use to me in my future career. . . ." The resident said, "I can't go around giving out all of my information and not have some left for tomorrow." Johnson said, "Well, all right, I'll ask you a question." And then he described a case he had had the post-mortem on. . . . It was a case of a kid who was in shock, was dehydrated, was in alkalosis, and so on, and the problem was how you would go about replacing his water supply. It was all on a very empirical technical level; he wanted to know how much to give of this, that, and the other thing, what dilutions to use, where and how to give these things, etc. He already seemed to know quite a bit and wanted the resident to iron out the conflicts in what he knew. The resident said, "Well, there are two or three ways of doing it. I prefer such-and-such a way, but the other ways are all right too. It depends, different people like to do different things." He went on to describe exactly how he handled such a problem. Both Johnson and another student who were there wrote down all the details of the procedure in their little notebooks.

(Junior Pediatrics. October, 1955.)

We see the students expressing the clinical experience perspective in incidents embodying their concern over whether or not they have properly absorbed the lessons of clinical experience. One of the important things the student is supposed to get from clinical experience is the ability to recognize diagnostic signs: the distinctive rash of measles, the heart murmurs characteristic of the several varieties of heart disease, and so on. If the students are to acquire this kind of knowledge, they must do it during their clinical training, for they have never before had the access to examples of these things coupled with the coaching of more experienced teachers. Students occasionally show concern about their ability to see and hear important kinds of signs, concern over whether they gained the clinical experience school is giving them. This is clearly an instance of acceptance of the importance of clinical experience, and is indirectly a judgment of the school, in the sense that if the school were really doing its job the students would have absorbed this experience and be able to apply it. An instance such as the following shows the way students worry over their inability to perceive diagnostic signs:

During ward rounds, the resident listened to a patient's heart and then had all the students listen. He said to a couple of them, after they finished, "Did you hear it?" Heath, when he was asked this, said, "Well, I heard something." The resident nodded, indicating that he didn't want to talk about it just this minute. Phelps, after he listened, said, "What are we supposed to hear, Jim?" The resident said, "We'll talk about it in a minute." When everyone had listened, we went out into the hall, and Jim questioned a couple of people about what they had heard. They, of course, differed considerably. Baer said the heart was shifted to the right. Jackson said it was shifted to the left. Phelps said it hadn't shifted at all. Finally Jim dispelled the suspense by saying, "What he's got is a pericardial friction rub. It's a pretty common post-op finding, and you'll never hear a more classic friction rub than this. If you didn't hear it, come back later today and listen to it again. It's just like the book describes." There was a good deal of discussion among the boys as to whether they had heard what they were supposed to have heard. None of them seemed very sure. Heath said to Jim, "I heard what you're talking about. But the noise sounded just like breath sounds to me." Jim said, "Well, that's easy to take care of. Just ask him to hold his breath, then you'll be able to see that the sound continues, so it isn't breath sounds."

(Junior Surgery. January, 1956.)

A somewhat different form of the same thing is found in the few incidents in which students insisted that the observer make use of opportunities to get clinical experience, even though the observer had no intention of practicing medicine. It was as though they felt such experience to be so important that anyone who had the chance to get it should take advantage of it.

A staff member demonstrated a patient with enlarged lymph nodes and had the fifteen members of the class take turns palpatating these nodes. Several of the students, while waiting their turns, told me that I should get in line and feel the nodes too. One of them said, "Go ahead. Get up there and feel those nodes. How are you going to know what happens to us unless you go through the same experiences?"

(Senior Medicine. March, 1956.)

All these kinds of observations, taken together, describe a student perspective that insists on the importance of clinical experience for a practicing physician, judges school activities by the amount of clinical experience they provide, and assesses a student's progress with reference to the amount of clinical experience he has acquired. They also describe the actions students take in acting on this perspective.

If we accept incidents having characteristics of the kind just described as individual expressions of the clinical experience perspective, we can now turn to demonstrating that use of this perspective is one of the customary ways students have of dealing with the problem of how to organize their activity and decide what is important in their apprentice training. First, we note that use of the perspective was widespread. Figure 5 indicates that statements or activities expressing this perspective were observed in every one of the eighteen clinical departments on which students spent time and with regard to most of the major activities carried on on these services. Four major activities are considered: 1. ward rounds; 2. lectures, discussions, and conversations with the staff; 3. working-up patients in the hospital or clinic; and 4. participating in therapeutic or diagnostic procedures. There were eighteen services on which students had training although, as noted in the chart, certain activities were not relevant on some services (i.e., students on emergency room service did not have ward rounds). We see, first of all, that items of evidence embodying use of the experience criterion by students were collected on all eighteen of the services considered. We conclude, therefore, that use of this criterion is not peculiar to the situation in a few departments of the hospital or to students in a given year, since it is found in services covering three school years. We also see that of the sixty-eight possible combinations of activities and services, use of the experience criterion was observed in forty-eight. Though the coverage is not complete, this indicates that this kind of judgment was not confined to any one activity. We can thus conclude that use of the experience criterion was widespread and not to be accounted for by any peculiar situational factors.

Second, we note that use of the perspective was frequent. Our field notes contain one hundred and eighty-one separate expressions of the perspective by individual students or groups of students, each incident taking one of the forms listed above. It should be remembered that almost all of our observations were made while participating with groups of students ranging in number from five to fifteen. Since expressions of this kind were observed in all departments of the hospital, it is reasonable to assume that the actual number occurring during the period of our field work was much larger; had we been able to observe all two hundred students in the clinical years simultaneously, the number of recorded incidents would be many times larger.

Finally, Table XXIV emphasizes two characteristics of our data which indicate that the clinical experience perspective was customary

ACTIVITY	3rd Year Medicine K.U.	3rd Year Medicine Menorah	3rd Year Medicine VA	3rd Year Surgery K.U.	3rd Year Surgery VA	3rd Year Pediatrics K.U.	3rd Year Pediatrics Mercy	4th Year Obstetrics K.U.	4th Year Obstetrics General	4th Year Medicine	2nd Year Physical Diagnosis	4th Year Psychiatry	4th Year ENT	4th Year Neurosurgery	4th Year Urology	4th Year Orthopedics	4th Year Anaesthesiology	4th Year Emergency Room
Ward rounds	X	–	X	X	–	X	X	X	–	–	X	0	–	–	–	–	0	0
Lectures, conversations, and discussions with staff	X	X	–	X	X	X	X	X	–	X	X	X	X	X	X	X	X	X
Working-up patients in hospital or clinic	X	X	X	X	–	X	X	X	–	X	X	X	X	–	X	X	0	X
Participating in therapeutic or diagnostic procedures	X	–	–	X	X	–	–	X	X	–	X	X	X	–	–	–	X	X

Symbols

X = At least one instance observed.
– = No instances observed.
0 = This activity not carried on.

Fig. 5 – Distribution of Observed Instances of Use of the Experience Perspective by Students

and collective in character. First, the expression of this perspective in any item of evidence might have been directed by the field worker; that is, he might have asked a student, "Did you like that lecture because the lecturer gave you a lot of stuff from his clinical experience?" On the other hand, the student might simply have volunteered the opinion that the lecture was good for that reason. Although both items would constitute evidence of the perspective's use, we feel more secure if some substantial proportion of such items were volunteered, for this would give us grounds to believe that students made use of the perspective in the course of their ordinary activity. If we know only that they answered "yes" to direct questions, we would have grounds for worry over whether this was not simply a verbal response which came into play only when the field worker broached the subject.

Table XXIV presents the 181 items of evidence classified according to whether their expression was volunteered or could have been suggested by some question of the observer. Since only four items could be classified as having been directed by the observer, we are justified in concluding that use of the experience perspective is part of the everyday activity of the students. The largest number of volunteered items consist of comments made by students to the observer. Though these were frequently unsolicited, they were often made in response to general questions by the observer. A sizable number of these questions were asked in an attempt to check the distribution of use of the experience perspective, but they were phrased in a vague way. For instance, the observer would ask after a lecture full of "practical" tips on the treatment of some disease, "How did you like that?" Though such a question in no way indicated use of the experience perspective as an answer, students answered in those terms. The second largest category of evidence consists of statements students made to each

TABLE XXIV

Evidence for the Existence of the Clinical Experience Perspective

		VOLUNTEERED	DIRECTED	TOTAL
Statements	To observer............	83 (47%)	4	87
	To others in everyday conversation	52 (29%)	–	52
Activities	Individual	13 (7%)	–	13
	Group	29 (16%)	–	29
Total	....	177 (99%)	4	181

other in everyday conversation. The remaining items of evidence consist of observations of student activities. Individual activities were largely efforts to get instructors to emit "pearls." Group activities might be instances in which a whole class collaborated in such an effort or observations of a class taking many notes on a "practical" lecture or sleeping through one that was "impractical." The group activity category undercounts the actual number of individual acts, since each entry in it combines the acts of several students; the field notes, however, often fail to distinguish the individuals actually involved in the activity so that the only practical solution was to count each group activity once.

The same table allows another argument to be made for our proposition. All the observed items consisting of statements students made to one another can be thought of as "public." That is, the statements were made in the presence of other students who, if they had disagreed with the statement, might have argued the matter. Students were willing to argue with one another over disputed points; many other issues provoked intense argument. But these public statements either went unchallenged or were agreed with. We may conclude, therefore, that the experience perspective was shared by students and its use was considered legitimate by them.

Discussion of the evidence that students customarily used the experience perspective would not be complete without mentioning the small number of negative items of evidence. As compared to the one hundred and eighty-one positive items, the six negative items do not cast much doubt on our conclusion. These consist of student statements or activities indicating great interest in matters that students typically regarded as impractical. For example, students were observed to be very interested in a lecture presenting newly discovered research findings which had as yet no practical clinical importance. At the level of the individual statement, negative instances took a similar form. One student, for instance, said the only kind of surgery he liked to watch was brain surgery; he found it "really interesting," though most of the other students felt that such surgery did not allow them to see anything which would add to their own clinical experience.

We have now demonstrated that students do assimilate and make use of the clinical experience perspective, a perspective suggested to them by the faculty and by the organization of the hospital. This conclusion will be further supported by analyses to be presented later, in which it will be shown that the perspective is used with regard to other matters: preferences among kinds of patients and choices of internships.

The Medical Responsibility
Perspective

Medical responsibility — the responsibility of the physician for the welfare and ultimately the life of his patient — is also presented to the student, as we have seen earlier, as an important and valuable thing to have. The student is told in many ways that the exercise of such responsibility is the hallmark of the real physician. We now turn to demonstrating that students elaborate this idea into a perspective on school work, using it along with the perspective based on clinical experience to answer the question of how their work can best prepare them for a future of medical practice.

As the student struggles to find his way in the bewildering maze of medical school, two areas of activity seem most involved with questions of medical responsibility. The first consists of examining and diagnosing patients. The main responsibility here is that of arriving at a correct diagnosis on the basis of a thorough and accurate examination. A person exercises responsibility in this area when his findings and diagnosis are accepted, without being repeated or checked on, as the basis for the patient's treatment. The second activity consists of performing diagnostic and therapeutic procedures containing some element of danger to the patient. These range in degree of potential danger from such relatively minor procedures as venipuncture to major surgery.

Students find some answers to the question, "How can I best make use of my apprentice training to prepare for medical practice?" in the perspective they develop around the concept of medical responsibility. This perspective may be summarized in the following statements:

1. It is important for a doctor to have had the opportunity to exercise medical responsibility.

2. School activities are good and worth devoting one's effort to insofar as they provide opportunities to perform procedures and engage in other activities which constitute an exercise of medical responsibility. School activities are bad insofar as they allow one no opportunities of this kind.

3. One must make a determined effort to get as many chances

to exercise responsibility as possible, for the school functionaries do not pay much attention to students' problems of getting to do this.

4. Being allowed to exercise responsibility, and handling one's opportunities to do so skilfully and well, are important signs of one's personal worth and hence have symbolic value beyond the actual experience involved.

We conclude, from an examination of our data, that students hold this perspective and organize their behavior in ways that are congruent with it.

Our attention was not called to the hypothesis that students used the perspective by any dramatic incident; rather, a series of small incidents, of which the following is perhaps the one in which the theme is most explicit, suggested that students had a great interest in being allowed to "do things":

The resident asked Johnson if he had ever done a lumbar tap. Johnson said, "No, but I have seen them done." Carl, the resident, said, "Well, come along, you are going to do one right now, unless you don't want to if you don't think you can handle it. I'll be right there. You might as well do it right now as later." So Johnson said he would be glad to. He turned to me and said, "Now that's the way they do things around here; they just throw you in cold; they say that's the best way to learn anything is just to do it." When we arrived at the patient's room a nurse told us that the patient was a hospital employee whose supervisor would want the resident to do the tap instead of the student. Carl said, "Well, if that's the way they want it, we'll do it that way." Johnson was pretty disappointed and Carl said, "I'm sorry, but there's no sense kicking up a fuss; we might as well do it that way, but you can assist me."

The next day, in the course of a discussion of internships, Johnson referred to this incident. He said, "You see, like what happened with that lumbar tap yesterday, that's likely to happen all the time while you are here in medical school. I'll be lucky if I get to do ten or twelve of those all the time that I'm here . . . You are always being cut off from those experiences for one reason or another." He went on to indicate that it was very important to have practice in these procedures so that you would know how to do them when you began practice.

(Junior Medicine. October, 1955.)

The students' frequent use of the term "responsibility" in connection with similar incidents led us to suspect that it embodied a generalized conception of great importance for them. From the first month of our field work, therefore, we searched for information on this topic.

Many kinds of observations made in the field can be interpreted as expressions of the medical responsibility perspective. We now discuss the significant features of those observations which led us to see them in that light, the features which allow us in later tabulations to count any incident having one or more of them as expressions of the perspective.

We found the most direct expression of the responsibility perspective in the relatively rare statements by students that they wanted responsibility given to them because this was necessary training for medical practice.

Charles had come early that morning to draw bloods and then had done a circumcision. He said that since they were only on the service about ten days he wanted to get in on as many circumcisions as possible, because he felt that this was something he would be called on to do in general practice. He said that he was glad to have the experience.

(Senior Urology. October, 1956.)

Similarly, there were many incidents in which students made a judgment on the training they were receiving on a particular hospital service by referring to the amount of responsibility given them. This was typically expressed in a statement about how much one "gets to do" on the service — i.e., what procedures one is allowed to do.

One student told the observer and several other students about his experience in the Emergency Room: "It sure is interesting. They get all kinds of cases in down there. They are very busy. There's so much to do that the intern really lets you do a lot." The other students were listening very interestedly. He went on: "Yeah, I got to sew up a couple of lacerations, and I did a couple of pelvics too. You know, none of us have ever done them before. But some woman came in with acute PID (pelvic inflammatory disease) and the intern said, 'Go ahead and do a pelvic on her.'"

(Senior Surgical Specialties. October, 1956.)

The many casual complaints by students that their time in the operating room was "wasted" because they "never got to do anything" illustrate the same theme. Students often made this point by comparing their experience at the Veterans' Administration hospital with that received in the university hospital.

I had lunch with three students. In the course of comparing their experience at various hospitals in which they received training, one said: "We just came back from the VA. We were there on surgery and it's a whole hell of a lot better than surgery over here, let me tell you. They let you do so much more over there. Here the place is all cluttered up with student nurses and interns and residents and you don't get to see anything or do anything. You're just on the ward. It was a lot different over at the VA. I wish I could have stayed there the whole time."

(Junior Pediatrics. November, 1955.)

Some students hold jobs as externs in private hospitals around the city, in which they function as a kind of junior intern; they frequently tell tales of all they have "gotten to do" as externs.

Jenkins told a couple of students and myself that he had sewn somebody up the other night over at the private hospital he externs at. He was in the Emergency Room; somebody had come in with a face wound and he had sewed it up. Star said, "Those wounds are tougher than those that are in other places; you have to do a better job." Jenkins said, "Yeah, I know but I did it all right."

(Junior Medicine. October, 1955.)

In each of these instances, students judge the value of a service by the amount of responsibility they are allowed or, more specifically, by the number of "things" — procedures involving the possibility of error and consequent harm to the patient — they are allowed to do. We find further instances of students expressing the responsibility perspective in those incidents in which students either complained about being denied responsibility or expressed pleasure at being allowed to exercise it.

Several students were sitting in the laboratory in which they did lab work on patients. One of them complained: "Do you know I haven't done a pelvic examination all the time I've been here [on the medical service at the university hospital]? I sure as hell won't get to do it over at the VA hospital."

(Junior Medicine. October, 1955.)

I went with Temple and another student to have coffee. I had just met them and explained that I was interested in how they became doctors. Temple, who was in the early weeks of his junior year, said, "I remember my experience this summer. I took general medicine as an elective. The first time I did a lumbar tap was something great. I had seen it done, but I hadn't ever done one."

(Junior Medicine. October, 1955.)

Again, students sometimes made special efforts to be allowed to perform various procedures. One student explained his success in this to the observer and several other students:

Walters said that he had gotten to do a whole lot of things, that the residents had let him do a great many things. For instance, he had done and repaired more episiotomies than anyone else in the group. Many of them had not gotten to do any and he had done three or four and repaired them. He said, "You've just got to push these residents a little, that's all. If you tell them that you want to do something, well, then they will let you do it, quite frequently. But if you don't ask them they won't even think of letting you do it — it just doesn't occur to them. I just made it a point to ask if I could try doing this or that or the other thing and usually they would let me do it. I've gotten to do a pudendal block a couple of times." The other students said, "You have? They let you do that?" Walters said, "Certainly they did. But I had to ask. They never would have offered to let me. I just went ahead and asked them and they did. They were surprised sometimes when I asked them but usually they let me try and when I did all right then they let me do it again."

(Senior Obstetrics. May, 1956.)

What is of interest in this and similar incidents is not the student's success, of course, but the effort he makes to get responsibility and, implicitly, the evident importance he attaches to it.

Student use of the responsibility perspective can also be seen in those instances in which, offered a choice of alternative activities, they choose the one most likely to give an opportunity to exercise responsibility.

During the morning, while we were on rounds, the resident came in and announced that a visiting doctor would be here at two o'clock to make rounds with everyone on medicine. He asked Carter, "Have you ever done a paracentesis?" Carter said, "No." The resident said, "Well, I'm going to do one this afternoon on that patient of yours with the distended abdomen, so if you would like to come along and help I'd be glad to have you." Carter said, "All right, but how about these rounds this afternoon?" He said, "I think we can do it at one, meet me up here and we'll do it."

At one o'clock the resident told Carter and me that he couldn't do the procedure now because he had to go to a residents' meeting and that they could do it at two if Carter didn't mind missing a few minutes of the visiting doctor's rounds. Carter hesitated and the resident said, "You don't have to come along, you know. I just thought if you would like to I'd be glad to have you help out, if you want to." Carter said, "I think I'll come along, I'll catch up on the rounds later."

(Junior Medicine. October, 1955.)

Student use of the responsibility perspective is also implied in their distaste for kinds of work which, while medical in nature, do not allow any opportunity to take responsibility. Though there are other reasons for student dislike of what they call "scut work," the absence of any tincture of responsibility contributes strongly to their antipathy for routine lab work and similar student duties. Later we will analyze in more detail the debate between students and faculty over lab work. Here we simply note that the lab work students do is felt by them to be futile and meaningless because, as they think, no patient's life or welfare is likely ever to depend on the results they produce.

One student described his experience in the Emergency Room to another student and the observer: "You know what that intern down there did last night? I had to stay over last night, and he woke me up at two o'clock to run a white count and differential on a kid that had a pain in his belly. They thought it might be appendicitis. That's a big nuisance to try and do one of those at night too. You have to run all over the hospital getting equipment and everything. When I finally got it done I brought it down to him, and I was kind of excited because I thought it showed something pretty positive. But he just gave him some aspirin and sent him home. He didn't even bother to say thank you to me. Now, I don't mind doing something like that, but if they're not going to pay any attention to the results, even when they're positive, why did he bother to wake me up? There isn't any sense to that."

(Senior Surgical Specialties. November, 1956.)

Because student's frequent complaints about doing lab work often contained reference to the fact that any unusual findings they turned up in admission lab studies were often duplicated by the hospital's main laboratory before being accepted as valid, we felt justified in interpreting complaints about lab work (and other kinds of work defined as "scut") as instances of student use of the responsibility perspective.

So far, the material presented has indicated simply that students used the responsibility perspective in organizing their daily behavior as students. The material we now turn to goes to this point, but different implications of the concept of medical responsibility come to the fore. We have so far been concerned only with the primary meaning of medical responsibility for students — that a doctor-to-be needs a chance to exercise it. We turn now to one of the subsidiary meanings of the concept.

When an organization's hierarchy clearly reflects the operation of a value, as the organization of the teaching hospital so clearly reflects the value of responsibility, participants in that organization are likely to gauge their own worth by the amount of that value they possess. In a society dominated by the concept of pecuniary gain, as Veblen showed, the measure of personal worth becomes the amount of money one has at his disposal and the mark of honor the ability to dispose of wealth freely. In a society dominated by religious values, piety or possession by the gods (depending on the kind of religion) might form the basis of self-esteem. In an organization dominated by the medical values we have been discussing, we would expect participants to make use of those values in judging themselves.

If the exercise of medical responsibility is seen as one of the key traits of the full-fledged physician, and if opportunities to exercise it are given more frequently to students and house staff as they move up to higher positions in the hospital hierarchy, then the experience of exercising responsibility should be a crucial influence on the student's assessment of himself, reflecting as it does the presumably considered judgment of his superiors on his abilities, expressed in the objective form of privileges granted or withheld. Students, then, would be expected to show, both in words and actions, that they interpret the amount of responsibility given them as public certification of their personal worth and are accordingly cast down or buoyed up by the denial or granting of responsibility. Many observations indicate that this is the case.

Students occasionally explain this very directly:

Two students and the observer were discussing Pediatric Clinic. In the course of the discussion Dayton argued that they actually were given a good deal of responsibility, but Croft disagreed. Dayton said, "Gee, don't take away the little responsibility they have given us. That's what you're doing, the way you're talking. I like to think that maybe I could do something wrong. It makes it seem more important if I do something right. . . ." Later on in the discussion, Croft agreed that they did get some responsibility and added, "I'll tell you one thing, it's a pretty good thing that we do have some experience like this where people look up to us with a certain amount of respect, where we do get a certain amount of prestige and are treated like doctors by some of these people, because we do need a little of that ego-building or else I don't see how you would ever get through medical school. It's a pretty damned long grind. I don't know if I could take it if I didn't have some of that kind of thing going on all the time. . . ."

(Junior Pediatrics. October, 1955.)

Students express the same idea more indirectly when they point out that what they do really contains elements of responsibility, even though this might not appear to be true on superficial inspection. By pointing to the importance of what they are allowed to do, students minimize the damage done to their self-esteem by the obvious fact that there are so many things they are not allowed to do.

I asked Croft how they spent their days on pediatrics. He explained their schedule, and then said that "occasionally the residents let us do something, like letting us do a cutdown. We do a lot of those down here. You probably didn't see much of that in medicine, but it's not easy to get into a kid's vein and very frequently we have to cut down on one. But actually we aren't given much responsibility, so we don't have too much to do; that's the truth of it." Dayton said, "Well, I don't know, I think that we have quite a bit of responsibility in the clinic." Croft said, "Do you? Everything we do is checked by a resident. . . ." Dayton said, "Well, I don't even always talk to the resident. A lot of times when I'm pretty sure what's going on I just go in to him and say, 'This patient has such-and-such. Do you want to take a look at him?' and he'll say sometimes, 'No, that's all right, just go ahead.' And it is a responsibility because, after all, you might miss something on the physical examination, and it would be pretty important; and that is a responsibility to know that your examination is going to be the one that stands and it might be because of you that something is overlooked." Croft said, "Well, I never thought of it that way. But after all, if it was that important, it would be pretty obvious, wouldn't it?"

(Junior Pediatrics. October, 1955.)

Other students pointed to actual mishaps they had been involved in, as evidence that the work they did as students contained elements of responsibility.

Several students were discussing their work in the operating room. Morrison said, "You know, I did something pretty bad the other day. I put too much traction on the retractor I was holding and broke a vein. Jesus, there was blood all over the place. Pennon [the surgeon] took it pretty calmly, and I'm not sure that it was my fault. But that's a hell of a thing to have happen." Carson said, "I'll say. I know that I'm damn careful with those retractors. If it's just one of the small ones up near the skin, well, you can pull as hard as you want on one of those. But when they give you one of those deep ones to hold on to, where you've got organs and everything, then I don't pull at all, I just try and hold it steady where it is. Of course, that's not too easy to do when you are standing there for two hours or so. Your hand gets numb, and your arm, and there's a tendency to yank on the thing."

(Junior Surgery. January, 1956.)

This discussion of the dangers inherent in holding retractors gains importance when we realize that students typically dislike holding retractors on the grounds that there is no responsibility involved in this activity; they ordinarily refer to retractors as "idiot sticks," implying that an idiot could handle one.

In a different mood, students make a great deal of those incidents in which their examination of a patient reveals something that has been missed by a staff member, resident, or intern. In telling such stories, they implicitly argue that they are very worthwhile medical people, deserving of a great deal of responsibility since they handle what they are given so well.

One of the students said to the observer, "Remind me to take you around later to have a look at the luckiest man in the world. A guy down the hall here. He had boils, and his local doctor couldn't do anything with them. The doctor suspected diabetes, and when he ran a urinalysis he found a terrifically high amount of sugar so he sent him in here for a diabetic work-up. Actually, the guy didn't have diabetes at all; it was a laboratory error. But in the meantime he came up here and got a pretty thorough work-up. The student who was examining him did a rectal and found a polyp way up in his rectum. These things are kind of dangerous because they turn into cancer pretty frequently. They biopsied the thing and sure enough it did have peculiar cells in it and was a pretty sure thing to turn into cancer so naturally they operated and removed it and probably saved his life. The chances are that it never would have been discovered until it was too late otherwise. . . . The resident didn't catch it and the staff member didn't catch it, but it was there all right, and they took it out and saved his life."

(Junior Surgery. December, 1955.)

Two of the students told me how they had diagnosed acute rheumatic fever on a kid in the Emergency Room yesterday when the intern had missed it. They were both very proud of this and said they had heard the murmurs and noticed the hot joints and the intern had not. They called it to his attention and he agreed they were right, that they had made the proper diagnosis and he had missed it. I said, "What are you trying to do — make that same smart diagnosis on every kid that comes in now?" Harlan said, "Well, you know that every sore throat is a possible case of rheumatic fever and a lot of them have been missed in the past, so it's a good thing to keep in mind. Better to think about it and be wrong than miss it."

(Senior Surgical Specialties. October, 1956.)

In these ways, then — by redefining activities as more responsible than ordinarily thought and by capitalizing on instances in which they use what responsibility they are given in proper fashion — students attempt to maximize by verbal means the amount of responsibility they do have.

Expression of the responsibility perspective is also found in all those incidents in which students react with resentment to the withholding of responsibility, feeling that in being denied responsibility they are being insulted in some way. This comes out most clearly where students are not allowed to perform procedures on "important" patients which they do routinely on ordinary patients; the implication that they are "not good enough" annoys them.

Heinz said, "Well, I'm going to have a circumcision now. The baby's father is on the staff here, so naturally I won't get to do it. I guess I won't get to do any at all, because this is the only morning I'm up for circumcision, and that's the only one they have, and naturally they have to have the senior resident do it — couldn't let a student do it."

(Senior Urology. October, 1956.)

One of the students' big gripes on OB is that they are not allowed to do anything at all on private patients, though they are required to sit with them, time their pains, do the lab work, and scrub in for the delivery. They are not even allowed to do rectal examinations on these patients and they do not do the actual delivery, only the auxiliary work connected with it. Donovan made a joke of this to the observer: "Say, we have a great opportunity here with the private patients. They're very good to us, not at all like what you hear about other patients. Why, I have even heard of cases where they let a student weigh and measure the placenta on a private patient. That's really something, isn't it?" [The point of his remark is that handling the placenta involves no responsibility at all.]

(Senior Obstetrics. May, 1956.)

The heavy-handed irony of these two examples also colors those student comments which point sarcastically to the fact that they are not yet allowed to exercise responsibility. In these incidents students gloat self-pityingly over their subordinate position in the hierarchy of responsibility of the hospital.

One of the students was scheduled to scrub in on a nephrectomy [removal of a kidney]. We worked all morning on the following joke. We were going to tell the other students that he had taken the kidney out all by himself and done a very neat job of it. The payoff to the joke was going to be that he had taken the kidney out all right — he had taken it out in an aluminum pan to the surgical path lab after the operation was over. He kept saying that that was probably all he would do, since he would be fourth assistant on this operation and there wouldn't be much for him to do in that capacity.

(Senior Urology. October, 1956.)

Several students were quizzing one another on a subject they were about to take up in class: traumatic injuries of the chest. Grant said, "There are various kinds of injuries — crushing injuries, perforating injuries. . . . " He named several other varieties. I said, "I suppose you know what to do about all of those, too." He said, "Sure, simple. Call a doctor." It has occurred to me since that this is a very suggestive phrase that highlights the student's position in the hospital. This is just what he must do if anything goes wrong — call a doctor, since he himself is not one.

(Junior Surgery. January, 1956.)

"Call a doctor," used as a joke in this way, appears frequently in our field notes.

Closely related to this kind of humor are those incidents in which students attempt to embarrass or harass faculty or house staff by refusing to exercise small amounts of delegated responsibility or otherwise participate in hospital procedures; in this way they wish to call attention to their belief that they are really worthy of greater amounts of responsibility and to what they believe to be the absurdities of the routine denials of that responsibility.

A staff member described what the students were required to do on the service; this was their first day and they didn't know the rules yet. One of the students asked whether they were supposed to scrub in on operations and the staff member said, "You can if you want to," and let it go at that. I said to Gordon, "Are you going to scrub in on any of these operations?" He said, "Not unless they make me do it. I've worked as an orthopedic nurse and I've seen all the orthopedic surgery I care to see. I mean, if it's just a matter of standing there and watching, I've done that already and I don't see any point in doing any more of it unless I have to. If they were going to let me do something beyond watch, that would be different, but they won't. So there's no point in it."

(Senior Orthopedics. September, 1956.)

In extreme and unusual cases students may deliberately misuse small responsibilities for this reason.

A student I was spending some time with was required to do a blood count on a patient he regarded as not being sick at all. He drew a syringe full of blood and carried it out to the nurses' station. In front of the nurse, he held the syringe up to the light, looked at it, and handed it to her, saying, "Here, you can have this now. I've already done my blood count and differential." The nurse looked at him and laughed nervously. He said, "Oh well, with somebody like her, what the hell difference does it make? She isn't likely to have any hematological trouble. We'll just fill it in with normal values. That will be all right." While the nurse giggled, the student took the chart, opened it up to the page where lab results go and said, "Let's see, her blood looked pretty good. I'll put down twelve grams of hemoglobin, that's about 77 per cent of normal." He wrote down these figures and filled in imaginary figures for the other values to be reported. I said, "Tell me, do people turn in lab results like this very often?" He said, "Sure they do. What the hell, she hasn't got anything that needs a blood count. It's just a lot of damn fool scut work. I'll show that goddam Jones." (Jones, the patient's doctor, was a member of the staff this student particularly disliked, feeling that he, more than other staffmen, tried to "Keep the students in their place.") [1]

(Senior Obstetrics. May, 1956.)

The students' pursuit of responsibility as a means of bolstering their self-esteem does not work, however, for no matter how many individual procedures are allocated to them they are still not doctors. If students valued the chance to do procedures solely for the chance given to rehearse techniques before entering practice they would continue to value them after being allowed to do them once. But they also value the chance to do procedures for the symbolic boost given their self-esteem, and when they find that the boost is only symbolic and leaves them just as much students as they ever were they return to feeling that their true worth is not recognized. For this reason, we see as expressions of this facet of the responsibility perspective those incidents in which students indicate that some element of responsibility they once wanted very much now no longer seems very desirable. For example, juniors uniformly complain that they are not allowed to do pelvic examinations, making clear that they resent the implication that they are not "ready" for this yet. But once they become seniors and work in the gynecology clinic their attitudes change quickly:

Warner said, "Another thing I don't like is that damn GYN clinic. Boy, I hate to do pelvic examinations." I said, "I'm surprised you dislike that so much. I thought it would be kind of fun for you guys." Berton went on to say, in the crude manner in which young men often talk among themselves,

[1] The student's statement, made in a moment of disgust, that laboratory results of this cavalier character are often turned in is not to be taken as evidence that such is the case. It is only evidence of his belief that students are assigned some work of no importance.

that when a person was called upon to do pelvic examinations every five minutes he no longer finds them interesting.

(Senior Obstetrics. April, 1956.)

Thus, even though their progress through school brings them increasing amounts of responsibility in the form of procedures they are allowed to do, students continue to complain through their senior year about not "getting to do anything," because whatever they are allowed to do quickly loses its symbolic value.

Finally, having the opportunity to perform a procedure or otherwise exercise responsibility also makes it possible to perform it improperly. We see as expressions of the perspective all instances in which students exhibit either concern over performing a procedure badly or pleasure at having done it well, interpreting either of these feelings as being related to the student's estimate of his own worth, based on his ability to handle responsibility.

All these kinds of observations, taken together, describe a student perspective that sees one of the most important functions of medical school as that of providing opportunities for the exercise of medical responsibility, viewed as a necessary part of any physician's training; this perspective judges school activities by the opportunities for the exercise of responsibility they provide and suggests that one's own personal worth can be judged in terms of the amount of responsibility one is allowed to exercise and how well one uses the opportunities he gets.

If we accept incidents of the kinds described above as constituting, each in its way, expressions of the medical responsibility perspective, we can now turn to demonstrating that use of this perspective is one of the customary ways in which students deal with the problem of how to organize their activity and decide what is important in their training as apprentices.

We see, first, that use of the perspective by students in their daily activities was both frequent and widespread. Instances of its use were observed on seventeen of the eighteen services students spend time on during their clinical work, psychiatry being the sole exception. Again, though the actual number of incidents observed has little meaning, this number was sizable; one hundred and eighty-eight such incidents were observed. Since we observed only from five to fifteen students at a time the number of incidents which probably occurred among all two hundred students in the clinical years and might have served as evidence must be much larger.

The character of our data also shows that students made use of the medical responsibility perspective in organizing their ordinary school behavior. Only eight of the one hundred and eighty-eight items of evidence were elicited by direct questioning. The other one hundred and eighty items consist of incidents in which the use of the concept was volunteered by students. (See Table XXV) Indeed, 68 per cent of these items are of such a character that they probably would have occurred had the observer not been present at all, being items of conversation between students (48%), or individual (14%) or group (6%)

TABLE XXV

EVIDENCE FOR THE EXISTENCE OF THE RESPONSIBILITY PERSPECTIVE

		VOLUNTEERED	DIRECTED	TOTAL
Statements	To observer	57 (32%)	8	65
	To others in everyday conversation	86 (48%)	–	86
Activities	Individual	25 (14%)	–	25
	Group	12 (6%)	–	12
Total		180 (100%)	8	·188

activities. All this goes to show that students made use of the concept in a routine, everyday way, and it was thus part of the culture with which they approached their school work.

Table XXV also allows us to argue that use of this concept was legitimate, as well as common, in the medical school. The incidents of conversation among students and of group activities, making up 54 per cent of all incidents observed, were public — that is, the concept was used in the presence of other students. In none of these instances did the other students offer any disagreement or indicate in any way that they felt use of the concept to be illegitimate, even though (as we have already noted) they were often willing to argue at length when they thought another student was in the wrong.

We must, finally, consider the relatively small number of negative instances which appear in our field notes. There are eight incidents which indicate that students do not use the responsibility perspective to organize their school behavior. Though the number is small and does not cast much doubt on our conclusion, these cases merit examination. In two instances, it is questionable whether the cases really deny the importance of the perspective, for in both students appear nervous at the thought of taking on responsibility and would prefer not to. For instance:

One of the boys asked Johnson about physical diagnosis in pediatrics, whether you got to do anything or not. Johnson said that the last time they were there the faculty must have heard that everyone was dissatisfied because they gave each fellow a patient and let him do the complete work-up. The other guy said, "You mean they let you make your own diagnosis and everything?" Johnson said, "That's right. We went back and consulted with them of course, but they let us handle the whole thing. I'm not too anxious to do all that kind of thing on my own yet. It's quite a bit of responsibility and I really don't think we know enough to undertake all that yet. It was even worse in surgery the last time we were there. We had a woman who needed to have a proctoscopic examination. They got her prepared and then the resident gave the proctoscope to me and said, 'Go ahead, you might as well get started now. You'll never learn unless you try.' That kind of scared me a little, particularly since this patient was thought to have a rectal stricture. You don't just want to go barreling in on someone who has anything like that." I said, "You mean he just told you to go ahead?" He said, "That's right. I had never even had one of the things in my hand before and here I was supposed to go and do that kind of examination on a patient. That's one reason I don't care too much for surgery in general. I don't like these spur of the moment things, you know. I like to have time to read up on something and have plenty of time to make up my mind about what is going on before I actually do anything. I just didn't have a chance there."

(Sophomore Physical Diagnosis. April, 1956.)

It can be argued that a student who feels this way actually does accept the responsibility perspective and organizes his school behavior around it. He is too frightened by the seriousness of the procedures he is called on to do to respond as eagerly as other students, and his actions are a mirror image of theirs.

The other six incidents are truly negative, consisting of statements by students that getting responsibility is really not very important, of statements which might be deduced from such a major premise, or of activities which implied such a position. Students were observed, for example, to be indifferent when denied responsibility or to argue that it did not make much difference whether one got to do procedures or not. It is noteworthy that in five out of six incidents the student was alone with the observer when this occurred; only once were students observed to argue to other students that a service was very good even though they got to do nothing in the operating room. This suggests that the widespread public agreement among students on the importance of responsibility masks some underlying dissidence. Although they all act as though responsibility were terribly important, many may well entertain other evaluations. The results of our interviews with a random sample of students are interesting in this connection. It should be remembered that these interviews were conducted away from the normal settings of everyday student activity and that no other students were present. Under these circumstances students are somewhat less likely to stay on the rails provided by student culture. When we asked, for instance, "Do you think that students get enough chance to carry out procedures such as lumbar punctures, passing gastric tubes, etc?" more than half the students felt they had sufficient opportunity to exercise this kind of medical responsibility. Similarly, when we asked, "How important is it to get this kind of experience?" less than half thought it was very important (see Table XXVI). In short, the near unanimity exhibited in behavior in the hospital does cover up a certain amount of disagreement held privately. But, to put it another way, these private reservations do not greatly affect overt behavior in the hospital.

TABLE XXVI

INTERVIEW FINDINGS ON THE IMPORTANCE OF MEDICAL RESPONSIBILITY *

Question 94: "Do students get enough chance to carry out procedures, such as lumbar punctures, passing gastric tubes, etc.?"

Yes	17
No	12
Total	29

Question 96: "How important is it to get this kind of experience?"

Very	12
Medium	10
Little	7
Total	29

* These questions were asked only of those students who had some clinical experience, i.e., the 29 juniors and seniors in our sample.

Responsibility, Experience, and the Medical Student

Medical students make use of two important medical values — responsibility and experience — in developing a perspective on the problem of what to study and learn of the mass of material they are presented with. But, in making use of these values of practicing physicians, they do not simply incorporate them, intact and unchanged, into their own ways of thinking and acting. Students of acculturation have often pointed out that culture traits change their form and meaning when they are transferred from one society to another. The changes that take place in the concepts of responsibility and experience when they are used by medical students point to the ways the medical student's world and problems differ from those of practicing physicians and re-emphasize our contention that student behavior must be understood in its immediate situational context.

The physician talks about his responsibility for his patients' welfare, the possibility that he may cause a patient harm and the necessity for relying on clinical experience when scientific knowledge provides no guidelines. But the medical student does not talk about such things, for he has no patients of his own, cannot legally exercise medical responsibility, and has no clinical experience to fall back on. The physician lives in a world peopled by his patients and colleagues; but the medical student's world contains, instead, his teachers and their patients. The physician wants to practice good medicine; the student wants to learn what he will need to know in order to practice good medicine.

Because the worlds and problems of students and physicians differ, the meanings they attach to such key concepts as responsibility and experience also differ. For the physician, responsibility is something he has and must exercise; clinical experience is something he has and uses. For the student, responsibility is something he wants but is often denied, as is clinical experience. The physician uses these terms in thinking about his entire medical career as well as immediate specific situations. The student may use them in thinking about the future but tends always to give them the connotations they have for him in school, seeing them as scarce commodities of which he may not get enough.

The important immediate effect of the existence of the responsibility and experience perspectives lies in their influence on the *direction* of student effort. Students, as we have noted earlier, may work very hard and yet frustrate the faculty's desires by working at quite different things and for quite different purposes from those the faculty thinks worthwhile. In the area we have been considering, the perspectives students collectively adopt give their efforts an intensely practical and short-run character. Students who identify what is important for them in schoolwork as the acquisition of experience and responsibility tend to reject (whether consciously or simply from lack of having considered them) such alternative descriptions of possible directions for the expenditure of effort as the acquisition of scientific knowledge for its own sake, intellectual curiosity, and similar less practically oriented descriptions. Since, as we shall see later, substantial segments of the faculty believe, at least part of the time, that these alternative directions are important while the student orientation is "practical" only in the short run, if at all, the dominance of the experience and responsibility perspectives creates the possibility of faculty dissatisfaction with students.

The fact that these perspectives are held collectively provides a base of social support for student actions that at times may violate faculty expectations. Were students not united in the use of these perspectives, they would presumably be less immune to faculty suggestions that they approach their work differently. Any individual student gains strength to continue along the lines suggested by the perspectives from his knowledge that all his fellows believe and act similarly.

Because of the differences between the meanings which faculty and students attach to the concepts of responsibility and experience, the student is placed in a situation of considerable tension and strain. The opportunities to gain responsibility and experience that he desires so much are often denied him, either because the faculty thinks other things are more important or because they are unaware of the meaning their action will have for the student. For instance, the faculty will place the patient's welfare above the student's need for responsibility and experience and not allow him to deliver breech babies. In this respect, the student is in the classic position of the job hunter who can neither get a job for lack of experience or experience for lack of a job. But the faculty may also deny the student an opportunity to do things because they think the matter unimportant, not realizing the impact this may have on the student's assessment of his own worth.

While we do not wish to take the student's part, it should be pointed out that he is at a considerable disadvantage in trying to better his situation, as he sees it. Not only is there a tremendous gap in prestige and power between students and faculty, but in addition the faculty regard the students' desire for increased responsibility as unreasonable and therefore not a legitimate topic for debate. Since they do not understand how serious access to responsibility seems to students, the faculty do not give students a chance to argue the matter with them. Just as wildcat strikes occur in industry when workers have grievances which are not considered legitimate topics for arbitration under the existing contract,[2] students sometimes engage in petty cheating or harassment of the faculty as a way of "prosecuting grievances" that cannot be dealt with in more legitimate and formal ways.

The students' development of the responsibility and experience perspectives has certain other consequences which we should note. First of all, having developed a coherent way of thinking and acting with regard to problems of what to study makes it possible for students to carry on meaningfully in what might otherwise be a disorganizing situation. Many perspectives might, of course, accomplish this and thus save the student from the incapacitating panic he might experience had he no guidelines for organizing his activity in a situation which gives no clear-cut cues on how to proceed.

In another direction, adopting the responsibility and experience perspectives gives the student a "professional" and impersonal way of viewing events and experiences that might be very difficult should he continue to look at them with the eyes of a layman. Many occupations deal routinely with things that are shocking, horrifying, or revolting to lay people. Their members develop a technical vocabulary and point of view based on that routine acquaintance with the horrible and reflecting the specific occupational interest they have in it. Thus, a janitor does not experience the same disgust with garbage as the layman and an undertaker does not turn away from a corpse with a layman's revulsion.[3] Instead, they see garbage and corpses as technical problems to be dealt with in the appropriate way. The technical vocabulary and point of view furnish an alternative way of experiencing the event and spare the professional the anxiety or discomfort the lay perspective suggests as an appropriate response.

The medical student sees many things laymen customarily think of as "traumatic"; in particular, death and disabling or disfiguring disease.[4] The medical profession has a language and point of view

[2] See the discussion by Alvin W. Gouldner in *Wildcat Strike* (Yellow Springs, Ohio: Antioch Press, 1954).

[3] See Everett C. Hughes, *Men and Their Work* (Glencoe, Ill.: Free Press, 1958), pp. 49–52, 78–101.

[4] A somewhat different and considerably more detailed analysis of medical students' reactions to trauma will be found in the forthcoming "Sociological Calendar of a

toward these things which provide a technical and impersonal way of experiencing them. The student, as we have seen, is not yet a doctor and does not fully participate in the culture of the medical profession. But he too has his "professional" preoccupations, those associated with his present "profession" of student. The perspectives he adopts in the course of his student activities serve him in the same way as medical culture serves the doctor. He sees death not so much as a human tragedy as a problem in the use of medical responsibility.

Although we will later explore this point in more detail, we should note here that this does not mean that the student becomes cynical and unfeeling; it simply means that he has the reactions appropriate to one in his situation. These seem cynical to the layman because they do not include the simple horror he would feel or thinks he would feel in the face of death or disabling disease. But the student's reactions include some that are principled and moral, the very opposite of cynical. For instance, the student's insistence on assigning responsibility for bad results in the cases he observes reveals the use of a moral standard. But it is a professional rather than a lay standard, sophisticated and relative.

Medical School" by Renée Fox, particularly in those sections dealing with "training for detached concern."

Chapter 14

The Academic Perspective

Dealing With the Faculty

W<small>HILE</small> much of the behavior of the students is specific to
their relation to medicine, other aspects of it may be considered as
due to imperatives of the role of student, considered independently
of medicine. The teacher formally imparts certain knowledge to students who do not yet possess it. In modern educational institutions,
the teacher ordinarily also examines his students and grades them
according to how well they have assimilated the knowledge presented
to them. The examinations determine the course of the student's career in school; they also determine what happens to him after school.
For it is increasingly true in many occupations, and absolutely true
in medicine, that students cannot move on into practice unless and
until they have demonstrated their mastery of the required knowledge to their teachers. No alternative way of learning and of proving
one's proficiency is provided. One must, for a period of several years,
keep one's teachers satisfied with his progress in desired directions.

The students, as they become involved in a variety of situations,
each with its own special obligations toward their teachers, develop
an "academic" perspective. It is this collective response to their role
as students which we describe and document in this chapter.

Student relations with residents and interns are not greatly influenced by the academic perspective. Relations with the house staff
are informal, and the house staff are around the wards and clinics
much of the time. In contrast, students have a very formal relation
with the faculty, who appear ordinarily only at specified times for

formal academic exercises such as rounds and lectures. In consequence, the faculty appear to the students as distant and awe-
inspiring figures, whose evaluations are important. The faculty gives
grades, the house staff ordinarily does not. So it is the faculty toward
whom the students typically act in terms suggested by the academic
perspective.

Though students receive grades in the clinical years, they are not
routinely told what they are but can apply to the dean's office for
information. They do know that the grades are not numerical scores
based on the amount of knowledge displayed on some standardized
test, but rather a set of faculty judgments as to whether a student's
performance is superior, satisfactory, or unsatisfactory on a series of
characteristics. The characteristics listed on the grade card which the
faculty fills out (see Fig. 6) cover such a wide area that students
realize that they must do more than get a good score on an occasional
formal examination. They are reminded of their obligations as students by the many situations in school in which they perform for
observant staff members and in which they might reasonably expect
a poor performance to be noted and to have a bad effect on the faculty's evaluation of their work.

The most familiar of these situations is the written examination.
These are relatively rare. A general examination in medicine (taken
by all clinical students and by all members of the house staff as well)
is given at the end of each school year. Written examinations are also
given in surgical specialties and in some of the minor lecture courses.

Also familiar, and probably of more importance in the faculty's
eyes, are the oral examinations which are given at the end of a student's time in each of the major departments during the third and
fourth years: medicine, pediatrics, and surgery in the third year, med-
cine and obstetrics and gynecology during the fourth year. In them,
several members of the department faculty (including men with
whom the student has had no close contact during his time in the
department) quiz a few students at a time on material covered in lectures, reading, and ward rounds. The department of medicine varies
this slightly by requiring students to submit complete summaries on
all patients assigned to them during the quarter; questioning is then
built up around these cases. Faculty members may choose their questions from a very wide range of subjects and can phrase them more
ambiguously than in a written test. They can also, if they wish, pursue
a subject about which a student appears to be ignorant or evasive,

KUMC 212	Name				Course or Service					
PICTURE	Class				Term					
	Final Course Evaluation 1. Superior ☐ 2. Satisfactory ☐ 3. Unsatisfactory ☐									

FUND OF INFORMATION	1	2	3	PERFORMANCE	1	2	3	CHARACTER	1	2	3
Fund of information.				Reliability				Rapport with patients			
Comprehension				Application & Initiative				Poise			
Problem Solving Ability				Judgment				Ethical Standards			
				Originality				Likeability			

Would you accept this student as a house officer or graduate student in your department?		1	2	3
	Probable success in medical school			
	Probable success as a physician			

[REVERSE]

Staff member having most contact with student:

Remarks: (Please comment on superior or unsatisfactory student)

Fig. 6 – STUDENT GRADE CARD.

or temper the wind to the ill-prepared student. The student thus is brought face to face with some of the most august and remote personages of the faculty, with the consequent possibility that his performance will be hampered by fear or by ignorance of their favorite ideas and topics.

Some classes are run in conventional academic style, and a kind of Socratic teaching method may be used. The staff member teaches by quizzing students over material he feels they should know, trying to elicit through his questioning the set of facts or line of argument he wishes the students to understand. Since these classes seldom contain more than fifteen students, none can avoid this kind of classroom questioning. The discussions take on something of the character of an oral examination. The staff member may ask questions over a wide range of material and can pursue an evasive or unprepared student until he is satisfied that he has got the point or will make sure to get it the next time.

Experience in the hospital provides the students with a great many other situations in which they must perform academically under the close scrutiny of the faculty. The most common are ward rounds, surgery, clinic, and the many occasions on which faculty informally discuss patients, disease, and treatment with students.

Ward rounds are most important in the course in medicine in the junior year but also occur occasionally on other hospital services. We describe rounds in medicine as being the most fully developed instance of the phenomenon. Ward rounds take place each weekday morning from nine until eleven. The students, residents, and intern go around with one of the physicians in charge of the service to see the patients under their care. Each patient has been assigned to one of the students, who is expected to know everything important there is to know about the patient's status and the course of his disease. The staff member may ask the student for the pertinent facts in the case and also for diagnoses and possible courses of treatment. The student is expected to have read thoroughly on the patient's disease and to know what an informed medical opinion about the case might be. Further, he is expected to have kept up to date on the patient's progress, in order to be able to make the best use of his knowledge about the disease.

The students' major responsibility during rounds, however, is the presentation of cases newly admitted to the hospital. When a patient is seen for the first time on ward rounds, the student to whom he has

been assigned is required to give a summary of what he has discovered in the history and physical examination. He is also required to
know the results and significance of any laboratory findings. Finally,
he is required to give a differential diagnosis of the patient's condition and to recommend treatment on the basis of this diagnosis. The
attending physician will typically make the presentation of a new
case the occasion for a combination lecture and quiz of the students
on the basic disease involved or some other relevant problem. These
discussions may be carried on at the patient's bedside, accompanied
by demonstration of important physical findings; or they may be carried on out in the hall, where the patient cannot hear the discussion.
In either case the student is, in effect, being examined, even though
he receives no formal grade. He can give the right answer to the staff
member's questions, or not; he can demonstrate knowledge of the
disease under discussion, or not; he can demonstrate that he has done
an adequate examination of the patient, or not.

During the time the student is on surgery, he undergoes similar ex-
amination-like proceedings in the operating room. He is required to
act as assistant in operations performed on his patients and, though
he seldom does important surgical procedures, he is often called on to
perform academically in much the same way he does on rounds in
medicine. The surgeon thinks of surgery as an excellent teaching situation and often quizzes the student in great detail on the anatomy of
the region being dissected, the diagnosis of the patient's disease and
the method by which the diagnosis was made, and the surgical treatment being undertaken.

Similarly, when students are in clinic, they examine patients and
arrive at tentative diagnoses and plans of treatment. They then discuss the case with a member of the staff, who may find errors in the
facts they have collected in the examination, in the diagnosis based on
those facts, or in the plan of treatment they prescribe. In presenting
a clinic case to a staff member, the student may reveal his ignorance
in crucial areas. The importance of this situation for the student may
be somewhat decreased by the fact that many of the staff members
he deals with are not on the full-time staff of the hospital and school
and thus are not in a position to penalize him much academically for
his errors.

In addition to these routine contacts with faculty, a student assigned to one of the hospital wards may occasionally find himself in
informal and unanticipated conversation with a staff member, fre-

quently about one of the patients for whom he is responsible. In the same way that he is quizzed on rounds, in surgery, or in the clinic, the student may be subjected to what is in effect an oral examination on the particular case and the medical knowledge related to it.

A final situation in which students must perform for the faculty and display their academic prowess is the Clinical Pathological Conference (CPC). This hour-long conference, held each Saturday at noon throughout the year, is attended by all students on the Kansas City campus of the medical school, by interns and residents, and by many of the hospital staff. Cases which presented difficult diagnostic problems and ended in the hospital for autopsy are presented. A group of seven or eight students taking senior medicine is held responsible for discussion of the case. Each such group has this responsibility for two or three weeks in a row. A protocol giving the essential facts in the case is distributed, both to the students responsible and to everyone else in the hospital, on the preceding Thursday. During CPC several of the students are required to get up and deliver discussions of the X rays, the laboratory findings, and the electrocardiogram, and one of them is required to give a detailed discussion and differential diagnosis of the case. They are then quizzed on these discussions at some length. Finally, the pathologist reports on the autopsy findings, thus revealing publicly the extent to which the student's diagnosis was correct. Even though the faculty may not conceive of CPC as an examination, there is a strong element of performance before influential superiors in it.

Students, then, face a series of school situations in which they are obliged to perform academically for the faculty. The faculty assesses a student's ability and the amount he has learned largely on the basis of these performances. It is possible, though it seldom happens, for a student to be dropped from the school because of poor performance in these situations. Students, in the face of this recurring set of ordeals, develop a perspective on this area of their school activities which may be summarized in the following statements:

1. The faculty can prevent any student from getting through school or, less extreme, can make his passage through school difficult and uncertain, if he gives evidence of not having done satisfactory work.

2. The faculty can humiliate and even degrade a student when he gives evidence of not having done satisfactory work.

3. It is necessary, therefore, to make a good impression on the

faculty — to present them with either the substance or the appearance of learning.

4. It is, however, very difficult to tell what will impress the faculty as real learning; their reactions cannot be predicted in any logical or simple way.

5. No simple method of making a good impression will suffice, therefore; it is necessary for the student to be sensitive to faculty demands and modify his behavior accordingly, even when these demands seem foolish or likely to nullify the purposes of medical school.

We believe that students held the view expressed in these propositions and, further, organized their behavior around it; we refer to it, as already noted, as the academic perspective.

We first developed the hypothesis that students held and acted on this perspective when we observed, on almost the first day of observation in the teaching hospital, the peculiarly docile behavior of the medical students and their eager fishing for a correct answer.

Went to Jones' seminar on fluids and dehydration this morning. Here are my impressions of the class. He teaches purely by asking questions and trying to tease out answers. For instance, "What is dehydration?" He calls on a student, who says something. "All right, but what's the matter with that?" Or, "What does that mean?" Or, "How does that work?" The students were getting off on all kinds of wrong tracks and he let them pursue these into the ground. In particular, they seemed to want to get off on exotic kinds of things — biochemical reactions, ions in the extracellular spaces, etc., — whereas the right answer turned out to be that dehydration decreased the volume of blood so that the patient goes into shock. In other words, they were being too fancy. But this did not become clear till almost the end of the hour; he had let them wander around all the rest of the time. Jones' teaching was, I thought, kindly but cruel; difficult for a student to cope with. After asking his initial question, he called on one fellow to answer and kept him on the pan for about ten minutes, pursuing him with Socratic questions. Finally he asked someone else and went through the same routine. The students frequently misunderstood these simple Socratic questions, which was the cause of much of their trouble. They were clearly bothered by this, didn't know what to make of it. Jones frequently made fairly nasty sarcastic remarks. Thus he asked one student about something and the student replied, "Well, I'm not so interested in the blood, I'm more interested in the extracellular fluids," about which he then made a few apparently incorrect statements. Jones said, "Well, I'm glad you are. Perhaps that will lead you to learn something about it one of these days." Or when a student made an incorrect biochemical statement Jones looked at him in awe and said, "Now where did you ever learn that?" "In biochemistry." "You did? Well, things must have changed a lot since I last looked at that stuff." And so on. They took it lying down.

(September, 1955.)

This incident caused us to ask, from the beginning of the study, what the students felt it was necessary to do in order to get along with the faculty and suggested that the answer ran along the lines of the credo presented above. We remained on the lookout for further evidence that this was the case.

Several kinds of student activities and statements express the academic perspective. Any incident having one or more of the characteristic features we now describe has been used in our later analysis of the evidence for the customary character of this perspective.

One expression of the perspective consists of student statements indicating a feeling that one must please the faculty in order to finish school or avoid the delay of repeating a course or a whole year, no matter what is required to please them.

A faculty member had done something the students resented very much, something that emphasized his power over them. I sat and listened to a discussion of what they could do about this. One of the students said, "One thing you have to understand is that most of us here will put up with just about anything if we really have to in order to get through. We've spent too much time getting this far to start being crusaders about something like that. Whether we like it or not, we have to put up with it and we do. I remember in college there were guys who practically got themselves completely ostracized because of some crusade or another that they would get mixed up in. One boy practically made a social outcast of himself by writing letters to the school paper about the fact that there was not enough school spirit on the campus. Well, maybe that kind of thing is all right in college, but when you get to medical school you have put in too much time already. We have too much invested to throw it all away for some idea like that. We can't afford to have ideals like that while here. Maybe after we get out of here we can do things like that, but right now we are just trying to get through and we will do anything that we really have to in order to get through." The other students nodded their heads in agreement.

(Junior Pediatrics. November, 1955.)

Such incidents indicate the generalized feeling of subordination coloring students' views of their relations with faculty.

Another expression of the perspective consists of incidents in which students reveal a fear of making a bad impression on the faculty because of the consequences in low grades or humiliation. Anxiety over examinations constitutes the most typical expression of this theme.

A couple of students were engaged in one of their favorite pastimes: discussing their own health. March said, "You know what? Last quarter when we had orals? Two days before mine I got so upset that I vomited. I really got sick. I could feel all of that stuff swirling around in my stomach and finally I gagged myself and threw up. Well, it looked to me like it was about three gallons." Pearson said, "That's funny. I vomited too the day before orals."

(Junior Surgery. December, 1955.)

But many other situations are similarly regarded as providing an opportunity to make a bad impression on the faculty: rounds, discussion classes, CPC, etc. In each of these students are likely to be asked questions, and a wrong answer will indicate to the faculty that one does not know what one ought to and thus may be the occasion for a public humiliation by the teacher (as in the first incident cited in this chapter) or may conceivably result in having to repeat a course.

On the way to class Morrison said, "Well, is everybody ready for the inquisition?" I said, "What's that?" He said, "A lecture by Dr. Penn. Has everybody read his lesson?" Dr. Penn typically taught by quizzing students over an assigned chapter in the textbook.

(Junior Surgery. January, 1956.)

Such casual comments as this reveal the way students interpret their contacts with the faculty as partaking (at least metaphorically) of the nature of the inquisition, with extreme penalties for improper answers.

Further indication of the prevalence of this attitude comes from our interviews with a random sample of medical students. We asked them, "Can you think of any particular thing about medical school that has been traumatic?" In asking this question, we hoped to elicit statements about cadavers, autopsies, first experiences with death, and other matters students are exposed to which laymen often consider traumatic. But the students' answers pointed in quite a different direction — to the trauma of those situations in which they might make a bad impression on faculty members. If we include in the category *examination* orals, rounds, and CPC as well as written exams, we get the data contained in Table XXVII.

TABLE XXVII

STUDENT RESPONSES TO QUESTION ON TRAUMA IN MEDICAL SCHOOL

RESPONSE	JUNIORS N 15		SENIORS N 14		TOTAL	
Examinations	13	(61%)	13	(59%)	26	(60%)
All other sources of trauma....	8	(39%)	9	(41%)	17	(40%)
Total	21	(100%)	22	(100%)	43°	(100%)

° The total of responses is greater than the number of students because some gave more than one response.

Fully three-fifths of the traumatic experiences reported have to do with situations in which the fear of making a bad impression on the faculty predominates.

Incidents in which students state that it is important to make a good impression on the faculty also illustrate use of the perspective.

I had been talking with a student about an incident in which an intern made a diagnosis the staff had missed. He said, "That's a wonderful way for a medical student to make a good impression on the staff — if he's the guy who comes up with the right thing. You can make a big impression on them if you make a real smart diagnosis that they miss. Of course, you don't get too much of a chance to do that around here because these guys are pretty smart. But I saw it happen with a guy in our class over at the VA hospital." He told a story of a student who had diagnosed a rare complaint the chief of surgery missed. He said, "You can bet they talked about that for a while." I said, "I'll bet they did." He said, "That's what I'd really like to do — pull something like that at CPC when my turn comes up. Get up and figure out the diagnosis that the whole staff here missed."

(Senior Surgical Specialties. October, 1956.)

Though students occasionally state the point in this direct fashion, much more frequently we infer the presence of such a belief from observations of students' attempts to make such an impression. These attempts take several forms. The most obvious consist of hard work directed toward acquiring knowledge which can be easily put on display for the faculty. In the following incident a student skips a meal to prepare a presentation that will make a good impression.

A resident came into the lab on the floor, where I was sitting with some students, and said, "Which one of you is Terry?" Terry identified himself and the resident said, "You've got a couple of cases of liver disease, haven't you?" Terry said, "Yes," and the resident said, "Well, the visiting staff member you'll be making rounds with this afternoon is particularly interested in that, so if you have those two cases ready to present I think it would be a good thing." Adams said, "All right." He didn't go to lunch, but stayed up on the floor working up his presentation of these cases.

(Junior Medicine. October, 1955.)

A second form of this attempt to make a good impression is more modest. Here the student believes that his best efforts to make a good impression will not avail, so the safest thing is to make as little impression as possible.

At lunch, the boys were talking about CPC — how many times they would be up for it, who would be assigned the difficult job of giving the differential diagnosis, etc. Crane said, "I know — I'm just not lucky. I'm going to get stuck with the differential three times in a row." Harrison said, "Just think what a wonderful opportunity that is to make a real impression on everyone and show them how smart you are. It really is, Tom." Crane said, "I don't want to make any impressions on anyone. I don't want anybody to know who I am. Dr. Lackluster — that's who I want to be. Just so long as I get out of here. I don't want anyone to know who I am. I'm not smart enough to do that thing right."

(Senior Surgical Specialties. October, 1956.)

Perhaps the most noticeable form of attempting to make a good impression is the use of trickery of various kinds to give the appearance of knowing what one thinks the faculty wants one to know or having done what the faculty wants done, even though these appearances are false.

I was discussing one of the faculty members with the students, a man who had been giving them a hard time on rounds. One student said, "You really learn how to handle these teachers. That's one thing you do learn, so that even if you don't know the answer you can get around them. We certainly learn that very well even if we don't learn anything else."

(Junior Medicine. February, 1957.)

The mildest and probably most frequent kind of trickery students employ consists of an attempt to get clues to the right answer from the staff member without disclosing one's real ignorance. Though this does not always have the desired result, as in the following example, students are apt to fall back on it when their only alternative is to say "I don't know."

One of the students was assigned to scrub in on a thyroidectomy and I went to surgery with him. The surgeon taught by reviewing the anatomy of the region he was dissecting, quizzing Small about various pieces of tissue he was working on. He asked Small the name of a particular thing he was working on. I forget the names that were involved in this interchange, but first Small gave one name and then another. He was very obviously looking for some small clue to tell him whether one or the other or neither of these answers was correct. And the surgeon did not give it to him; nor did the intern or resident. Anderson, the surgeon, kept Small hanging as he switched back and forth from one guess to the other. No matter what he said, Anderson would say, "Are you sure about that? Is that going to be your final answer?" And every time he did this, Small would back down and change again. Finally the resident said, "C'mon, you'll have to make up your mind sometime and stick by it. There's no sense trying to bluff." He seemed a good deal less good-natured about it than Anderson. Finally Anderson got an answer out of Small and then told him that it was wrong. (Junior Surgery. December, 1955.)

Students also occasionally attempt to get "illegal" clues to a right answer. For example, at CPC the students are supposed to make a differential diagnosis solely on the basis of the facts given them about the case. But they will frequently try to find house officers who were around when the case was in the hospital and who might give them some further information; they will try to reason from the kind of cases recently presented what kind of case the faculty might give them this time; they may try to find out what books the pathologist who will present the case has checked out of the library recently; and so on.

Similarly, students who have failed to perform some assignment will use "illegal" means to give the impression of having done it. This occurs particularly with examinations of patients and laboratory work to be done on patients.

The students were discussing a teacher who had given them a hard time about always getting lab work into the chart on time. Horn said, "He put a finger in my ribs one morning about that. I hadn't gotten the lab work in on a patient. Actually, by the time he told me to do it the main lab had already sent their results back." One of the other students said, "You could have just looked over their figures and interpolated." Horn said, "I did, but first I went around and drew some blood from the patient in case [the staff member] came and asked him."

(Senior Surgical Specialties. October, 1956.)

A final kind of attempt to make a good impression is by no means as docile as those we have so far considered. Students may band together to strike back at the faculty member who is making it difficult for them to be or appear knowledgeable by demonstrating to him that they "know more than he does." The following incident is one of the rare cases in which this occurred. Students do not ordinarily make such an attempt because of the work involved, the danger of it back-firing, and the possibility of making an enemy of the staff member in such a way that he will keep them from completing a course; it occurs only under extreme provocation.

I had just joined a group of students on one of the medical services. They told me there would be a lot of fireworks on rounds. There were not, but I was amazed by the amount of detailed information the students pos-sessed about their patients and their patients' diseases. At lunch, I com-plained to the students about the lack of fireworks and wanted to know what was so bad about Dr. Custer. They said he had probably behaved because I was along. Archer said, "Usually, he just kind of picks away at us — just keeps pushing away until he finds out something that you don't know that he thinks you ought to know, and then he really lets you have it. Now that's ridiculous, because it means that he ends up spending a lot of time on things that aren't very important for us." Barton said, "That's right. You heard this morning how when Tommy knew all the lab values on that patient, he asked what the lab values were six months ago. Now, what difference does that make to us? What's the sense of us memorizing all those lab values? He could be spending the time teaching us more im-portant things about the nature of the disease or how you diagnose it or how you treat it — things like that. But he gets carried away on these little points and just wants to show how much smarter he is than we are. . . . "

Crown said, "He's a no-good son of a bitch, too." Barton said, "You know, the first day we came on this service I was really pleased with him. I thought he did a really fine job of rounds — teaching us and taking us around. He really taught us a lot and I thought we were going to have a wonderful six weeks." Crown said, "Yeah! And then the second day you found out different, didn't you?" Archer said, "We sure did. He started in on us then and he hasn't let up since. . . . I remember how we came down to lunch the second day and we couldn't talk about anything else but how rotten it was going to be from now on, and we were right. . . . "

I said, "In other words you decided he was really out to get you. Is that it?" Barton said, "I'm afraid that's right." I said, "Well, have you decided on anything to do about it? How are you going to handle him?" Archer said, "We talked about it quite a bit and we decided just to slam it right back at him. If that's what he wants, that's what he'll get. If he wants us to memorize lab values for every day in the year, that's what we'll do. We may have to give up learning other things, but we'll learn what he thinks is important, and just give it to him. Just fix it so that he can't find anything to pick at us about. Just have the answer to every foolish question he asks right at our fingertips. Don't give him a chance to get at us at all. It's the only way we can protect ourselves. . . . "

Here are a couple of examples of the kind of tactics the students used in addition to memorizing a great deal of information [which they did]. Dr. Custer's manner did not seem very "malignant" to me, but it was clear that the students regarded it as such. Every question he asked was answered either with a very full and carefully qualified account of the facts and theories on the matter or else was answered with some very obsequious form of "I don't know," phrased in such a way that Custer would have a hard time pursuing the subject. For instance, Donaldson answered one question like this: "Well, sir, I'm afraid I don't know the answer to that question. Probably I should know it and I certainly will look it up right away, but I don't know it now. It's really an oversight on my part." This, of course, left Custer unable to pursue the subject, and a couple of times he looked as if he would like to, but couldn't think his way out of the verbal net Donaldson had thrown around him.

Another funny thing came up when they were talking about the use of some drug in treating some disease that one of the patients might have. Donaldson announced that something or other was a contraindication for use of this drug. Custer said that he had not heard of that before and was Donaldson sure about it? Donaldson smiled very politely and said, "Oh, yes sir. I just read it last night in Goodman and Gilman. They state very specifically that that is a contraindication but they don't give the mechanism and I'm sorry I can't tell you what the mechanism is. I should be able to but I can't." Custer said that ideas about these drugs had changed a lot and many of the precautions originally urged had been unnecessary. He ended by saying, "In fact, a lot of the information that is around on those drugs is archaic." Donaldson smiled again and said, "I'm sorry, sir, did I understand you to say that Goodman and Gilman's information was archaic?" Custer smiled and said, "That sounds like a wise-guy question to me." Donaldson stopped smiling and said, "No sir, I certainly didn't mean it that way. I'm very serious. Do you think that their information is outdated?" The resident pointed out that the book had been revised in 1955 and Custer finally backed down, saying he did not know enough about the subject to say one way or the other.

There were many such exchanges through the morning. Several of the students complimented Donaldson on his excellent handling of Custer.

(Junior Medicine. February, 1957.)

This last incident illustrates still another kind of expression of the perspective: cases in which students judge faculty according to how hard they are to get along with.

We have seen that students will expend effort in several directions in order to make a good impression on faculty members. The perspective is expressed in another form in those incidents where we see that students tend to work less hard when there is so little faculty pressure to do so that they cannot make an impression by working or when they consider the faculty to have so little to do with their academic fate as to not be worth bothering about.

Carson was debating whether or not to go to an operation he was assigned to scrub in on. He said, "There's really nothing to see. It's so boring. I just hate going up there. The only thing is I hate to think about them noticing me not being there. This is our last day on the service and I don't want to call any attention to myself, not that way." Parker said, "Oh, hell, they don't even notice. They don't know who the patients are assigned to. They don't know whose patient it is when they come into surgery." Carson decided not to bother.

Parker and Thompson, on this same service, had taken to going out to play golf several times a week, figuring that no one would miss them.

(Senior Surgical Specialties. October, 1957.)

The same phenomenon was noticed frequently when students had their training at hospitals away from the medical center. They felt that their teachers in these hospitals would not be able to make much trouble for them or would not particularly want to and relaxed accordingly.

Similarly, students are often at a loss as to what to do because a staff member has not made his wishes clear, even though their assignment is such that they do not ostensibly need any expression of his preference. This is seen most clearly where a faculty member gives a student a very open question or unstructured assignment and the student tries to get more specific directions before responding. It is perhaps seen most frequently in psychiatry where the staff's approach makes it almost inevitable that students trying to find a way to please will not be able to discover one.

I asked a student what he got out of the psychiatric supervisory hours, in which students discussed their cases with a staff psychiatrist. He said, "Not very much, I'll tell you that. In fact, I find them completely confusing. I really don't know what she wants."

(Senior Psychiatry. February, 1956.)

Earlier observation of a supervisory hour with this student led to the observer recording the following impressions:

The psychiatrist does not respond to the overt meaning of what the student says. Instead he responds to what he thinks is the underlying meaning, usually some unconscious tendency to avoid painful topics, or some naïve and possibly disastrous oversimplification of what he has been told. Or the psychiatrist anticipates the likely meaning of something the student has started to say and responds to that. The student, on the other hand, wants to get through the hour as painlessly, with as little embarrassment, as possible. To do this he wants to do anything within reason that he knows how to do that will satisfy the psychiatrist. But he tends to think in concrete and immediate terms, the way he thinks about physical disease, and this simply does not mesh with the way the psychiatrist does business. For example, the student wants to put things into classifications and so he depends a great deal on the typologies of mental disease offered to him and wants to classify his patients as paranoid or schizophrenic or whatnot. The psychiatrist wants him to get away from these and use his understanding on the individual case. The student might be willing to do this if he knew how, but he doesn't.

This is what went on in this supervisory hour. For instance, the student wanted to know if his patient could be classified as a compulsive or a schizophrenic. The psychiatrist responded to this as a quest for a certainty on his part and, instead of answering the question, began to talk about the way these classifications were really not useful at all. The student kept trying to create the impression that he was trying to do what the psychiatrist had told him. For example, he said over and over again that he had followed directions and had not exerted any influence on the course of his patient's conversation, but had simply allowed her to talk.

(Senior Psychiatry. February, 1956.)

In these and similar situations in other departments, students will devote great effort to finding out just what is required in order to perform properly from the faculty's point of view. We see here the analogue in the clinical years of the freshmen's difficulties with faculty admonitions to "learn as much as you can" or "work to your own capacity." In both cases, students believe that the faculty do have something specific in mind and do not want to commit themselves without finding out what that something is; any other course of action would only waste time. Whether it be a matter of finding out what will pass muster on examination by quizzing the faculty about the kinds of answers that will be acceptable or of finding out what will constitute a passable senior paper, students attempt to learn what is required before they respond to faculty directives. Though examples from psychiatry are clearest, many other teachers' pedagogical style raises the same difficulties:

The way Dr. Bell ran the class was largely by asking questions of the kind I have heard students refer to as "What am I thinking of?" questions. For example, he asked if there was any particular syndrome they had ever heard of that could produce this particular set of symptoms. One of the boys said it sounded like Leriche's syndrome, which was the right answer. Here is a good example of the kind of questioning that went on. He said, "What are some of the signs you would find if the patient had this disease?" The students suggested a number of things: diminishing of the peripheral pulses, pallor of the extremities, lowering of the skin temperature, etc. To each of these Dr. Bell said, in effect, "Yes, that might be one of the things you would find, but what else?" And in each case it was clear that although these things were perfectly reasonable answers to his questions they were not the answers he was looking for. The students seemed very unhappy with this and he finally had to bring out the point he was after himself.

In the midst of one of these guessing games, one of the students smiled at Bell and said, "We're not getting the answer you want, are we?" This threw Bell a little. He said, "Well, you're giving very good answers. But no, it's not quite the thing I had in mind."

(Junior Medicine. January, 1957.)

We have seen in the earlier incident involving Dr. Custer how students tend to judge faculty members according to how well they treat students, that is, according to how little they take advantage of their opportunity to embarrass or humiliate students. All observations of students using this criterion to judge or describe faculty members can be interpreted as expressions of the academic perspective, since the use of such a criterion implies acceptance of the belief that faculty members have it within their power to be "nice" to students or not as the fancy takes them. Such observations include instances of students describing teachers according to this criterion, complaining about or praising teachers with reference to this criterion, horror stories of particularly vicious teachers, and so on.

The lecturer said in a very nasty voice, "What's the matter, doctor?" No one knew who he was speaking to. He said, "You back there, doctor, what's the matter?" One of the students, who had been looking at him all the time, said, "Me?" The lecturer said, "No, not you, the doctor next to you. What's your name, doctor?" The fellow had been looking at the schedule. He looked up and said, "Martin." The lecturer said, "Well, what is it, Dr. Martin, am I boring you? You seem to be sleepy." Martin said, "No, sir, I was just looking at the schedule." The lecturer said, "I see, it looked to me like you were falling asleep. O.K., doctor." After it was over, I said to Morrison, "Gee, I was surprised by the way he sounded." Morrison said, "He sure was malignant, wasn't he? He sounded like a grade five to me."

(Junior Surgery. December, 1955.)

(This use of tumor classifications to categorize faculty members — from benign through several grades of malignancy — is quite common among students.)

It is worth noting that the students pass the word about teachers in just these terms, describing teachers to one another according to how well or badly they treat students. This practice not only creates reputations for teachers but teaches students to use this criterion for judging them; gossip, in addition to passing along facts, imparts the perspective according to which those facts are important.

One sophomore said to me, "We saw Dr. Parker in action last week. He's tough." The other sophomore with us looked interested, as though he hadn't heard any of this before. The first student went on: "Everybody knows that Parker is the toughest one around. You really have to toe the line with him. . . . You're expected to know everything that's in the patient's chart, without looking at it. Say if it's October 26, he's likely to ask you what medication the patient received at what times and what dosage on October 12, and you'd have to know it. If you don't he really chews you out. He's really tough, that's the guy you really ought to watch. . . . You know Harmon [a junior student]? Harmon was telling me that he only got two hours' sleep the other night." The other guy said, "Two hours' sleep?" "Yeah, they called him up some time in the middle of the night, and he had to come over and see a patient and write up the case history and do a physical examination and do all that lab work and everything and have it ready for Parker in the morning."

(Sophomore Class. 1955.)

Finally, we see the perspective expressed when students reveal that they consider faculty actions difficult or impossible to understand and predict; that they consider it possible, perhaps even likely, that the faculty will act capriciously; that they consider it possible that the faculty will act maliciously or in ways that will gratuitously penalize a well-meaning and hard-working student. This theme appears in various forms. Students may attribute their difficulties with a female faculty member to irritability produced by her menstrual cycle. They may be provoked by the "unfairness" of unannounced examinations. They may complain that the examinations given are graded in an arbitrary way. They may suspect that faculty members will deliberately trip them up in examinations by asking hard questions to which they cannot "rightfully" be expected to know the answers.

Ireland was furious about being given an unsatisfactory grade on an examination. He really was having a temper tantrum. He said, "I am really furious with those people. Who do they think they are, telling me that my paper was unsatisfactory? Those questions don't have any right answer. Any fool knows that."

(Senior Medicine. March, 1956.)

Perhaps the neatest indication of the students' view of faculty as capricious and unpredictable can be found in their discussions of how students are chosen to give the differential diagnosis at CPC. Out of each group of seven or eight students assigned to CPC only two or three will be given this harrowing task. The heavily magical character of these discussions indicates that students cannot see any logic in the choices made.

Carter was talking about CPC. He said, "I saw Carney the other day. I told him I heard a rumor that Williams was going to pick him to give the discussion at CPC this week. His group is up. Boy, did he look scared." Harrison said, "I'll bet Williams does pick him, too." Grant said, "No, he won't. He'll pick Trout." They discussed this for some time. Finally, I said, "What makes you think he's going to pick either one of those guys?" Carter said, "Well, Carney is kind of short and I think Williams would like to give him the business. He's just the kind that Williams would like to do that to." Grant had some equally idiotic reason for thinking Williams would pick the other one. I finally said, "Well, that sounds very logical. I really would like to know how he picks them though, wouldn't you?" Carter said, "You bet I would like to know. I just know he's going to pick me when it's my turn. I'm just the type he likes to get his hooks into."

(Senior Surgical Specialties. October, 1956.)

All these kinds of observations, taken together, present the student's picture of themselves as at the mercy of a capricious and unpredictable faculty which can, at its discretion, impede or halt their progress toward a medical degree and which, therefore, must always be presented with the best impression possible of the student's abilities and knowledge, however this impression be made. Further, we see that students act in accordance with these premises, endeavoring to make good impressions and avoid making bad impressions.

Two provisos are in order. First of all, there is more to the students' picture of the faculty than this. This chapter is devoted to but one aspect of the teacher-student relationship: The teacher as examiner, disciplinarian, and controller of the students' academic fate. The students have, in other contexts, the highest regard for their teachers.

Second, although we have presented some extreme cases as examples, such violent expressions of the perspective as revolts against the faculty or acts of outright cheating are rare. Students express the perspective most bluntly and aggressively, furthermore, when the faculty are not present. The most common kinds of action attributable to this perspective are those which take place in the presence of a faculty member and consist in the students' routine efforts to discover what is on his mind and shape answers to fit this for the daily ordeals of rounds, surgery, and quizzes.

Accepting incidents of the kind described as individual instances of the expression of the academic perspective, we can now turn to evidence that this perspective is widespread and in common use, that it is accepted among students as reasonable and legitimate to view things in this way and act accordingly. First of all, we note that observations acceptable as evidence for this proposition were made in seventeen of the eighteen services on which students spent time during their clinical years. (The one exception, the Emergency Room, is easily accounted for by the fact that no faculty member holds the students responsible for their work in Emergency; such authority as is exerted is in the hands of an intern.) From this we conclude that this perspective was not confined to any one part of the hospital and was not simply a reaction to one or two unusual situations or personalities.

We note further that our field notes yield a total of one hundred and seventy-five items of evidence. Applying the same reasoning used previously and considering that we observed only a few students at a time, it is clear that the actual number of such instances occurring which we were not able to observe must have been considerably higher. This supports the conclusion that student use of the academic perspective was a commonplace feature of hospital life.

Finally, Table XXVIII emphasizes two characteristics of our evidence which make it likely that we have correctly described an operating reality in school life. First, only two out of the one hundred and seventy-five items of evidence were in any sense directed by the observer; that is, two represent a response in which the ideas we attribute to students were suggested by the observer and only assented to by the student, rather than being volunteered by the student as in the other instances. Second, in 77 per cent of the observed items of evidence the observer participated only as a bystander, and these

TABLE XXVIII

EVIDENCE FOR THE EXISTENCE OF THE ACADEMIC PERSPECTIVE

		VOLUNTEERED	DIRECTED BY THE OBSERVER	TOTAL
Statements	To observer alone........	40 (23%)	2 (100%)	42
	To others in everyday conversations	84 (48%)	– –	84
Activities	Individual	19 (11%)	– –	19
	Group	30 (17%)	– –	30
	Total	173 (99%)	2 (100%)	175

may be fairly considered to be events which would have been equally likely to occur had the observer not been present. Sixty-five per cent of the items involve interaction among students such that if the perspective were not commonly accepted as publicly legitimate other students present might have disputed its expression; no such disputation was observed.

We must now consider the six items of negative evidence found in our field notes. Although these negative cases do not cause us to give up our proposition that the perspective we describe was commonly held, they do indicate that it was not held with complete uniformity. Four of these incidents consist of students stating or implying by their actions that it is all right to answer questions in what seems the most logical and sensible fashion even though one runs the risk of creating an impression of ignorance. One incident described a student who gave the observer the impression of being much more interested in the subject matter of a problem he was discussing with faculty than in the impression he might be making. The final negative instance consisted of a denunciation of many of the premises of the perspective:

A student asked how I was enjoying the field work. I said, "It's a lot of fun. I have all the fun of being a medical student and none of the responsibilities. Just once in a while I get stuck when somebody doesn't know who I am and asks me a question." He said, "Well, I imagine you do as well as a lot of us with some of these questions where we just don't know the answers. You couldn't know any less." I said, "I haven't quite picked up the trick of answering a question when I don't know the answer, which a lot of people around here seem to be able to do." He said, "You mean talking in generalities without quite getting down to the point." I said, "Yes, most of you people seem to have that down to a fine art." He said, "I don't think it's such a fine art. We get caught at it too many times. In fact, I just don't do it anymore." I said, "It must have worked out sometimes because people keep on doing it." He said, "Maybe before, but it doesn't work here. Were you at that lecture the day the fellow got caught talking about dehydration? Dr. Crane asked him to define dehydration and he wasn't sure. So he kept talking in generalities and saying more and more things and everything he brought up, Crane would ask him about. I guess he figured he had a right to because the student had brought it up. He had him going for about half an hour." I said, "I suppose a lot of people learned their lesson from that." He said, "It certainly convinced me that it was smarter to keep my mouth shut and never volunteer anything, because if you don't know you're sure to get caught."

(Junior Surgery. January, 1956.)

The evidence of our field notes thus demonstrates that students customarily made use of the academic perspective. Instances of its use appear frequently and are spread throughout the many services on which we made our observations. In only two of these instances did the observer suggest use of the perspective to the students and in the majority of instances students were observed using the perspective in interaction with one another, so that we may conclude that they regarded its use as legitimate.

The most obvious consequence of the existence of the academic perspective is what appears to the faculty to be a serious misdirection of student effort. Students spend much energy in learning things for what the faculty consider a totally wrong and misguided reason: to please the faculty and thereby get through school. Students using this perspective, when placed in a situation that has the quality of an examination in which they may make a bad impression on the faculty, show no interest in learning the material they are dealing with for its own sake and concentrate instead on doing whatever is necessary to make a good impression.

We will see later that the faculty, although occasionally recognizing the motives that lead students to act this way, probably deplore the existence of this perspective and wish that students would be more "mature" and ignore the situational pressures that appear to make it necessary to concentrate on making a good impression. But, as in the case of the experience and responsibility perspectives, it should be remembered that the academic perspective at least makes it possible for students to deal with a problematic situation which might otherwise throw them into an incapacitating panic. Though this perspective is not the only one students could develop, and others might more nearly approach what the faculty would like to see among students, it provides a basis for sustained action and so prevents disorganized behavior among the students.

As in the case of the responsibility and experience perspectives, the fact that the perspective is held collectively has the consequence of providing a set of social supports for the individual student as he engages in behavior that runs counter to faculty expectations. The knowledge that his associates think and act in the same way strengthens any individual student's determination to do what the perspective specifies as necessary to get through school.

Since most contemporary schools share with the medical school the characteristic combination of teaching and examining functions in the faculty, we may expect that the academic perspective or some variant will be a ubiquitous feature of educational institutions. Insofar as faculty members have some influence on the fate of students beyond the fact that what a student learns in school may affect his life in some way, insofar as the faculty can hurt students by giving low grades or bad recommendations, we may expect that students will respond by attempting first of all to impress the faculty with what they have learned. Teachers quite commonly complain about this, as did the faculty of the medical school, but they should realize that it is probably an inevitable, though unintended, consequence of the power they wield over students through the use of examinations and grades.

Chapter 15

Student Co-operation

STUDENTS are bound together by ties of many kinds: those of friendship, those of class, race or ethnic background, those of home town or college. In this chapter, however, we consider how students are bound to each other by their common role of student with its attendant obligations and difficulties. In particular, we are concerned with the groups of students assigned together to a particular hospital service, sharing work and a faculty "boss."

Relations in these work groups pose several kinds of problems for students as they pursue their twin goals of gaining experience and responsibility while simultaneously attempting to make a good impression on the faculty. These problems grow, although not completely, out of the school situation which faces the students. In dealing with them, students develop a collective perspective covering the areas in which these problems arise.

First of all, students are assigned some work for which they are, in a sense, collectively responsible. A certain set of tasks must be done and some limited group of students shares the responsibility of seeing that it gets done. Even though smaller units of the work are assigned to individual students in various ways, the entire group is responsible for the entire task, so that what one person does not do must be done by another. The faculty never formally proclaims a dogma of collective responsibility, but students believe that if the entire task is not completed the faculty will be angry with the entire group involved.

The most important of these shared work situations arises in the clinics, where patients come for examination and treatment. They wait their turn to be seen by students. All patients who have appointments for a given half-day clinic session must be seen during that period. Though clinic personnel attempt to make appointments with no more people than can be reasonably handled, it often happens that there is more than enough work for the students to do. Some patients require extensive work-ups and others pose problems about which the student needs lengthy consultation. The workload is apparently calculated for a full complement of students working at top efficiency, but unforeseen contingencies may make it heavier than anticipated. The important point is that this workload, be it heavy or light, must be handled by the students assigned to the clinic. If one student should be absent or not work hard, the others will be faced with an even heavier load. When students share responsibility for a task in this way, they face the possibility that some student will "goldbrick" and thus increase everyone's workload.

A similarly shared work situation, though the pressures are not as great, exists on the hospital wards where students serve their clinical clerkships. Here the students assigned to a particular service share the responsibility for preparing the complete work-up — history, physical examination, and diagnosis — of each patient assigned to that service. Though every service has established routines for allocating patients to students designed to spread the workload in an equal way, there are always ambiguous situations in which it is not clear who is to work-up a patient or in which the established routine appears to create inequities. A lazy or unscrupulous student can try to manipulate ambiguities in the rules to lighten his own workload. Again, the total amount of work is the responsibility of the entire student group assigned to the service. Work that one student shirks or gets out of must be done by another. These problems of equitably sharing work for which an entire group is responsible constitute a major focus for the development of collective perspectives on relations among students in work situations.

A second focus for the development of a perspective is found in certain assignments which, although individually set, have possible consequences for all. Particularly, any assignment which specifies no maximum amount of work, though each student is held individually responsible for the work, creates the possibility that the student who does the most work will in so doing set a standard against which the faculty will judge all other students. A great variety of situations create this problem. A faculty member may suggest that students read up on a particular disease; the student who, out of a desire to make a good impression or because of genuine interest, reads more than any other student sets a standard with which the others may be invidiously compared. A student who puts a very lengthy history into a patient's hospital record may also be setting a difficult standard to meet, as may the student who includes a great number of possibilities in his differential diagnosis of a patient's disease.

A final focus for the development of a collective perspective on student relations consists of a variety of small problems which may be eased by student co-operation. These problems may arise out of school interests or out of the impingement of outside interests on school activities. For example, a student's outside activities may make him want to shift his night call assignment to some more convenient night; another student who also wants to shift or who is indifferent can switch with him. In addition to these matters of convenience, students may help one another avoid making a bad impression on the faculty by covering up for a student who has done something wrong, by checking into situations in which an associate appears to be having psychological or financial difficulties, and so on. Finally, a great deal of studying and learning occur through informal student contacts. Students may quiz each other on material they feel they should know. They may trade patients with one another so that a student will get a patient who has some disease he is anxious to observe at first hand. In a variety of ways, they may help one another through the daily routine of learning, doing, and dealing with the faculty, and may create problems for one another by failing to help.

Thus, the relations of students with each other produce problems. In facing them, students develop a perspective on this aspect of their school activities. This collective perspective may be summarized in the following set of rules and beliefs:

1. In situations in which responsibility for an assignment is shared by a group of students, every student must do his fair share of the work when he is able.

2. In situations in which one student's efforts may set a standard difficult for others to achieve, collective agreement about the amount of work to be done should be reached and abided by.

3. Collective limitation of work applies only to those activities in which the faculty sets a quantitatively undefined goal, in which the results of different students can be compared by the faculty, and in which limitation would not reduce the amount of

learning of facts and procedures the student thinks necessary for medical practice.

4. Students should co-operate as far as possible to make school assignments more convenient to carry out, in learning medical information and procedures, and in helping fellow students avoid making a bad impression on the faculty.

We believe that students held the view expressed in these propositions and organized their behavior around it. The perspective can conveniently be referred to as the "student co-operation" perspective.

The material we present on this perspective will in some ways suggest a characterization of these student groups, although not definitely demonstrating it. Briefly, student work groups are formed by faculty fiat rather than student choice; students are assigned to them according to an impersonal scheme which takes little or no account of any personal preferences students may have for certain work associates. The members of these groups hold the beliefs described about the virtue and necessity of student co-operation and on that basis work out specific modes of co-operation appropriate to the particular work situation in which they find themselves. Because the administration typically assigns students to a group on an alphabetical basis, a single group may remain together through several changes of service; if the whole group is disrupted, some nucleus of it will probably find themselves together in the new arrangement. Though students cannot carry specific patterns of co-operation with them when they move from one service to another, some co-operative measures — how, for instance, to deal with the problem of allocating patients in a clinic — have wide applicability. A group which stays together also becomes aware of the peculiarities of individual members and learns what particular measures may be required to deal with deviants or with members whose personal problems or situations require special modes of co-operation from others. Thus an "old" group will co-operate more readily, with less necessity for discussion and conscious working out of plans, than will a group newly constituted. Nevertheless, the new group will soon have patterns of co-operative activity.

A check of our field notes reveals no one incident to which our first interest in this hypothesis can be traced, although a memorandum written after two months of field work reveals some concern with it: "As students, they are faced with the problem of setting reasonable limits to the boundless task they are presented with, and of establishing informal co-operation to ease the strain. The way they do this, and the degree to which it continues through the clinical years, deserve study." Apparently, though we were aware of the problem early, we took it for granted and made little effort to explore it, simply recording in our field notes such evidences of student co-operation or lack of it as we observed. A reawakening of a conscious interest in the problem came with the second year of field work, when study of the freshman class indicated the importance of this theme in their lives and suggested a closer look at it in the clinical years. In the remaining time in the field we made a more conscious effort to gather material on student co-operation, but the hypothesis in its present form was not developed until we were long out of the field.

Many kinds of observations we made contain expressions of the student co-operation perspective. Incidents having the characteristic features we now describe have been used in our later analysis of evidence for the customary character of this perspective.

One expression of the perspective consists of student discussions in which an attempt is made to allocate work on the hospital wards or in the clinic in some equitable fashion. Every time a group of students moved to a new service they engaged in long and detailed discussion of how they could adjust the new work assignment so as to provide a fair amount of work for each member. We refrain from citing such an extended example and instead present an incident in which students decide how to allocate new patients coming in to the hospital when other contingencies have produced inequities:

Dearborn and Martin were talking about who would take the two new patients who were coming in and about who would do the blood counts on them. Martin said, "Well, I'll tell you, Harry, seeing that I have two new patients coming in, I'll let you do the blood counts." Harry said, "Now wait a minute, Jack, how many patients do you have now? After all, we've been here getting patients for over a week while you were over at Psychiatry." Jack said, "I only have two patients now." Harry said, "Well, I have three." Martin agreed that this being the case he should do the work.

(Junior Pediatrics. November, 1955.)

Disagreements were sometimes less amicably settled, although the norm of fair division of the work was brought into play:

There was some discussion between Parsons and Anderson about a patient named Green. Parsons said that Green had been assigned to him as a new patient but he didn't think he should get him as a new patient. He thought that whoever was up for an "old patient" (i.e., a patient referred from elsewhere in the hospital with an established diagnosis) should get him and that was Anderson. Anderson objected, saying that he had more than his share of patients already. They argued back and forth about this and finally had to go to the resident for a decision.

(Junior Surgery. January, 1956.)

Once some agreement has been reached about the proper allocation of work among the members of a group, they are expected to abide by it and not use subterfuges to avoid their share and thus increase the work of other members. We also see as expressing the perspective all items in our field notes in which this norm is seen operating, but in our later tabulations this seriously underestimates the force of the norm. When students do abide by this rule, there is no outward evidence of it except the fact that they get their work done, which they might well do for other reasons. Therefore, our evidence on this point consists largely of instances of deviance, where other students complain that a student has violated this norm. For example, this norm operates most clearly in the clinic where the students feel that they must remain until all patients have been seen, so that the absence of one man shifts his workload on to the shoulders of his colleagues. Though we find an instance or two of a man showing up for clinic when he does not feel well and has stayed home instead of attending his other classes, most of our material consists of complaints about those few men who systematically violated the rule:

The boys complained a lot about Noland, particularly about the fact that, according to them, he seldom shows up for clinic. Wilder said that Noland comes and sits over in the delivery suite half the time he's in school and never shows up at clinic at all, which makes it harder on the other guys because they get that many more patients per man. I asked Morgan why everyone complained about Noland so and he said, "Clarence has just been goofing off on this service. He really has. . . . He goofs off in clinic and makes it hard on the rest of us, so we resent it."

(Senior Obstetrics. May, 1957.)

Obviously, such an incident must be viewed in two ways. Noland's failure to do his share is a negative instance of our proposition that students customarily use the co-operation perspective, an instance in which a student does not abide by the agreements about student co-operation which we assert exist. On the other hand, the reaction of Noland's colleagues constitutes an important verification of the proposition. (We consider the negative cases to our proposition later.)

We also see students organizing their relations along the lines sug-

gested by the student co-operation perspective where they are observed to limit their activities collectively when one person's efforts
might set a quantitatively high standard others would have difficulty
meeting. Such collective limitation of effort covered a wide range of
activities; for example, students often were confused as to how long
and detailed a medical history they should take on their patients, and
their casual conversations about this problem had the effect of creating a standard of length:

Chalmers had to write up a history he had just taken. We went down to
the student lab. Sawyer was there and Chalmers showed him his rough
version of the history, which he was going to copy out in ink. He said,
"Look at this, the history of the present illness takes up about four pages.
Isn't that something? I can't seem to get them any shorter." Another student said, "I think my trouble is I don't write big enough. I write so small
that my histories never take up much room."

(Junior Surgery. January, 1956.)

In the same way, students might agree not to get a given assignment
done before an agreed time:

Wanting to plan my time in the field, I asked the boys whether there would
be anything going on over the weekend on the service they had just started
on. Horn said, "I guess not. We've each got a patient to work up and we
might get new patients by Monday, but still I don't think I'll work mine
up till Monday morning. It looks like we'll have plenty of time then. No
sense hurrying through it now. There'll be plenty of time on Monday to
get all the patients worked up." All the boys agreed that they would not
work up their patients until Monday.

(Orthopedics. September, 1956.)

Toward the end of our field work we seized the opportunity to make
a detailed and systematic check of our hypothesis. In this case, we
were able to get an all-around, detailed view of something we had
only seen in parts: the process through which limitation of work effort was collectively arrived at:

While we were waiting for rounds to start, Heller said, "Say, what about
these case summaries we are supposed to turn in?" [The students were
required, on this service, to turn in elaborate summaries of each case assigned to them, including their own findings from the history and physical
examination, important laboratory findings, a discussion of the possible
causes for these findings, references to relevant literature, and a discussion
of modes of possible treatment.] Oliver said, "Just how many of those do
we have to turn in anyway? Do you have to have them on every single

patient you've had?" Larson said, "I guess so." Oliver said, "I'll tell you what I'm going to do. I'm not going to turn in any on some of those crocks I've had." [A "crock" is a patient with vague and untreatable psychosomatic complaints, but no discernible physical pathology.] He said, "And I'm not going to turn in any on patients that belong to any of the staffmen except the ones that teach us. . . ." Larson said, "Yeah, I don't think we ought to have to write them up on patients of other doctors." Another guy agreed with this and still another repeated that they shouldn't bother to write them up on crocks either. Later in the day, I asked Hart, "Are you going to write up a case summary on every patient you've had?" He said, "Well, just about. Of course, not all cases lend themselves to being described in that form equally well. For example, if you had a patient with a broken leg, and I have had one like that, there isn't any question about making a differential diagnosis on anything like that — so the whole form is kind of silly for people like that." I said, "Are you just going to leave them out?" He said, "I think I will."

The students all brought their completed summaries to school the next day. While we were waiting for rounds to start, I asked Lord how many summaries he had. He said, "Five." I said, "Is that all the patients you've had?" He said, "Oh, no. I've had more than that, but I didn't do any of the patients that belonged to other doctors, and then there were a couple of crocks I'm not going to turn in either. I wouldn't even know how to write them up on that sheet, and it just wouldn't make any difference anyway." I said, "Who told you you didn't have to turn them in?" He smiled and said, "Well, we were sort of talking about it. . . . There just wouldn't be any sense in doing it." The next guy I asked was Heller. I asked him how many case summaries he was turning in and he said seven. I asked him if that was all the patients he had and he said, "No, I've had more than that, but I didn't bother to write them all up. I had a couple of crocks who didn't have anything the matter with them at all, so I didn't bother to try and make a differential diagnosis on them. I just forgot about those, and then I had a patient with a fracture and of course that's not a problem of diagnosis either, so I kind of forgot that one too." I said, "Who told you you didn't have to hand those in?" He said, "I don't know. Nobody did — it just doesn't make sense, does it? I mean, why would I write up the fracture case? There isn't anything else it might be. We were talking about it and sort of decided there wasn't any sense in handing those in."

Later in the morning I asked Larson how many case summaries he had prepared and he said seven or eight. I asked him if that was all the patients he had had and he said no, he had some more but had not written them all up, especially the crocks — he had just left them out. He said the fellows had been talking about it and he had decided that was the sensible thing to do.

Still later I overheard Oliver and Hart talking. Oliver asked Hart how many summaries he had. Hart said, "Ten. I didn't put all the cases in. I didn't put the crocks in and some other things that just didn't fit. And there were some patients that belonged to other doctors that I didn't use either." Oliver said, "Gee, I've got ten too. I didn't hand in any of those kind either."

I got around to Miller, the last man in the group, the next morning. I asked him how many summaries he had and he said, "Not as many as there ought to be." I said, "What do you mean?" He said, "Well, I haven't prepared one on every patient I've had while I've been here. That's for sure." I said, "Oh, which ones did you leave out?" He said, "Well, I had a patient who had an earache — otitis media — I didn't bother with that one. And there were a couple of crocks and some I just didn't get finished, that's all."

At coffee that morning there was quite a conversation about the case summaries. Someone said they noticed that Lord had not turned in very many. He said he only turned in five. Each of the others told how many he had turned in (the figures agreed with what they had told me earlier). They began talking about which ones they left out and all agreed that they had left out crocks, patients belonging to other doctors, and patients with simple diseases that did not present any diagnostic problems or things like broken bones.

(Junior Medicine. January, 1957.)

This detailed account illustrates clearly the way students arrived at collective definitions of a proper workload and also suggests that student culture operates in somewhat veiled ways, so that students sometimes may feel they have arrived at a decision of this kind on their own when in fact the decision was made by the group.

We see the student co-operation perspective at work when students co-operate to make each other's work easier, more educational, or less likely to make a bad impression on the faculty, or when their discussions indicate that they feel this is the proper way for a student to behave. Students frequently co-operated in rearranging their assignments so as to be more convenient. For instance, a man might agree to trade nights on call with another man for whom this would prove personally convenient. The following conversation is typical of the kind that eventuates in such deals.

At coffee, some of the juniors were talking about the preceptorships they would have next year. One of them said he wanted to be located near Kansas City, so that he would be able to see his wife once in a while. He said, "If anyone gets near Prairie Village, I'll trade with them." Another guy said, "I'd like to get located near Great Bend. My wife's relatives live about twenty miles from there and I'd like to trade with someone to get near there."

(Junior Surgery. January, 1956.)

Similarly, students co-operate by passing on tips on how to safely cut down one's work through technical finagling:

Watson said that Brush had invented a one test tube complete blood count (CBC) and showed it to him and taught all the other guys in the group how to do it. He said the great thing was that it only required one test tube full of blood and many fewer operations to get done.

When I walked by the lab later, I saw Brush in there and went in. He was finishing up a urinalysis. I said, "Say, Buddy, I hear you've invented a brand new quick way of doing a CBC." He said, "Oh, yes, I've been doing that quite a while now." He explained the technique and added, "The whole thing is done in sixty seconds — it's really a whole lot easier and isn't cutting corners too badly. Besides, if there's anything really serious they send it down to the main lab anyway and they do it the right way, so what's the difference?"

(Senior Obstetrics. May, 1956.)

Students also co-operate to provide learning opportunities for each other. One form of this we find in our field notes is the informal teaching session, in which one student plays teacher for another in a subject he has more knowledge of and so helps him prepare for a similar quizzing by the faculty:

The main topic of conversation at lunch was Mr. Brubaker, a patient we had seen on rounds that morning. Bennett, whose patient Brubaker was, said that he was at an absolute loss to figure out what the matter was with this guy. He certainly didn't know what the original disease was, but he thought that Brubaker must have had a myocardial infarction later on. By this time Turner had joined us and said he didn't think it was an infarction, he thought it was an aneurism. They argued back and forth about this and finally Turner said, "Well, what are you going to do for him, anyway?" Bennett said, "I don't know, I haven't got any idea what they are going to do for him." Turner said, "Well, don't you have a plan? Are you just going to sit around and wait and let him get sick and stay sick?" Turner more or less took the role of the staff member at rounds and really quizzed Bennett.

(Junior Medicine. October, 1955.)

In the course of such a conversation the more knowledgeable student will pass on a great deal of information. Students also help each other to learn by trading patients in order to let a fellow student get a more varied experience or by giving up their own opportunities to "do things" for another student who has had less such experience.

One of the guys came down to see the two students with whom I was spending the day in the Emergency Room. He said that he had a minute or two off and came down to see whether we had saved any lives or not. He asked Wright how many lacerations had been in and Jerry said he had sewn up two and John had sewn up one, and that he hoped more would come in. He would let John do them because he (Jerry) had had a lot more experience with that, working in various hospitals around town.

(Senior Surgical Specialties. November, 1956.)

Students, finally, co-operate with one another in order to help a colleague avoid making a bad impression on the faculty. They will, for instance, do another man's work for him when circumstances make it impossible for him to do it himself; in this way they protect him from the adverse judgment the faculty would otherwise make:

We were finishing up the morning in clinic and someone noticed that there was still a chart in Lloyd's box but that Lloyd had left for lunch already. Star said, "What shall we do about it? We can't just let her sit there." After discussing the matter with the other guys, Star and the others decided that they just could not leave the patient sitting here and the chart in Lloyd's box, but had to do something about it. Star finally said he would take care of her.

(Senior Medicine. February, 1956.)

Students often keep close track of one another, in order to know when it may be necessary to help someone in this fashion. A person's absence from school becomes an occasion for concern, the other students wanting to know what the trouble is and whether they will be required to act on his behalf:

Harrison did not show up for clinic and the boys wondered where he was. Finally Parker told us that Harrison's aunt had died and he had gone home for the funeral and wouldn't be back until tomorrow. (In other words, his absence would be officially excused, so it was O.K.)

(Senior Surgical Specialties. October, 1956.)

An occasional student develops neurotic symptoms, which become a major concern of his associates, who will attempt to help him in whatever way they can:

At lunch, Star said, "Gee, you know Hines isn't here again today. I'm beginning to worry about him. It's gotten so that he only comes about three mornings a week. He generally shows up for clinic but outside of that he's hardly ever here. . . . Maybe we ought to go down and see how he's doing — if he's really sick or something." Jones said, "I know. You know, he lives down there all by himself and, goddam it, he's so withdrawn already that I don't really think it's good for him to live that way. I think we ought to check up on him."

The next day Hines failed to show up for clinic and the other students really got worried. Everyone commented on his absence and speculated as to whether he had gone into a depressed state or what. Someone remembered him talking about being real despondent and two of the guys finally planned to go see what was the matter after lunch. They also began discussing possible ways of preventing a recurrence of this trouble.

(Senior Medicine. March, 1956.)

The student co-operation perspective is expressed in student statements that they hope their group will remain intact when they move on to a new service; such statements seem to us to imply a dependence upon established patterns of co-operation that would be disrupted by a change in the group's membership:

The students got their instructions about reporting to the VA hospital. Thirteen students were going, including the five in this group. Thorpe said, with a certain amount of serious concern, "I wonder how they're going to split us up? Do we get to keep our same group? I sure hope so." Bell said, "Well, I don't know, but I sure hope it works out that way." There were several more comments and all the guys seemed concerned that they should be assigned together and get to work together.

(Junior Medicine. October, 1955.)

Finally, we have seen as an expression of the student co-operation perspective certain observations of deviant behavior by students and the reactions of their associates to their deviance. A student's associates might consider atypical behavior to be either "odd" or "wrong." Students were very tolerant of unusual behavior of many kinds, as long as it did not violate the rules we have considered in this chapter and thus make school more difficult for others. We participated in groups which had student members who were considered "odd" or "peculiar." Some had eccentric mannerisms or were given to what their associates considered wild exaggeration. Some were withdrawn and difficult to get to know. Some liked to study and would spend all of their free time in the library, ignoring the daily recreations of the others. None of these students became the object of anger or reprisals from the other students.

We also came to know two students who were regarded as deviant in a more serious sense. These students were considered untrustworthy and dangerous; it is no exaggeration to say that their associates hated them. What was characteristic of the behavior of these wrongdoers, as distinguished from the behavior of "odd" students, was that they frequently and apparently intentionally broke the rules contained in the student co-operation perspective and gave additional evidence in their talk that they did not feel bound by these rules. Both these men had made their reputations for non-co-operation long before we met them and their deviance was so firmly established that when one of them failed to show up for clinic, for example, his associates automatically interpreted this as an attempt to "goof off" at his colleagues' expense; when an "odd" student failed to appear in clinic, his associates expressed concern and wondered whether he needed help.

All these kinds of material may be seen as instances of use of the student co-operation perspective. We find evidence that the perspective was widespread in the fact that observations which can be interpreted as evidence for it were made on seventeen of the eighteen services on which students spent time. The one exception was Psychiatry, and this can be accounted for by the fact that there was little necessity or opportunity for student co-operation on that service. Students were assigned there in groups of two, which obviously cut down possibilities for co-operation, and were assigned very little work, which did away with the need for co-operation.

We note further that our field notes yield eighty-seven instances of use of the perspective. Considering that we saw only a few students at a time, it is clear that the actual number of incidents occurring which we were not able to observe must have been much greater. Furthermore, as mentioned earlier, many positive acts of abiding by the rules contained in the perspective could not be counted as evidence for they might have been tied to quite different perspectives. Most of our evidence, therefore, was taken from incidents occasioned by acts of deviance and incidents in which agreements were in the process of being arrived at.

Finally, Table XXIX exhibits certain features which make it likely we have described an operating reality in school life. First, none of the eighty-seven items was directed by the observer; every item containing evidence on the point contains it through the student's, not the observer's, doing. Second, 78 per cent of the items did not involve the observer in any way and presumably would have occurred in the same way had we not been there. Sixty-eight per cent of the items involve interaction among the students; if the perspective had not been commonly accepted and publicly legitimate, its use would have been challenged by students participating in the interaction.

The negative instances to be found are of several kinds. First there are items describing the failure of the top two known "wrongdoers" to abide by the rules. These cannot realistically be considered to cast doubt on the existence of the perspective but do force us to revise our conclusion somewhat. We can no longer say simply that the students held this perspective but must be explicit about the fact that certain deviants did not hold it. The existence of two deviants raises the possibility that there were others whose existence we did not discover. While we cannot, of course, be positive that there were not many more, we consider it unlikely. The deviance of these men caused so much commotion in the groups they belonged to that it is improbable that others could have existed in these or the other groups we observed without our hearing of them. Furthermore, students who were not members of work groups containing these deviants knew of their existence both from experience in the preclinical years and from gossip in the clinical years, which we also heard. Had there been other such deviants, we probably would have heard them gossiped about in the same way. Therefore, we feel that we are still safe in concluding that the great majority of students held the student co-operation perspective.

A second class of negative instances consists of those items in which erring students are taught the rules by their associates. Since these errants did not repeat their errors, we may safely attribute their failure to co-operate to ignorance and need not revise our hypothesis to take account of these incidents.

TABLE XXIX

EVIDENCE FOR EXISTENCE OF THE STUDENT CO-OPERATION PERSPECTIVE

		VOLUNTEERED	DIRECTED
Statements	To observer alone......................	18 (22%)	—
	To others in everyday conversation	32 (36%)	—
Activities	Individual	9 (10%)	—
	Group	28 (32%)	—
Total	....	87 (100%)	0

Finally, we discover three incidents in our field notes in which students who appeared usually to abide by the rules contained in the perspective broke those rules when they felt they were unobserved by their fellows.

The residents in the clinic had suggested to me that students would cheat in the clinic by taking a patient's chart out of their pigeonhole and putting it in another student's. [Patients were assigned to students by having their chart put in a pigeonhole with the student's name on it.] I saw this happen this morning. Flaherty took a chart out of his box, looked at it, and said, "Oh, Johnson wants to see this one. I know he does." He took the chart and stuffed it in Johnson's box after looking around to see if anyone were watching him. He gave me a sly smile, indicating that Johnson didn't know anything about the patient and did not want to see him.

(Senior Medicine. March, 1956.)

We may safely assume that many more incidents of this kind occurred than we observed; by the nature of the act, it was likely to be carried on secretly. The fact that incidents like this occurred suggests a further revision of our hypothesis. Unfortunately, we cannot check this revision systematically. We suspect, however, that there is a marginal area in which such acts can be thought of as jokes or tricks that one student plays on another and in which they can be justified in this way if they are discovered. If this hypothesis is true, it does not so much cast doubt on the customary use of the student co-operation perspective as it cautions us that some of its major terms are sufficiently ambiguous to allow a good deal of leeway for individual variation.

This review of the evidence contained in our field notes indicates that students use the student co-operation perspective customarily, in the sense that its use is frequent, widespread, and was observed to occur in spontaneous (i.e., unaffected by the observer) student interaction.

The existence of the student co-operation perspective has several consequences. Of most concern to the faculty, of course, is the collective limitation of work in those areas students consider nonessential or where one hard worker can set a difficult standard for others to meet. This facet of the perspective helps the students set upper limits to the level of their work effort and thereby decreases their opportunities for learning.

This finding has considerable import for the understanding of the phenomenon ordinarily referred to as the "restriction of production." Research has shown that industrial workers typically set collective quotas for their production; if they exceed them, they are likely to be punished by their fellow workers in more or less subtle ways. It is apparent, of course, that in industrial plants the interests of workers and management are likely to be widely divergent. They do not want the same things and, indeed, their interests may actually conflict. Restriction of production — quota-setting — can easily be seen as simply a specific manifestation of this more generalized condition of group conflict.

But we find the same phenomenon of the collective setting of a ceiling on work efforts in the medical school, which is not character- ized by any such generalized divergence of interests between students (the educational analogue of the workers) and faculty (the educa- tional "management"). In the long run, faculty and students desire the same results: that the school should turn out competent, well-trained physicians. There is no disagreement or conflict on this point. This suggests that collective setting of work levels can take place without such generalized conflict and that other conditions may be equally productive of the phenomenon.

The case of the medical school indicates that, even in the absence of conflict, the superiors in a hierarchy may set tasks that subordinates find unmanageable, may create situations in which subordinates feel it necessary to defend themselves, or through ignorance of the sub- ordinates' perspective unwittingly do damage to the subordinates' interests. If any of these occur, subordinates may find it necessary to set collective standards.

The perspective also enables students to facilitate their learning. The injunction to trade off patients in order to get a more varied clinical workload and the pattern of informal quizzing over medical facts both provide increased opportunities for learning beyond what the organized curriculum makes available.

The existence of the perspective also seems to solve certain admin- istrative problems for the medical school. Students co-operate to share workloads in the clinic and on the wards in an equitable fashion, and this no doubt has the effect of making those hospital facilities operate smoothly, particularly where, as in the clinics, much of the work is done by students.

Finally, the perspective provides social support for students en- gaging in activities the faculty might view as improper.

Students and Patients

T_{HE} student spends much of his time in the clinical years interacting with patients. This activity comes closest to the things he will do once he is a "real doctor" practicing medicine. It is, in fact, the closest approach the student makes to the core drama of medicine while he is in medical school.

Students have well-formed ideas about the patients they meet in the hospital, well-defined expectations of how patients ought to act and what kinds of people they ought to be. But they have no unitary perspective towards patients, no consistent and interrelated set of attitudes covering their interaction with patients. Rather, students' ideas and expectations exhibit a great variety, reflecting the variety of sources students draw on for them. Some ideas are part of student culture, being applications of perspectives that students create when they face the problems of choosing an appropriate level and direction of effort in school, problems that arise when the faculty or environment do not dictate a choice. Some ideas are taken directly from the medical culture that dominates the hospital environment, being applied to those interactional problems with patients in which there is no marked difference between the student's problems and those of a practicing physician. Still other ideas arise with reference to problems that do not affect the student in his capacity either as student or prospective physician. These ideas are drawn from cultures associated with other roles the students play, cultures that have no connection with their status as medical students; in particular, we refer here to cultures associated with sex and social class. In this chapter we describe students' interaction with patients, the variety of views of patients students hold, and the roots of these views in the various cultures students participate in.

Students' views of patients draw heavily, though not exclusively, on student culture — on the set of perspectives we have described. To the degree that this is so, it supports our view that medical students' behavior can best be understood by seeing them primarily as *students*, as people who must operate within the limitations and with the disabilities of that role in pursuit of goals defined as proper for occupants of that role. The material to be presented also makes the point again that students acquire, in the course of their training, a technical vocabulary expressing the point of view and interests appropriate to the role of student. In so doing, they acquire a way of dealing with matters that might prove disturbing should they continue to look on them from the point of view of the layman.

Student-Patient Contact

Students' contact with patients occurs in a few typical kinds of situations. These differing situations occur more or less in sequence, although there is a good deal of variation for some student groups, depending on the way the Dean's Office arranges their schedules. This sequence of situations of patient contact, ideally, presents the student with technical and interactional problems of increasing extent and complexity. We describe this sequence in its ideal form, recognizing that for many students it will not be quite like this.

The student meets his first patient face-to-face in his second-year course in physical diagnosis. A group of four or five students meet in the clinic once a week with a staff member, and one of them takes a history from and performs a physical examination on a clinic patient. This responsibility revolves among the members of the group so that each one performs an examination approximately once a month. These examinations are ordinarily performed in the presence of the staff member and other members of the group, so that the student is insulated from many of the potential difficulties of interaction with patients. However, several times during the year the student must work-up a patient on the hospital wards for presentation to the entire class. In this case, he operates without benefit of the staff member's presence, but his only problem is to perform the examination adequately enough to get the information required for his diagnosis.

The third-year student typically meets his patients when they are hospitalized for diagnosis and treatment. He comes into contact with them repeatedly during their hospital stay. He performs a complete examination upon the patient's arrival in the hospital. He presents the patient to the staff and other students during rounds, describing the case in detail, demonstrating outstanding physical findings, and suggesting a diagnosis and plan of treatment. He checks daily on the patient's progress, quizzing and re-examining the patient frequently. He enters into a casual but continuing relationship with the patient. The major problem patients present for the student on the hospital wards, then, is to maintain this continuing relation in such a fashion as to be able to get the necessary information for the job he is assigned.

The fourth-year students (and third-year students in pediatrics, to some extent) see their patients in the outpatient clinic rather than on the wards. Like the third-year student, he performs a complete examination without a staff member being present. He may then demonstrate the patient to a member of the staff, although frequently he simply describes the case to the staff member, who may not have any actual contact with the patient. In this setting, then, the student is the sole dispenser of medical information — diagnosis and recommendations — to his patient. It becomes his responsibility, as it is not on the wards, to tell the patient what the diagnosis is and what measures must be taken to deal with the disease. The student is also the only medical person to get the necessary information on which diagnosis and treatment can be based.

The clinic situation produces a further set of problems. Clinic patients are not in the hospital and are not under the constant observation or control of hospital personnel. They do not always note and report, on return visits, the things the student has asked them to report on. Hospitalized patients take the medicine they are supposed to take when they are supposed to; they eat the diet the doctor has prescribed; they do, in general, what they are supposed to do. But clinic patients do these things only if they remember to or want to, and they frequently fail to follow the student's medical orders. In short, the clinic presents the student with the additional problem of attempting to control patients' behavior when they are not under direct supervision.

Students meet patients in this variety of circumstances. Their interaction with patients poses or impinges on certain crucial problems. Students develop attitudes toward patients by applying premises acquired elsewhere to this interaction and these problems. We turn now to a consideration of student views of patients. In preparation for a later analysis, we divide these views according to the culture on whose premises the student draws in building the particular attitude under discussion.

Student Attitudes Toward Patients
Drawn from Medical Culture

Medical students look forward to being practicing physicians, and in the course of their experience in the hospital they acquire many ideas which are part of the general culture of the medical world. It is true that some perspectives we have included in student culture are drawn from medical culture — such as the emphasis on clinical experience and medical responsibility — but these are used by students with a particular emphasis on the application of the notion to the peculiar problems of the student's position. Other aspects of medical culture, however, get no such distinctive student phrasing but are taken over more or less intact. Students draw on some of these ideas in organizing their thinking about patients and interacting with them. Insofar as the problems patients present to students are the same as a physician would meet, insofar as students and doctors are in the same boat in dealing with the patient, students make use of ideas from medical culture.

We must make clear that we have undertaken no study of medical culture in its own right, either as it appears in the teaching hospital or elsewhere. Consequently, when we identify the sources of some of the student ideas about patients we are about to consider as medical culture, we necessarily speculate, albeit on the basis of experience in the medical school. In any case, with regard to our later analysis it is important to show the kinds of ideas that are *not* rooted in student culture, for we intend to compare student ideas about patients rooted in student culture with those that are not, whatever their source. With this proviso in mind, we turn to consideration of those ideas that appear to us to have their origin in the culture of the medical world.

As we have noted earlier, the concept of medical responsibility pictures a world in which patients may be in danger of losing their lives and identifies the true work of the physician as saving those endangered lives. Further, where the physician's work does not afford (at least in some symbolic sense) the possibility of saving a life or restoring health through skilful practice or losing them through ineptness, the physician himself lacks some of the essence of physicianhood.

This perspective, which we believe to be an important one in medical culture generally, furnishes a basis for classifying and evaluating patients; those patients who can be cured are better than those who cannot. Furthermore, those patients who cannot be cured because they are not sick in the first place are worst of all.

Students, participating vicariously in the medical drama of life and death, sometimes make such a classification of patients. "Crocks," for example, are not physically ill and, though students may occasionally feel sorry for them, are not regarded as worthwhile patients because nothing can be done for them:

Prince decided that the patient was not really sick but just had a lot of trouble in his personal life that was making him sick. After the patient left, he said, "I feel sorry for a guy like that. He's really got a problem and there isn't going to be much we can do for him, I don't think, unless maybe we send him to psychiatry clinic and I don't think that'll help him very much. . . . We'll do the best we can but I don't think we'll be able to help him too much. We sure see a lot of these cases up here. . . . I don't think he's a goldbrick. I think he really does have pain and discomfort. It's just not a kind that we can deal with very well, I'm afraid."

(Senior Medicine. February, 1956.)

Obese patients, too, are frequently seen as essentially incurable and not worth bothering with:

Two of the students were discussing the kinds of practices they would have when they got out, and the way they would treat various diseases. One said, "I'll tell you the way I would treat obesity. I would just tell them that I will give them a diet and if they follow this diet they will lose weight. If they don't want to follow the diet, then I will just tell them that I don't want to have anything more to do with them. It's all a matter of will power. I'd scare the hell out of them about all the diseases they could get from being overweight. If that didn't do it, I would just get rid of them." The other student agreed.

(Junior Pediatrics. January, 1956.)

Students also draw on what appears to us to be medical culture when they worry about the dangers to their own health involved in seeing a steady stream of unscreened patients, some of whom may have dangerous communicable diseases. This kind of danger is well-known and is one to which students are exposed in exactly the same way as a practicing physician. Students consequently participate in the anxiety generated by the appearance of a "dangerous" patient:

Morrison came into the clinic office to tell a staff member about a patient they had both seen previously. Her chest X ray had been interpreted as indicating active tuberculosis. Morrison said, "I used to have a negative skin test for t.b. but I probably won't anymore." He asked the staff member if he wanted to go listen to the patient's chest, saying that certain important sounds could be heard best from the back. The staff member said, "That's the only way I'm going to listen to her from now on — from the back." Later on Morrison told one of the residents about his contact with this patient. He said, "I sure hope she didn't spread any of it to me. I've always had a negative skin test but I'll bet it's going to turn positive now."

(Senior Medicine. February, 1956.)

Students appear to be drawing on medical culture, as best they can, when they think about patients in terms of the problems they will have to face with patients in actual practice. There are many problems students are insulated from while they remain students, problems which will erupt into full activity once the student begins to practice. Students sometimes look ahead to their future practice and wonder what they will do about these problems. Their discussions seem to bear the flavor of medical culture, if only in the character of the problems raised:

The staff member described the case of a patient who would die very shortly of an inoperable tumor. Hunter asked, "What do you tell patients like that? Do you tell them the truth or do you keep it from them?" The staff member gave a long and complex answer, pointing out that frequently patients figured it out for themselves or, on the other hand, didn't want to know anything about it. In either case the physician had no decision to make about whether to tell or not. Hunter was not satisfied and posed this question: "What would you do if you had a patient like that and you knew he didn't have his affairs in order?" He was trying to state the case where the patient would have to be told so that the staff member would explain how it was done.

(Junior Medicine. January, 1957.)

Student concern over how one handles a problem like this, a problem they do not face as students, seems a clear instance of students drawing on medical culture for their thinking about patients. So do student concerns over how to run the business end of a medical practice, how to avoid or deal with malpractice suits, and so on. Finally, student ideas about what kinds of patients one wants in one's clientele and how patients of particular social classes should be handled seem to have this same source:

I was having a Coke with Craig. He said, "I'll tell you one thing, you'll never catch me doing any charity work." I said, "Someone's got to do it, don't they?" He said, "I have some pretty bizarre thoughts on that subject. The way I feel is if they can't pay for it, they don't deserve to get it. . . . Not all of them, but you take the kind of guy who thinks it's more important to make the payment on his television than to pay his doctor bill. He figures that if he doesn't make the t.v. payment they'll come and take the set away. But the doctor can't take back the shot of penicillin he got. So he lets the doctor wait. Now a guy like that I would just have no sympathy for at all."

(Junior Surgery. January, 1956.)

A student described his observations of the difference between the university medical center and a private hospital in town to me. Among other things, he said, "The fact that these doctors are strictly in private practice probably makes them different, too. You learn that you have to cater to the patient and his disease here a little more than you do at K.U., where they don't bother about that kind of thing so much." Another student mentioned this difference: "They don't order all the tests and things here that they would order on a patient at K.U. Over there they are likely to have everything done they can think of, because they have a more academic way of doing things . . . Here they take more account of the fact that people have to pay for these things usually, so that makes a big difference too. This is more like the way medicine is practiced by most people."

(Junior Medicine. January, 1957.)

It can be argued that medical culture lies at the basis of students' concern with the problem of managing interaction with patients so that patients will be pleasant and co-operative. Students view this as a pervasive problem of medical practice and one which they will have to solve adequately in order to have a comfortable work life:

A staff member spoke informally about the school's policy of seeing to it that students have contact with patients early in their medical education. One of the students said to me, "You know, what he was saying about the human relations approach and patients and all that. I'm glad they do it this way. I think it is much more important to learn how to get along with patients. I mean, the scientific part is important but I'm glad they emphasize this too."

(Sophomore Pathology. April, 1956.)

On this view, patients can be seen as people who may possibly create embarrassing or difficult situations for the doctor, and they can be classified according to whether or not they do this or how likely they are to do this. The student's interaction with patients in the hospital partakes in part of the style of the doctor's interaction with his patients, and some of their comments and ideas about patients reflect this facet of medical culture:

Stone said, "It's pleasant to have a patient like Mr. Green for a change. He's such a friendly guy." Somebody else said, "Yes, he's not like some of these crocks we get around here. He's really friendly. . . . He's been very nice to me."

(Junior Medicine. September, 1955.)

In the same way that unfriendly patients are disliked, patients who are friendly and co-operative are thought well of:

I asked the students how the patients had been at another hospital at which they had done some of their work. Young said, "They treated us very nicely. They were all very co-operative. We never had any trouble examining them or working them up. I think sometimes you can have more trouble about that over here than over there." Heinz and Krause agreed to this.

(Senior Surgical Specialties. October, 1956.)

Students think of psychiatric patients as particularly likely to present difficulties of this kind:

A student said to one of the staff members in the clinic office, "Boy I really don't know what to do with this one. I think she's a real schizophrenic." He described her bizarre behavior and quoted a number of pretty crazy statements she had made, such as claiming to have invented the theory of relativity before Einstein. The staff member went to see her. The social worker said to Prentiss, the student, that the woman needed psychiatric care. Prentiss said, "I wouldn't even think of mentioning that to her. . . . Not me." The social worker suggested that Prentiss might try to establish a therapeutic relationship with her himself. He said, "I don't think it would work and I certainly don't want to have any more to do with her if possible. Frankly, I'm afraid of her. She scares me to death." The social worker said, "Well, do you think you could do that?" Prentiss said, "I don't know, but I'd rather not try."

(Senior Medicine. January, 1956.)

Many students dislike pediatrics for similar reasons. They feel that children are particularly unco-operative and difficult to examine and would rather avoid what they consider to be the inevitable scenes that accompany pediatric practice.

Perhaps the most difficult scenes come about when patients have no respect for the doctor's authority. Physicians resent this immensely; the students would resent such behavior more if they were not so ambivalent about their own status. They would prefer that patients accept them as physicians yet know that they cannot themselves claim this status. Although they may at times "feel" like a doctor, they know perfectly well that they are not and cannot claim the authority of the medical role. In the anxiety they exhibit over how patients will receive them in their pseudomedical role, students draw on medical culture both for the definition of what constitutes a full-fledged physician and for the feeling that patients should respect incumbents of medical statuses.

Anxiety over the patients' reaction to the intrusion of a medical student is widespread before any actual patient contact occurs:

I attended the first meeting of the Physical Diagnosis class this morning. Every time they were offered a chance to ask questions, students raised questions about how they should behave with patients. Should they refer to themselves as "Doctor" or not? Should they tell the patients they were students? And so on.

(Sophomore Physical Diagnosis. November, 1955.)

Though such initial worries are allayed by the suggestions and reassurances of the staff, the feeling is likely to return, particularly where ambiguities in the situation cause patients to suddenly discover that their "young doctor" is not a doctor after all:

A student was comparing the private hospital he's assigned to with the medical center. He said, "One thing I don't like over here is something that Dr. Barron does, and it's kind of a problem in general. Occasionally Barron will walk into a patient's room with us and say, 'Well, I've got the students along with me this morning.' Now if you've been in there the night before and introduced yourself as Dr. Horn, and not exactly lied, you know, but just kind of hinted that you were really a doctor — I mean, in other words, you don't tell him you're a student and this guy comes along and tells them that you are — well, they lose all their respect for you right away and half of them don't ever want to see you again after that. . . . Now at K.U. it's different. Everybody who comes in there knows that it is a medical school and there will be students around examining them and all that. So it doesn't affect your relationship with the patient. But your patient relationship sure goes to hell when they thought you were a doctor and then find out that you're only a student."

(Junior Medicine. January, 1957.)

A final set of student ideas about patients that seems to be drawn from medical culture consists of variations on the theme that some

patients are bad because they are directly responsible for the existence of their own (or of their children's) illness. It is our impression
that many physicians feel little sympathy for patients who become
diseased as a consequence of their own actions or neglect and that
they think that patients who do not follow medical advice more or less
deserve what they get. Students occasionally express similar thoughts
about patients and, though we cannot be completely sure that these
are rooted in medical culture, we assign them to this category.

Students, for example, add to their indictment of the crock the
charge that the crock is responsible for his illness because he enjoys
it and the attention it brings him:

The boys took me to see a patient who claimed to have a great many pains
in a variety of places. They proved to themselves that she was not "really
sick" by curing one of her pains with an injection of sterile water. Harris
said to me, "She's a real crock." I said, "What's that?" He said, "I don't
know exactly how you'd define it. I guess you'd say a neurotic. Always
moaning around like that and carrying on. . . . The kind that gets a pleasure out of being sick all the time, so they have to have pains and do."
(Junior Medicine. September, 1955.)

This attitude finds somewhat subtler expression in cases where the
student has to persuade a patient to follow medical orders or spend
money on medical treatment; students often find that without special
effort on their part patients will not do these things:

Garrity said, "This was one patient I really knew what to do for. In fact,
I knew what to do two weeks ago when she first came in, but I couldn't
persuade her to do it . . . It was pretty obvious what she had and what she
needed was some radioactive iodine, but she said she couldn't afford it. It
only costs three or four dollars and she had to have it, but I can't force her
to spend her money on it if she doesn't want to, so I tried to persuade her.
I guess she was feeling a little worse this time and that convinced her. . . .
Usually you don't have to talk them into it. You just let them go home and
get into a little trouble from their disease. That will usually convince them
and they'll be back begging for whatever you told them they needed."
(Senior Medicine. February, 1956.)

In all these judgments of patients, then, students appear to us to be
drawing on medical culture. Once again we note that we have not
studied medical culture itself, so that our attribution of these ideas
to this source is necessarily speculative.

Student Attitudes Toward
Patients Drawn from
Lay Cultures

Some student attitudes toward patients have no connection with student problems related to preparing for practice or overcoming the academic obstacles in the way of graduation. Nor are they related to problems which students share with other medical personnel. Neither student nor medical cultures provide the base from which these attitudes are projected. Instead they seem to draw on various lay cultures for their content. In expressing them, the student is acting in some latent identity which finds its home in a nonmedical organizational setting. The major cultures on which students seem to draw in developing the attitudes we are about to discuss are social class culture, sex culture, and lay culture about pain and disease.

Social class culture probably lies at the root of students' disgust with patients they consider immoral or immodest. Despite the legendary rowdiness of medical students, the men we studied accepted the major tenets of conventional middle-class morality and were shocked and offended by patients who violated them:

After medicine clinic, the boys, as usual, were comparing their morning's experiences. O'Brien said, "I really had a prize today." He began to laugh in an embarrassed way. I said, "What was it?" He said, "A twenty-three-year-old girl, fat as a pig. I asked her what her trouble was and she said she had a backache. I asked her where it was and before I knew what was happening she pulled up her skirt and dropped her pants and showed me. Boy, I've never had anything like that happen before. It was the damndest thing I ever saw . . . I asked her if there was any time that it hurt more than other times and she said it always hurt more right after humping, only she didn't say that." Krause said, "Well now, there is a nice frank young girl. You didn't have any trouble taking a history from her, did you?" O'Brien said, "No, but I'd just as soon do without that kind. It was really weird."

(Senior Medicine. March, 1956.)

Students similarly dislike patients whose disease shows that they have been acting "immorally":

Bruce said, "Well, here we go again to clinic. I'm really kind of getting to dislike that clinic. All those women with discharges and bleeding. So damn much of it is gonorrhea and, you know, I don't like to have much to do with people like that. They're really not very nice people, you know."

(Senior Gynecology. May, 1956.)

Class culture also seems to furnish the basis for occasional complaints that charity patients did not act properly "poor" or submissive. Students complained, for instance, that they had seen a clinic patient driving a Cadillac, which apparently violated some half-formed sumptuary rule. Or they might complain when patients chafed at the way they were treated in the clinic:

The patient's wife complained a great deal about having to wait so long before they were seen and about other aspects of the way the clinic was run. The student handling the case said to me later, "How do you like the way she was carrying on? I sure would have liked to give her a piece of my mind. Isn't that terrible? After all, they're getting their medical care for free when they come up here, and when you get something for nothing you have to put up with a little bit of waiting. If they want any fancier treatment they can pay for it. If they can't pay they can just wait and keep their mouths shut."

(Senior Surgical Specialties. October, 1956.)

There exist fairly well defined sex cultures in this country: sets of understandings shared among males and among females, having to do in large part with behavior toward members of the opposite sex and, in less-explicit form, with relations between members of the same sex. Students appear to draw on these understandings for certain kinds of comments they make about their patients.

If there is such a thing as male culture, one element of it certainly consists of an injunction always to have an eye out for a pretty girl. Obviously, this runs afoul of the medical injunction that a doctor must never abuse his position of trust in his dealings with his female patients. Medical students never, to our knowledge, abuse this trust, but they remain male enough to look at and comment on their female patients:

I was talking with some of the students when a very pretty girl in a maternity smock walked by. White said, "We never get any that look like that in GYN clinic. I don't know why. I sure wouldn't mind doing an examination on someone like her." I said, "What's this? I thought you guys had got all over that and just took it in your stride. You know, didn't bat an eyelash." Barton said, "When that happens, I'll be old and gray, believe me. I'm still young enough to enjoy looking at something like that."

(Senior Obstetrics. April, 1956.)

Intra-sex avoidance and prudery are also evident:

Tyler said, "There are still some parts of the examination that bother me a lot." Kerr was listening interestedly. Tyler said, "For one thing, I don't like to examine external genitalia on men." I said, "Why not?" He said, "I don't know. I guess there is some kind of connotation of sex there or homosexuality or something, but that does bother me." He looked at Kerr and said, "You know, I've worked out a new routine on that. I always wear a rubber glove when I examine external genitalia." Kerr said, "I've always done that." Tyler said, "It fits very easily into the routine. The next thing you do is a rectal anyway and you have to wear a rubber glove for that. So I put the rubber glove on, have him stand up, examine the genitalia, and then have him turn around and bend over and I do the rectal. It is very smooth that way and I like it a whole lot better." Kerr said, "Sure, that's the best way to do it."

(Junior Medicine. November, 1955.)

It is an open question whether sex culture or medical culture plays more of a role in the students' perception and handling of the problem of protecting female patients' modesty during the physical examination. Clearly, the medical profession has developed a set of techniques for dealing with this problem, and students learn these; for this reason, we might have discussed these attitudes earlier in talking about the role of medical culture in students' views of patients. However, the students' concern over patients' modesty seems to be a hangover from their days as laymen, and this view is reinforced by the observation that students are also embarrassed by having to invade patients' privacy with potentially embarrassing questions; though these questions (such as those about past venereal disease or the use of alcohol) go beyond matters of sex, they are clearly part of the larger family of medical actions that patients might interpret as incivilities, actions that are in consequence embarrassing to perform:

I watched Meyers examine a woman. Later on we talked about what had made him uneasy during the examination. Then I asked him, "What do you think made her feel most uneasy?" He said, "Well, with women, any time they have to get undressed, it upsets them. It always makes women nervous when they have to take their blouse off. A man, well, you can just strip them down and examine them, but you have to protect the woman's modesty. You notice she was always trying to cover herself up and when I examined her breasts, for instance, well — not that it bothers me, it doesn't embarrass me, but they get embarrassed and that makes it a little harder to do the examination and it's something you just have to deal with. What I try to do is just be as businesslike and matter of fact about it as possible and that way, you know, let them know that this is strictly business. But ordinarily we try not to do things that will embarrass them."

(Junior Medicine. September, 1955.)

A staff member was teaching students how to take a history. They were to take their first history from a live patient that day. One student said, "I have a question. On this sheet here they say that we ought to ask about alcoholism and syphilis, how do you do that? Do you just ask it right out?" The staff member explained that this was necessary information and you just asked the questions.

(Sophomore Physical Diagnosis. November, 1955.)

Common knowledge indicates the existence of widespread lay cultural notions about pain and death which are systematically violated in the medical student's experience. These violations occasionally cause the student discomfort. In particular, students dislike having to cause patients pain. In the lay world, the rule of civilized behavior is that one avoids causing pain to others; but medical students regularly have to perform procedures which hurt patients, ranging from relatively minor pain-producing actions like venipuncture to such major trauma as the urethral dilatation of a male. Students sometimes feel queasy when they must hurt patients in these ways and are particularly upset when pain is caused by their own ineptness:

I was sitting around talking with Brooks, Kern, and Burton. Brooks said, "Did I ever tell you about the time I blew up a Foley catheter in a man's urethra?" Kern said, "You did? My God, that must have hurt!" Brooks said, "Yeah, last year. I put it in and I thought I had it all the way into the bladder. . . . I started to blow it up and the patient didn't say anything for awhile. Finally he said, 'It hurts a little bit down there, Doc.'" Kern said, "A little bit. Boy, if it was me I would have hit the ceiling by that time. He must have been the stoic type." Brooks said, "Yeah, he was. Boy, I sure felt terrible about that."

(Senior Surgical Specialties. October, 1956.)

Students are also sometimes upset by the fact of death or by what laymen would consider hideous and depressing sights one sometimes encounters in a hospital: infants born with grotesque anomalies, patients with extensive brain damage, and so on. During these upsets, students act essentially on premises contained in lay culture.

I asked Perry whether there were any kinds of patients he preferred. He said, "There are a lot of things around here you have to get used to and you get used to them pretty quick. I thought I would not like it having patients that might die, but I've had patients die on me now — I went to a post-mortem this morning — and it doesn't really bother you too much. I guess you kind of get calloused about it. Especially little infants. When they die there's just no feeling about that anymore than I suppose there would be when old people die. I'll tell you the kind that bother me are some of these kids that we've had in here. Like that kid who was up on the third floor, seventeen-year-old kid, big good-looking blond kid. He dived off a diving board and hit his head on the bottom of the swimming pool and he was paralyzed from the neck down and I imagine he'll stay that way for the rest of his life. Now something like that really seems like a terrible waste, and that's pretty unpleasant to see." Moore said, "Yeah, those things depress me too. I don't like that at all. We've had two or three kids here like that who have fallen off things, fallen off bikes, and who landed on their heads and done serious damage to their brains. They're just never going to be the same, and that's pretty unpleasant to see."

(Junior Pediatrics. October, 1955.)

A number of students mentioned that the death of a patient bothered them, particularly when the patient was near their own age and died in a way they might conceivably die themselves.

These empathic responses to pain and death appear to be rooted in lay culture, as are the attitudes and actions drawn from class and sex cultures.

Student Attitudes Toward Patients Drawn from Student Culture

The great bulk of student views of patients, as we shall see later, draw on perspectives which are part of student culture. These perspectives contain ideas which are applied to interaction with patients. This application produces several classifications and evaluations of patients, each classification being made in terms suggested by a perspective from student culture. Let us consider in turn the several perspectives from student culture which students use in thinking about their patients.

We have discussed earlier the student perspective which emphasizes the importance of gaining clinical experience. Students draw on this perspective for their ubiquitous distinction between patients who are "really sick" and patients who are not sick at all. They feel, in accordance with the clinical experience perspective, that their best patients are those who have a "real" disease, a disease producing organic pathology from which the student can acquire the knowledge his books do not contain. This view implies a classification of patients ranging from those who have no discernible pathology at all through those having common or minor diseases to those having serious diseases which one seldom gets a chance to see. Students apply this perspective in a great many specific ways.

For instance, students complain a great deal when they are assigned patients who are not, in their terms, "really sick." Such patients take up the student's time but leave him with no more knowledge than before he saw them. Though students seldom make an explicit connection between this view and the clinical experience perspective, the actual connection seems obvious; the dislike for patients without physical pathology makes sense if one believes that the function of medical school is to provide an intimate knowledge of such pathology through firsthand experience. What students do make explicit is their preference for "sick" patients and their impatience with the other variety:

I watched one of the students work-up a patient in clinic. He told me that he was sure that the patient really had no disease, but just pain brought on by tension and worry. I said that I was surprised by how quickly he had arrived at that conclusion. He said, "You kind of get into that way of thinking around the clinic here, in fact, in the whole hospital. You see so many people who really don't have much the matter with them, except problems that make them worry and make them tense and consequently sick, that you can begin to smell it after a while, before you have any good reason to make a diagnosis like that. You see an awful lot of them up here." Another student overheard this and said, "I'll say. I spent my whole morning working up two crocks." The first student said, "I'm not too sympathetic to these people, especially to these old ladies — or young ladies — that kind of hurt all over, you know."

Later on, the three of us went out to lunch. The second student said, "Boy, they sure slipped it to me today. Dr. Jones was passing out charts for new patients and he put one in my box and then gave me another while I was standing there, so I had to work up two new patients and they were both crocks. It's enough to spoil your whole day." The first student said, "What's the matter? No pathology?" The second one said, "Not a thing. There isn't anything the matter with either of them."

(Senior Medicine. February, 1956.)

Like most students, these men use the term "crock" to refer to patients who disappoint them by failing to have pathological findings. While the word probably has the vulgar etymology readers may already have suspected, it is used in a more technical sense in the hospital. It refers to the patient without pathology, but includes a number of other ideas as well. (We analyze the imagery involved in more detail below.) Students frequently use the term in its restricted sense:

A student defined the term "crock" for me as follows: "The real true crock is a person who, well, I guess you could say is a psychoneurotic, somebody who you do a great big work-up for and who has all of these vague symptoms and you really can't find anything the matter with them."

(Junior Medicine. September, 1955.)

Similarly, students express pleasure when the luck of the draw provides them with patients who have physical disease:

I went with Sullivan to watch him examine a patient in the clinic. He said, "Boy, I've had one interesting case already this morning. Some real pathology — a guy with a possible myocardial infarct. I wonder what this one is." He looked at the chart and noticed immediately that the patient was short, but weighed 170 pounds. He immediately suspected that she was simply overweight and her pain was really "in her head." When he examined her she reported a sharp pain in her chest which sometimes radiated into her shoulder and neck. He questioned her about it and then went out to look for a staff member. He said, "Well, this is probably just another crock, but it's possible she had a myocardial infarct too. Boy, that would really be something — two of them in one morning. I haven't seen so much pathology since I came up here to the clinic."

(Senior Medicine. March, 1956.)

Students often use the term "interesting case" to describe the patient with pathology:

I asked Walters how he liked Pediatrics. He said, "It's pretty interesting." Pointing to the chart he had been reading, he said, "This is an interesting case here." Then he showed me the chart of this kid who had haemophilia. He read off a lot of lab results and showed me a lot of notes he had made about this kid and went on at some length about the way the diagnosis of haemophilia is established.

(Junior Pediatrics. November, 1955.)

What constitutes an "interesting case" differs from student to student, depending on his prior experience, for a case is "interesting" precisely as it affords an opportunity to gain clinical experience with something one is unfamiliar with. The experience of making positive physical findings reported in the next example is a case in point:

I was sitting in the student lab with Burnett. Martin came in and Burnett started to tell him about an interesting new patient he got. He described the patient as having a big knot in his rectum which had been misdiagnosed by an osteopath as hemorrhoids; when the patient had begun to suffer more alarming symptoms after the osteopath's treatment, he came to the medical center. I remembered that the resident had told Burnett he was lucky to be getting such an interesting case. Burnett told Martin that the patient had a real mass in his rectum. He asked, "Do you want to come down and feel it?" Martin said, "Well, I don't know. If you want my expert opinion on it I guess I'll be glad to give it to you." Burnett said, "The thing is, I've done so many rectal examinations and this is the first time I ever got any positive findings. I thought you'd be interested to actually feel something in a rectum."

(Junior Surgery. January, 1956.)

In other words, the "interest" of the case depends on how much new clinical experience it gives him. For this reason, students also prefer to be assigned patients whose disease they have not seen before in one of their own patients:

Prentice and Farmer were discussing who ought to get the patient they had just been shown in clinic. Farmer said, "I'd kind of like to have him because I haven't had a hemorrhoid case." Prentice said, "Well, I've had two so I'm not particularly anxious to have another one. We can just trade. I'll take the next one." Farmer said, "Gee, that's nice of you." Prentice said, "Oh, that's all right. It wouldn't do me much good to have another one."

(Junior Surgery. January, 1956.)

In the following conversation, students compare their luck in getting a wide assortment of patients:

Kern said he had been assigned a new patient. I said, "What is it?" He said, "Oh, it's another case of ulcerative colitis. That makes two of those I've got." Stone said, "That could be a real easy one to do. You've got your differential all worked out already for the first one." Kern said, "Yeah, but still I'd like it better if I'd get something a little different. I've had three myocardial infarctions and now two of these colitis cases. I'll be an expert on those, but I won't know a damn thing about anything else." Stone said, "Well, all of my patients have been different, I must say. I haven't got any complaint about that." Kern said, "I sure wish I'd get a diabetic or something for a change." I said, referring to a student who had complained about the number of diabetics he had been assigned, "That's Jim's department, isn't it?" Kern said, "Yeah, he seems to have a corner on diabetics." Stone said, "And Johnny has all the psychiatric cases."

(Junior Medicine. October, 1955.)

Finally, students make use of the clinical experience perspective when they complain that some of the services to which they are assigned give them too narrow a range of patients to work on:

One of the students' jobs on OB is to see women for routine checkup during the early part of their pregnancy. I watched North as he saw several of these women. He did not have to examine them, but only take their blood pressure and ask them a few routine questions. After he had seen three or four of them I realized how deadly dull this was. Each woman was asked the same questions: any dizziness, any nausea, any this, any that, etc. It was really dull. Finally I said, "No kidding, Bill, doesn't this drive you nuts?" He said, "You know it, brother. It really does get on my nerves. Same damn thing time after time and even when you do find complications it's always the same old complications. After all, how many things can go wrong? It's not like medicine clinic. Up there you never know when someone was going to walk in with something strange. We did get a lot of crocks but we got a lot of interesting patients, too. Here it's all the same."

(Senior Obstetrics. May, 1956.)

A second student culture perspective on which students draw in forming their views of patients is that which emphasizes the importance of getting a chance, as a student, to exercise some measure of medical responsibility. This perspective operates most clearly in the ideas that students express about the difference between private and charity patients. Over-all, it is true that students get less opportunity to "do things" with the private patients of staff doctors than they do with those patients who come to the hospital on a charity basis. This is not to say that students are completely denied access to private patients, but simply that they are likely to have fewer opportunities to work on them. This is most obviously the case in obstetrics, where students do not deliver the babies of private patients but only those of charity patients; students also believe that they have more opportunities to "do things" on charity patients than on private patients in surgery and other departments of the hospital.

Students make use of the responsibility perspective in assessing the situations that arise out of their exclusion from some aspects of the treatment of private patients and accordingly tend to view private patients as less desirable in this respect. They resent this exclusion, even though they may occasionally see it as more extreme than it actually is:

I was sitting with a group of students waiting for a lecturer to arrive when Thompson came in and started complaining about this patient who wouldn't let him examine her. He said, "I just don't know what to do. It makes me mad as hell. I guess she doesn't intend to have a student do anything to her. I can't do too much about it." Kern said, "Well, I'd just go right ahead and examine her. To hell with her. If she didn't like it, it would be too bad." Star said, "No. Now you know they tell us not to do anything the patient doesn't want done. Is she a private patient, Paul?" Thompson said, "Yeah, she's one of Dr. Brown's patients." Kern said, "Well, that's a different story. If she's a private patient, I guess you'll just have to go on along with her. It sure would get me mad." I said, "What's this about private patients? Why do you have to go along with her because she's a private patient?" Kern said, "The clinic patients aren't anybody's patient in particular. They don't belong to any of the doctors. This is a teaching institution, and a state institution, they just have to put up with us whether they like it or not. But the private patients are Dr. Brown's, or someone else's on the staff, and they could go to another doctor if they wanted to, so they have to be treated a little differently. You can't lose a patient for Dr. Brown, you see. Clinic patients, it just doesn't make any difference."

(Junior Medicine. October, 1955.)

The problem of limited access to patients is, as we have noted, chronic in obstetrics, where it is further complicated by the fact that certain kinds of patients (even when they are charity patients) cannot, for medical reasons, be delivered by students. In particular, patients who are having their first child and cases in which there is an abnormal presentation of the baby are delivered by residents rather than students. Students are likely to complain about all these kinds of denial of the opportunity to exercise medical responsibility:

I asked Small, "Were you up most of the night?" He said, "Yes, I'm afraid so. Goddam it, they got me up at three-thirty. And I've really been having bad luck with the cases I get. I've had a whole flock of private patients and naturally I wasn't allowed to deliver them. And I had a bunch of primips [women having their first child] and I didn't get to deliver them. This one that came in last night was a clinic [charity] patient and a multip [woman who has already had a child], and I really thought my time had come. But it turned out that it was a breech, so I didn't get to do that either. I don't think I've delivered more than two or three babies since I've been here."

(Senior Obstetrics. May, 1956.)

We should note in passing that, despite complaints of this kind, one of the major reasons students like obstetrics is that they get the opportunity there to play the main role in a clear case of the medical drama — the delivery of a baby — even though this opportunity is often denied them.

Students also draw on the academic perspective in forming their ideas about patients. Students can make a good impression on the faculty by giving an adequate presentation of a patient which omits no pertinent findings and thus provides a sound basis for a diagnosis or a plan of treatment. Similarly, they can make a bad impression by making a presentation in which important findings are not included. These findings, on which the impression the student makes partly depends, come from laboratory work, from the physical examination of the patient, and from the medical history the student takes from the patient. The student may fail to make these findings, either because of his own lack of experience in conducting the examination or because the patient fails to tell him something which later turns out to be important. Students accordingly view patients as persons who may either help or hinder their attempt to impress the faculty with their knowledge and ability.

We see this in the many expressions of student anxiety over performing an examination properly found in our field notes:

I had watched a beginning third-year student do a physical examination on a middle-aged woman the previous day. I asked him about it, saying, "What made you most uneasy about it?" He said, "Well, the thing that bothered me most, maybe you noticed, was the eye examination. It's very hard to do. You shine that light in through the pupil and you can see behind right into the eye; then you have to trace out all the nerves and blood vessels and see that they are all right. I was very nervous about that." I said, "I noticed it took you quite a long time to do it." He said, "Yeah, I'm not very good at it yet. Another thing is when you look in the ear. This one wasn't so bad but some people have curved canals in their ears and you have to poke in pretty far in order to be able to see the ear drum and you can't hurt them too much. Then, the neurological examination made me very nervous. It was the first time I'd ever done it and I didn't do it at all well."

(Junior Medicine. September, 1955.)

Students who are new at the game of examining patients engage in a variety of activities that express anxiety that they will forget something important. For example, they perform the examination and take the history with a mimeographed sheet of instructions set out in plain view. They phrase their questions to patients in technical language the patient cannot understand, out of a fear of getting the question wrong.

Students overcome these fears as they become more skilled, but run into a new difficulty which they similarly interpret in terms contained in the academic perspective. Some important findings can only be known if the patient remembers or chooses to tell them to the student examining him. The student faces the ever-present danger of a patient telling the staff member or resident some important fact he has neglected to tell the student. Such an occurrence inevitably, the student feels, places him in a bad light.

I went along while the students made rounds with Dr. Hale. Downs presented the case of Mrs. Cole, describing her difficulty as one in which her hands turned various colors whenever she put them in cold water or was chilled. Dr. Hale said, "Now there is one other circumstance in which these phenomena appear, isn't there?" Downs said he didn't know. Hale said, "That's emotional stress. Now Mrs. Cole, the first time this appeared you were quite emotionally upset, isn't that right?" She said, "Yes. . . ."

Later in the morning Downs said to me, "That's a funny thing about Mrs. Cole. She never mentioned that the first time she had those symptoms it was caused by emotional stress. Never mentioned that to me at all and then she pops out with it there on rounds. It's embarrassing. I felt kind of funny about that whole thing in there. You'd never think that I had been reading up on her all last night. It didn't look like I knew what was going on, did it?"

(Junior Medicine. October, 1955.)

This anxiety, rooted in the notion that one must make a good impression on the faculty, achieves its most institutionalized form in students' evaluation of patients according to the ease with which an adequate history can be extracted from them. By this criterion, the adverse judgment of private patients we have noted earlier is reversed, for they are regarded as much more likely to be good history-givers:

Crown and Strong were talking about how they liked to get private patients. I said, "What's so good about private patients?" Crown said, "They're more intelligent, I think. They can give you a better history and tell you things that you need to know. They can come right to the point and answer your questions the way you ask them and you can just put down what they say. They know what's expected of them. . . . Take a patient like that old fellow Burns. He just can't give you a straight history. He wanders around so much when he talks, you can't get him to come to the point. You just ask him a simple question and he rambles on and on for hours. It's just too difficult to work with people like that."

(Junior Medicine. September, 1955.)

Similarly, students dislike charity patients, who are likely to be, they feel, unable to give an intelligible history; charity patients are, in simple antithesis, "unintelligent" or "dumb." Students voice this idea most frequently in explaining how necessary it is to talk down to charity patients for fear of being misunderstood. Many students, however, feel that this precaution is wise with patients of all classes and do not restrict it to poor ones; by talking down to patients, they minimize the risk of missing some finding and possibly making a bad impression on the faculty:

Brown and I were talking about how needlessly "fancy" medical language was. He said, "You know what gets me? The way guys use those words when they're talking to patients. You know, they'll ask a patient whether he's ever had diplopia. If they're lucky, the patient will say, 'No, but I see double sometimes.' They do that all the time. I've heard guys ask patients whether they have hematuria — how the hell does the patient know? He doesn't even know what the word means. There are some patients who are pretty sharp and will understand you, but usually when I'm talking to a patient I try to bring everything down to fourth-grade level, like I was trying to explain something to my little son. Then I know that they will understand it."

(Senior ENT. October, 1956.)

Finally, we can make a somewhat hazier case for the argument that students draw on student culture in forming their views of patients when we consider their idea that patients should not take up a student's time without giving him something worthwhile in return. The "something worthwhile" they have in mind is something that gets its worth in the context of their medical education. Students consider that their time is extremely limited and that they have enough to do that is important for them educationally without being burdened with time-consuming tasks which give no tangible return in added knowledge or skill. They consider further that some of the activities they are required to carry out with patients do indeed "waste" their time by offering none of these rewards.

We have made this a separate category because many of the incidents we find in our field notes contain very little clue as to the nature of the reward which is lost in these "time-wasting" activities. Students simply complain that a patient has taken up a great deal of their time for nothing. Yet our previous discussion indicates that the rewards students look for in patient interaction are typically defined with reference to student culture. We therefore regard student expressions of this attitude as drawing on student culture perspectives unless there is clear indication that this is not so. A few examples will clarify the nature of our inferences in these cases.

Patients with certain diseases remain in the hospital for a long time, but for the bulk of this time are not in an acute (and therefore "interesting") phase of their illness but rather are convalescing. Coronary patients, for example, usually spend several weeks in the hospital, although there is very little change in their condition or treatment after the first week or so. But the student to whom such a patient is assigned must continue to visit him daily and keep track of laboratory reports in the event a staff member should decide to discuss the case on rounds. The student continues to be assigned other patients so that this long-staying patient means that he has an extra workload; the same patient, however, produces no new increments of information or clinical experience:

On rounds this morning we saw a patient of Crown's who has been in the hospital for seventy-five days. When we left the patient's room, Crown said: "That's one of them. Seventy-five days that guy has been here, ever since I've been here. He's one of those patients of mine who never goes home. Of course, one went home yesterday, now I've only got eight. . . ." I said, "Pat, you're always moaning. You either have too many, or you haven't got enough and you aren't learning anything." Several of the fellows laughed at this. I said, "What is the right number of patients that would just suit you guys, anyway?" Finch said, "I think about four would be just right. If you had about four at any one time, if they would turn over, not too quickly, you know, but be here long enough so that you could learn something about each one's disease, but they wouldn't be around any longer than was useful to you. Say, maybe one would go home every three or four days and you would get a new one and then you would have maybe four or five all the time. That would be just right."

(Junior Medicine. October, 1955.)

Patients who die in the hospital are usually autopsied, and the student to whom the patient was assigned must prepare a lengthy report on the autopsy findings, correlating these with the patient's clinical course. Students frequently feel (rightly or wrongly) that they learn little from this time-consuming exercise and so are apt to look with disfavor on terminal cases although, as the second of the following pair of incidents shows, in some circumstances terminal cases may actually take less of the student's time and correspondingly be regarded as "good."

I had coffee with several students in the coffee shop. Bruce was angry because he had an autopsy to attend. He said, "I hate to get patients like that. She came in with (he gave the name of the disease but I don't remember it) and you know people who come in with something like that aren't going to last very long. She only lasted about a day and now I've got to go and spend a lot of time standing around at the autopsy."

(Junior Surgery. January, 1956.)

Freeman said, "Well, I was assigned a patient. But it's O.K. He's really a terminal case and I don't think he'll last very long at all. I can just transfer him right down to the morgue and get rid of him. I think he's in hepatic coma so there won't be any history to do." Carillo said, "Well, that's good. It won't be too much work." Freeman said, "No, I don't think so. The only thing is I'll probably have to go through the post [mortem]."

(Junior Medicine. February, 1957.)

Finally, patients who short-cut what would normally be a time-consuming process are highly prized. Our notes on obstetrics contain several instances of this. Women vary greatly in the time they take to give birth to their children, some taking twenty-four hours or more while others deliver minutes after arriving at the hospital. To the student, the only worthwhile part of the entire performance is the actual birth, but he is required to keep the woman under close observation for the entire period before the delivery. Patients who delivered quickly were prized, and students assigned such patients were considered very fortunate:

I went over to the students' quarters in OB about ten-thirty tonight to see what was going on. Johnson woke up when I came in and I asked him what had happened. He said, "Art got a patient: She delivered on a cart in the hall — I think it was the quickest delivery they ever had here. It couldn't be much quicker." A little while later Art came in, laughed, and said, "You know that patient of mine?" Johnson said, "The one who delivered in the hall?" Art said, "Yeah, she's gone home already." He laughed and rubbed his hands together gleefully. Johnson said, "Gone home already! How did that happen?" Art explained that she had been on her way to another hospital but things started to happen too fast. He said, "She still wanted to go there, so when she was ready they took her over. She was here three hours altogether and I got a delivery and no patient to look after or write progress notes on." Johnson said, "Boy, are you lucky. Wait till Green hears about this one. That's the kind he usually gets."

(Senior Obstetrics. May, 1956.)

In all of the above ways, then, students draw on the perspectives which make up student culture for their views of patients.

A Note on Patient Types

The observant reader will note that while we have divided students views of patients into a great many varieties and subvarieties, the students themselves make do a great deal of the time with a few simple typologies. They speak of "crocks" or "interesting cases," they describe patients as "intelligent" or "dumb," they distinguish between charity and private patients. Most of these categories students commonly use have no single unambiguous referent. Rather, many of the attitudes we described merge into one evocative image. "Crocks," for instance, are not only patients without any disease, from whom the student acquires no clinical experience; they are also patients whom one can probably not cure and patients who are likely to create scenes.

Nor do these composite student images call for the consistent and unequivocal evaluation of the patient. Private patients are considered more likely to be able to give an adequate history and help insofar as possible with their own cure; but charity patients are more accessible to the student.

Finally, students do not automatically apply a label to a patient simply because he has the proper characteristics of the type, seen in the abstract. Circumstances of the particular situation and the nature of the student's previous experience have an important influence on the view he takes of any given patient. The simplest illustration of this is the way a patient who has diabetes, for example, will be much more "interesting" to a student who has never been assigned a diabetic than to one who has already had several.

We point out these characteristics of student typologies of patients in order to make what we think is an important technical point. The typologies students use have in themselves no intrinsic, unchanging meaning but are amenable to a wide range of interpretations. We cannot study medical students' terminology alone and expect to acquire knowledge which will allow us to understand or predict their behavior with patients or their attitudes toward any particular patient. Nor can we find meaningful distinctions between students who use this or that term to refer to patients and those who do not. What is of interpretive value is the dimension or dimensions referred to or implied by any such term, the kind of problem or problems to which the term alludes. Our argument here has been essentially that the dimensions of student attitudes uncovered in the analysis we have just made are relatively stable and that what is predictable about student behavior is that students, in their interaction with patients, will make use of some such dimensions as these, whatever terminology they use.

The Dominance of Student Culture

We have argued that the behavior of medical students is best understood by referring to their position as *students* in the complicated organization of the medical school, as occupants of a student status with its particular limitations and disabilities. We have documented this point by describing the system of perspectives students share: student culture. In this chapter we have presented the range of attitudes toward patients we observed students expressing in the school and have traced these attitudes to their roots in the several kinds of cultures students participate in.

If it is true that students' behavior is primarily a function of their position as students in the medical school, then it follows that their views of patients should be drawn primarily from student culture or, to put it another way, in thinking about and acting toward patients they should operate mainly in ways congruent with the perspectives we have identified as student culture. We can test this conclusion by seeing how many of the incidents in our field notes, in which students make reference to patients or act toward patients in ways that reveal their attitudes, show students making use of premises contained in student culture and how many show students expressing attitudes drawn from either lay culture or medical culture. Table XXX shows the results of such an analysis.

TABLE XXX
THE CULTURAL ROOTS OF STUDENT ATTITUDES TOWARD PATIENTS

	STUDENT CULTURE	MEDICAL CULTURE	LAY CULTURE	TOTAL
Number	145	46	37	228
Per Cent............	64	20	16	100

Almost two-thirds of all incidents observed showed students drawing on the perspectives contained in student culture for their views of patients. This is three times the number of incidents in which students were observed drawing on the premises of medical culture, the next largest category, and almost twice as many as the combined total of the other two categories. Table XXX lends substantial weight to our assertion that the student role is the most important of the several roles that the student plays while he is in school.

It should be remembered that our attribution of student attitudes to medical and lay culture are in some measure hypothetical, for we have not actually studied these cultures but simply inferred their presence from the character of student ideas. Therefore, the relative percentages of these two categories may not be very meaningful.

A further breakdown of the items classified as showing students drawing on student culture for their views of patients indicates that these modes of viewing patients were collective and customary in the same way as the perspectives from which they were drawn (see Table XXXI). None of the items contained in this analysis were directed by

TABLE XXXI

EVIDENCE FOR THE CUSTOMARY AND COLLECTIVE CHARACTER
OF STUDENT CULTURE-BASED VIEWS OF PATIENTS

	VOLUNTEERED		DIRECTED
To observer alone............	57	(39%)	–
To others in everyday conversation	75	(52%)	–
Individual	6	(4%)	–
Group	7	(5%)	–
Total	145	(100%)	0

the observer; in none of them, that is, did the observer suggest the use of the category to the student. Furthermore, more than half of the items report incidents in which these student culture-based ways of viewing patients were expressed in conversations between students or between students and other medical personnel. Another 5 per cent of the items report group activities. In each case, the collective character of the acts gives grounds for concluding that these views of patients (more accurately, the premises on which they were based) were customary among students and were shared collectively.

Chapter 17   # Student Autonomy

We have just shown how the students face the typical situations of their clinical years and have described the perspectives from which they come to view them. An unexpected feature of this phase of the students' training is the autonomy they exercise in setting their levels and direction of effort. But in what sense do they have autonomy? And why is that autonomy not severely limited by close association with residents and interns in the wards and clinics?

Let it be clear that the autonomy of the students is restricted to the matter of level and direction of academic effort. It stops abruptly where the welfare of patients is at stake. Patients are examined by qualified physicians as well as by students. The procedures performed on patients by students are supervised by their superiors. Diagnoses and plans of treatment proposed by students are evaluated by the faculty or the house staff.

However, in deciding what they will study and how hard they will work, the students do have considerable autonomy. On this matter the faculty can only suggest and provide appropriate models for the students to emulate; they cannot fully supervise. As we have shown, the student's situation is not always that of the practicing physician. He perceives imperatives and interests peculiar to his situation as student. He tailors his plans of action to fit that situation.

In theory, the students might have been so deeply constrained by the faculty's perspectives that they would have used their bit of autonomy to carry out the faculty's wishes beyond the point of necessity. In fact, they often use it to act in ways the faculty do not approve — evidence of some deep-lying differences between student and faculty perspectives. Indeed, the students' perspective proceeds from assumptions quite different from those of the faculty about the nature and purposes of medical education. These assumptions naturally result in specific situational perspectives which differ from those which the faculty, given their own assumptions, might logically desire the students to have. These disparities are presumptive evidence of student autonomy.

We do not have systematic data on the perspectives of faculty members on the level and direction of student effort. In what follows we make use of what faculty members said to students in the presence of observers, some material from interviews with the faculty, and comments made during the seminars in which we discussed our preliminary findings with the faculty. We think a good deal of confidence can be put in these fragments of data, partly because we seldom heard anything contradictory and partly because, as we shall see later, the faculty perspectives we describe (albeit briefly) embody one pole of a debate over the proper ends of education that has been going on since Erasmus.

One clear difference between the assumptions on which faculty and student perspectives are built can be found in the answer to this question: Are the four years of medical school the beginning or the end of a medical education? The faculty answer to this question appears in the university catalogue:

> The attainment of a medical education is a dynamic and lifelong process. The medical degree is granted at the end of four years of study in recognition of the fact that the student has acquired sufficient information and medical skill to be able to assume the responsibility for the free selection of his own future medical education. It does not mark the end of an educational experience, but only the beginning of the independent acquisition of knowledge.[1]

This is not merely a statement in a catalogue. It is a belief held strongly by many faculty members, to our knowledge; we suspect that if we had the data we would find that all faculty members assent to the idea. This belief and its corollaries have consequences for the way faculty members view and handle their teaching assignments.

The faculty believe that medicine has grown so complex and that so much is now known about various diseases, their treatment, and

[1] Bulletin of the University of Kansas, Vol. LIX, No. 10 (October 1, 1958), 158.

the principles of basic medical science underlying these that four years of medical school are simply not enough time to learn it all. The staff seem to feel that students will not be adequately equipped to practice medicine when they leave. Their worry increases every time a student nearing graduation exposes himself as not knowing some important fact the faculty thinks absolutely necessary in order to practice medicine properly.

Since this is their view of things, the faculty naturally do not think it worthwhile to try to teach the student all the things he would need to know to set up in practice. Many things the students would like to have training in are regarded as too technical for them at this point and are reserved for later advanced training. The fact that residencies in general practice have been set up at the medical center is indicative of the faculty position.

The faculty recognize, of course, that a great many of the students who graduate will never have any residency training and may be so located geographically that they will have very little opportunity for training of any kind once they finish their internship. Even in these cases, they feel, school should be the beginning of a man's medical education, not the end. The graduating student should realize how little he knows and how much he has to learn and should continue to study on his own, keeping up on latest developments in various fields through assiduous attention to medical literature and through attendance at postgraduate courses. The faculty, in all these ways, show they do not consider the four years of medical school final preparation for medical practice itself.

The students see the worth of medical school training quite differently. While they would all agree that four years of medical school is not enough to know all there is to know about any particular field of medicine, many would still insist that it is training enough to start out in medical practice. They think that enough is known about a great many diseases to make them able to handle them successfully themselves or to recognize them in time to send the patient to the proper specialist. Consequently, they feel that while what they learn in medical school may not be the end of their education, it certainly marks the end of the most important phase of it.

The students have worked hard, from their point of view, during their four years in school and are as inclined to maximize the importance of what they have learned as the faculty are to minimize it. Instead of considering that these four years are only the preparation for their real learning, they prefer to think that these have been the years of real learning and that what follows will be more like frosting on the cake. They conceive of the "extra" things further training would give them as details which are of particular interest and necessity only to the specialist in given fields. With regard to any given specialty, the bulk of the students do not see themselves as possible members of it and therefore see no need to learn all these extra details.

This is not to say that most of the students have firmly decided that they will themselves have no further training. A majority of the students have not decided, even by graduation, whether they will take residency training or not and, if so, in what field. They agree that it is necessary for a man who is going to specialize to have additional training. But they argue, nevertheless, that a man is equipped after four years of medical school and an internship to handle a good deal of what he will see should he go into general practice then and that what more he needs to know he can pick up, so to speak, on the job.

In short, there is a significant disparity between the assumptions students and faculty make about the place of the four years of undergraduate training in a medical career. The faculty think it only the beginning of a lifetime of training, but the students think it is, at least, the end of one important phase of their training. These varying assumptions underlie some of the more specific disagreements between faculty and students, the existence of which indicates clearly that students do exercise some autonomy in setting the direction of their academic effort.

The most obvious specific disagreement stemming from this disparity in assumptions arises with regard to the kinds of procedures students are allowed to do on patients. As we have seen, students feel that it is important for them to get experience in doing diagnostic and therapeutic procedures and in handling the medical responsibility associated with such activities. This belief is clearly related to the assumption that medical school represents more than just a beginning of a medical education. Many students might say, "If we don't get the chance to do these procedures now, under supervision, we will have to learn to do them on our own, without supervision, later." Similarly, the student feeling that time ought not to be wasted on things they already know (as they feel it is wasted in doing admission laboratory work on patients) is related to this same assumption: since their time in medical school is so valuable it should be spent on those things which they will have to deal with themselves when they are out in practice.

More generally, those patterns of student action and belief we have described as the responsibility and experience perspectives imply a view of the medical career as one in which some major part of one's professional education must be got now because there will not be time to get it later. They envision themselves as entering practice immediately after completing an internship and being thrust immediately into the most compelling and demanding medical situations. If one must, let us say, remove an inflamed appendix in an emergency operation during his first year in practice — and this is the kind of emergency they envision arising — how will he do it without having had some experience with the procedure earlier?

The faculty side of these specific disagreements equally clearly arises from their assumption that medical school is only the beginning of one's professional education. They cannot understand why students make such a fuss over being allowed to "do things." If the students do not do lumbar punctures this year, they will do them next year; if not during medical school, then during their internships. What, the faculty asks, is the hurry? They see the educational process extending, ideally, through all the years of a man's medical practice. There will be plenty of time for him to learn things. They think, furthermore, that the man who has just completed his internship is not really likely to get into all the dramatic situations that he envisions. Few appendices are so inflamed and few communities so isolated that the patient in need of appendectomy cannot be transported to a place where a well-trained man can handle his surgery adequately.

The faculty think, furthermore, that the students' demand to be taught "practical" things, immediately useful in practice, is short-sighted. The "practical" way of treating diabetic coma today, for instance, may not be the best way ten years from now, for new scientific discoveries may have revolutionized the approach to the problem. If a physician will continue to educate himself through close attention to medical literature and postgraduate programs, what he most needs to learn now are the basic scientific principles and discoveries on which such new treatments will be based; knowing these, he will be able to grasp new discoveries in diagnosis and treatment quickly and incorporate them into his everyday practice.

A second set of assumptions on which the faculty and students display a great difference has to do with the role of the general practitioner in medical practice today. Partly because the school we studied emphasizes the training of general practitioners and partly because so many of the students have no clear vision of their professional futures when they graduate from school, the students tend to think of themselves as prospective general practitioners, even though they may have more or less detailed plans in other directions. Both faculty and students thus think of the four years of school as training for general practice and the judgment of what is appropriate behavior in school (for both faculty and students) follows from the conception one has of the role and proper functions of the general practitioner.

The views of both faculty and student on this question are complex and sometimes contradictory. Both views mix together two notions of the situation the general practitioner will find himself in: 1. The general practitioner located within easy reach of a metropolitan center with a large complement of highly trained specialists, and 2. the general practitioner located far off from such a center (as the local phrase has it, "out in western Kansas"), who has no access to the services of specialists. Let us refer to these as the city and the country G.P.

Even when thinking of the same kind of situation, faculty and students may disagree. For the faculty is likely to think of the general practitioner as having access to a variety of specialists and consequently not needing to do many things completely on his own. They tend to believe that the city general practitioner should function primarily in dealing with minor injuries and diseases and in directing patients to the proper specialists. They tend to want to restrict his role and channel as many of his patients as possible to men with more specific training in the diseases those patients are suffering from. They think the general practitioner, with his limited training, should refer a great deal so as not to try to treat things that are beyond what his training has equipped him for.

But the faculty, in another mood, realizes that many of their graduates will be country general practitioners who will not so easily be able to refer their patients to specialists and who will have to treat many things that might better have been handled by a specialist. When they look at the matter in this way, the faculty is inclined to concentrate on drilling a few basic points into the students' heads. They are continually bothered by the dilemma that this is what must be done although it is not the best thing. So each gives what he regards as the basic minimum of training in his specialty, but fears that the students may mistake this basic minimum for the much larger amount of knowledge necessary to practice that particular branch of medicine successfully. They are afraid that students, having had this minimum of training, will then think of themselves as qualified to handle all kinds of things, many of which must (in the faculty view) be sent to specialists if the patient is to have any chance at all of good treatment. They fear, in other words, that this elementary instruction will give the students the illusion that they know a great deal more than they do and will have the effect of causing some students to engage in medical activities far beyond their knowledge and capabilities.

The students seem on the surface to agree with the faculty, since they too subscribe to the idea that the general practitioner should do nothing beyond his capabilities; but they do not agree on what a general practitioner is in fact capable of. The students are also more likely to place this hypothetical general practitioner in the country situation where he has no access to specialists. This means that they see the range of things the general practitioner may be called on to do, whether he has the capability or not, as extremely wide.

Again, although the students say that the general practitioner should only do those things and handle those cases his training has adequately prepared him for, their notion of adequate training differs considerably from that of the faculty. Where the staff surgeons are apt to consider that only a man who has had a complete residency in surgery should do such procedures as appendectomies or tonsillectomies, the students are likely to think that a man can have considerably less training than this and still be properly prepared. They agree that he would still need some training beyond what he gets in medical school, but some think that this can be picked up during internship or a short postgraduate course.

Some evidence on this point can be found in our interviews with a random sample of students. We asked them whether a general practitioner should do any of the following operations: tonsillectomy, appendectomy, and herniorrhaphy. Faculty members had indicated to some students during the period of our observations that they regarded these operations as too dangerous and difficult for anyone without specialized surgical training to attempt. But many students disagreed. Of our sixty-two interviewees, twenty-four thought it proper for a general practitioner to perform all three operations, nineteen more thought at least two of the operations within a general practitioner's abilities, and eleven thought he could do at least one of the three. In short, fifty-four of the interviewees (87%) disagreed with the faculty in some measure. Nor is the size of this percentage due to the freshmen and sophomores, who are relatively unfamiliar with clinical procedures, being in favor of the general practitioner doing these operations. Rather, it is the students in the clinical years who are more likely to disagree with the faculty on this point.

The students consider it likely that, if they should end up practicing in some small town in western Kansas, they will of necessity have to perform procedures and handle cases that are "too difficult for them" by faculty standards. They envision many emergency cases in which the pressure of time will force them to perform such operations as appendectomy. Furthermore, they feel that they will not be able to practice successfully if they insist on referring all patients with complicated diseases to some far-off medical center, fearing that to do this would alienate members of their small community. This may or may not be so; but the students believe it, and the belief affects their behavior in school.

A man who thinks it likely that he will do some surgery in general practice (were he to go into general practice) will tend to be dissatisfied with the training in surgery given him by a faculty whose primary aim in the course is to teach him the mistakes that a poorly trained doctor can make in attempting surgery. Other chronic sources of friction are likewise deducible from the premises of this argument.

Indeed, the responsibility and experience perspectives find some of their roots in this set of assumptions. If students do not think of medical school as simply the beginning of their education it is in part because they envision a practice whose demands upon them will not wait for their education to continue to some ideal point.

A final set of assumptions on which students and faculty differ greatly has to do with the question of what constitutes a "serious" approach to the work of medical school. Faculty and students agree completely that a student should be serious about his work but differ in their notions of what it means to be serious. Students think they are being utterly serious when they attempt to concentrate on learning what seems to them, on the basis of their admittedly limited experience and incomplete knowledge, to be necessary for the actual practice of medicine. The faculty think of "seriousness," however, as a character trait expressed in single-minded devotion to one's present work. They think their students are not serious when they decide that some work deserves their full attention while other work can be safely slighted. Furthermore, they think students not serious when they take other criteria than medical importance into account in organizing their conduct toward patients and faculty.

The student perspectives described in earlier chapters run counter, on certain points, to faculty notions of a serious approach to medical education. One implication of the responsibility and experience perspectives is that some kinds of work and knowledge are more important than others and that some kinds of work (which have no clear relation to medical practice) are probably not important at all. Thus, students think it is a waste of time to do admission laboratory work on a great number of patients. Since they do not believe they will do such work when they are out in practice, they cannot see the utility of doing so much of it now. They think it is probably a waste of time to study rare diseases when there are many diseases so much more common about which they still do not know everything. This tendency of students to regard some kinds of work and experience as unimportant strikes the faculty as frivolous.

Related to this is the faculty propensity to think that students, for any of a variety of reasons, do not work as hard as they might. Some faculty members, realizing that most students are married and have children, feel that they are not as likely as earlier generations of students to spend evenings and Sundays in the hospital, except when required to. Others occasionally glimpse students playing pool or bridge when they might be studying or decide that they do not see many students in the library. The failure of students to work on things that seem to them too rare or specialized to warrant attention is frequently interpreted by the faculty as laziness or "goofing off."

The faculty point of view shows itself clearly in the ambiguous meaning, for them, of the term "responsibility." We have already seen, in an earlier chapter, that both faculty and students use "responsibility" in a very specific way to refer to the responsibility of the physician for the life and death of his patient. But the faculty use the same term in a much more general sense, to refer to a person's trustworthiness in meeting obligations of any kind and to his ability to do the best possible thing in any circumstances without direct supervision;

they do not restrict their use of the term to situations involving patients or the welfare of patients.

We became aware of this second meaning of the term for faculty members when we reported our finding that students felt they were not given enough responsibility. The faculty responded that the students did not act responsibly enough with what little responsibility they had and so could not be trusted with any more. As an example, they charged that students often do not bother to read up on rare diseases that are to be seen in the hospital. Giving another example, they said that students are likely not to do some kinds of work unless they know that the faculty will check up to see if it has been done; and so on. These, they said, are the actions of irresponsible youths, not of responsible men. A responsible man would see the actions demanded by the situation and perform them without being told.

The faculty also find the students not serious when they act on the academic or student co-operation perspectives; that is, when students noticeably act in ways that are attempts to please the faculty and when they act in order to limit the amount of work they are collectively held responsible for. They think that a truly serious student would know that they are best pleased when he is independent in his search for knowledge and consider the students childish for doing such things as trying to find out what answer to a question posed on rounds or in an oral examination will most please them.

In short, students and faculty also disagree on what constitutes a serious attitude toward medical education. Students act on their own assumptions, not those of the faculty; the perspectives of student culture, not the differing perspectives of the faculty, dominate their behavior in school. Insofar as students' ideas and activities express fundamentally different assumptions and perspectives, we can say that they have autonomy in setting the level and direction of their academic effort.

The perspectives of the faculty are clearly congruent with a major trend in educational philosophy and practice. Educational systems of all kinds suffer a continuing dilemma: Shall they consider their work as terminal, after which the student will learn no more, or shall they consider that they are teaching the student how to learn, a training he will continue to apply in later years, conceivably to the end of his life? One historic resolution of this dilemma is to assume that the school cannot predict just what the student will need to know later on and must therefore, even while giving him some knowledge to be put to use immediately, concentrate on training him to teach himself after he leaves the school. The medical faculty evidently accepts this philosophy, a common one among contemporary teachers in graduate and professional schools. As for the dilemma itself, it may be greater in medical schools than in others. The students, having spent four years in a college of liberal arts and sciences, are especially anxious to move from the general to the particular, from the theoretical to the practical, and to bring school to an end so that practice may begin. Yet it is in the nature of the medical profession (as of others which require long training) that the techniques one learns at the end of the long years of school are constantly subject to changes which are, in part, based on advances in theoretical knowledge and which can be understood fully only by return to a more general view. This makes the determining of the terminus of formal training an arbitrary judgment dependent upon the length of the perspective from which one views medical knowledge and medical practice. The faculty man tends to the view of Ulysses, seeing medicine as

> . . . that untravell'd world, whose margin fades
> For ever and for ever when I move.

The students, approaching the end of an already too long road, take a shorter view. They are willing, like Telemachus, to settle down and get on with practical affairs.

Residents and Student Autonomy

An important member of the cast of the student's daily drama is the resident. The resident comes to the school to be trained in a medical specialty or specialties. He has graduated from medical school, completed an internship, and is legally empowered to exercise medical responsibility. In the medical hierarchy of the hospital, he stands just underneath the members of the faculty, above the intern, in command when the faculty is not present.

Residents teach students in several ways, described below. In addition, they are substantially senior to students in the hierarchy of clinical medicine students become part of when they begin their work in wards and clinics. Insofar as students become involved in the management and treatment of patients, the residents are necessarily interested in seeing that their work is done conscientiously and well.

Residents are ordinarily assigned to one of the hospital services, a ward or clinic dealing mainly with patients whose diseases fall within the purview of the resident's specialty. Each such service has a staff "chief" to whom the resident is responsible. Many, but not all, services have one or more interns who, as part of their rotating internships, spend some time on a succession of services, assisting the resident in his medical duties. Finally, a service may have a small group of students assigned to it; the students' responsibilities on the various services they participate in have been described earlier. From the standpoint of the resident, it is important to note that students are much more involved in some services than others. Some services, at one extreme, may be responsible only for an occasional lecture or two while other services have students on hand at all times. Likewise, some residents always have students who must be taught, whose work with patients must be supervised, and so on, while other residents do not have this benefit or burden (for it can be evaluated in either way).

At the beginning of this chapter we raised a second question about student autonomy. Students in the clinics and on the hospital wards, though their contact with the faculty is often confined to such formal occasions as ward rounds and classes, are usually in much closer contact with the residents. Residents do not have offices elsewhere, and their main duties are ordinarily carried on in the places where the students work; consequently, they have more opportunity than the faculty to see what students are actually doing. Furthermore, they are much nearer the students in rank in the hospital hierarchy, more likely to have vivid memories of their own recent pasts as students, and therefore more likely to be privy to the students' thoughts (uncensored by the realization of the effect those thoughts might have on the faculty).

Since they are likely to know what the students are doing and why, we can expect that residents probably are aware of the ways in which students diverge from faculty expectations. If they chose, the residents might be able to undermine these autonomous actions of students, either through direct disciplinary measures or by reporting them to their superiors. The residents either do not do this or do not do it effectively because, as we have seen, students do have considerable autonomy with respect to their academic activities.

Even though residents and students work in close proximity, and despite the fact that residents stand above students in the medical hierarchy, their relations are such that they have little direct effect on one another. Residents and students have most importance for each other as people who can affect one's relations with the more important and more powerful faculty. That is, the resident is concerned with students as people who can affect his relations with the faculty and the student is concerned with residents as people who can affect his relations with the faculty. The residents' activity is important for an understanding of student autonomy only because they can affect the amount of autonomy the student has vis-à-vis the faculty. Residents themselves have no direct interest in controlling student activity. But their relations with the faculty must be known if we are to understand why students are able to act autonomously. In this section we consider the role of teaching and supervising students in the resident's conception of his work, the degree to which residents are likely to attempt to interfere with student autonomy, and the outcome of such attempts.

The resident has essentially three kinds of demands made upon his time, energy, and ingenuity. One demand he makes upon himself: to be a student and learn more medicine. A second demand is that he administer, or help to administer, various wards and services (including their medical supervision). A third demand, or expectation, is that he teach and oversee the work of the medical students.

The resident expects that he will get something out of his residency "for himself." He expects to receive a certain amount of formal training — through classes, conferences, and various meetings — and anticipates doing less routine work from which he will learn more than he did as an intern. He expects a certain amount of guidance from the faculty in medical and administrative matters; but he also expects an opportunity to learn from experience while engaging in administrative duties and a schedule that will allow him to balance his work, sleep, and studying. During some periods spent upon certain services the resident has few administrative and teaching duties and can maximize his student role. He can also devote himself mainly to learning when he has a very good (or "responsible") intern to assist him in his administrative work, one in whose hands he can leave some of his own responsibility and work. If the resident thinks the intern is not ready for such a delegation of authority, he must slight his own studies and spend his time doing those jobs he feels the intern is not yet ready for.

Administering, or helping to administer, the ward occupies a great deal of the resident's time and thought; it is one of the things his superiors expect of him and hope he will do well. Even his own learning activities must be fitted in and around his administrative work. He can, of course, learn a great deal in the course of running a ward, and indeed he tends to equate administering a ward with learning medicine by administering the ward. But sometimes this work leaves him little time or energy for learning; if his ward is understaffed, his expectations as a student must go unsatisfied. Sometimes the patients he sees in the course of his administrative work are of types already so familiar to him that he can expect little fresh clinical knowledge from them. His service chief (a faculty man legally responsible for all patients on the service) may judge him in part as an administrator, according to whether the service is well run, whether his nurses and interns are doing careful or sloppy work. The residents know that they are being so judged; when the service chiefs make rounds they criticize and evaluate his work and may embarrass him by caustic or reproachful comments.

Finally, residents are expected to teach and supervise the work of students. They must give scheduled classroom lectures to students assigned to their services; they supervise the clinical work done by these students; and they informally contribute to the learning of students in numerous, and almost undefined, ways — such as answering questions while at a patient's bedside or providing a model for the student to follow in handling patients and in managing procedures.

How do the residents view this obligation? Residents often wonder whether teaching students can add substantially to their own learning; it can certainly detract from the time available for studying and running a ward. Students who are "on the ball," who ask good questions, who keep one on one's toes, can make life more interesting and make some residents go to their own books for answers. But medical tradition is such that great emphasis is put upon learning from one's own experience by seeing patients and working with them; and by learning from superiors. Residents do not regard their own teaching as a stimulating experience which forces them to reorganize their own thinking.

In addition, the resident, like the students, rotates around the services (though not so widely around the hospital); he is sometimes just a beginner himself at precisely those times when a new group of students arrives on the service. So he not only has less to teach them than he might when he is more secure in his knowledge, but he has less inclination to teach.

Most important for the effect of residents upon student autonomy is this question: How do residents rank the importance of their triple functions as learner, administrator, and teacher? Although, as in the case of the faculty, we do not have systematic analyses of the residents' perspectives, we feel convinced by the data we do have that they put teaching and supervising students in last place. We are strengthened in this conviction because it accords with what might be expected on the basis of sociological theories of hierarchical organization. Typically, the middle strata in such organizations look up rather than down, are more concerned with pleasing their superiors than overseeing their subordinates, except when the performance of subordinates figures in the evaluations made by their superiors. They are not likely to devote much energy to enforcing standards on their subordinates when there are other ways of maintaining their position. The residents, the middle stratum in the medical school, act like the middle stratum in this model. Several kinds of evidence bear on this point.

First, residents were not often reprimanded, at least while we were observing, for not doing a good job of teaching; at the same time, we did observe residents being reprimanded for failures in their administrative-medical work. Second, when medical emergencies occur they automatically take precedence over teaching responsibilities; residents often failed to meet their classes when patients required their attention. Third, when residents meet each other, at coffee breaks or in the halls, and exchange communications, they rarely talk about students or about their own teaching; and when they do it is mainly to complain about or jibe at poor work done on the service rather than stupid questions asked during rounds or in the classroom. They talk, in fact, mainly about "interesting cases," particular procedures, what they have learned at conferences, their superiors, occasionally about good or bad interns, and about a variety of social matters. But they do not often speak of students and teaching. Fourth, residents in some fields believe that their specialties are so technical and specialized that students simply do not yet know enough to be able to learn anything.

Finally, the observer asked four residents to rank the relative importance of teaching, administration, and their own learning. Without exception, they ranked teaching last. Unfortunately, there was not sufficient time to pursue this line of questioning with more residents, but we believe that most of them would have answered similarly. We believe this because of the other kinds of evidence described and because it is likely, on the basis of our general knowledge of many-leveled hierarchies, that they would be more concerned with their own ambitions and with pleasing their superiors than with supervising their subordinates.

On the basis of the several items of evidence we have just discussed, we think it likely that residents consider teaching and supervising students the least important of their functions. Whenever one of their other functions makes demands on their time and energy, they will hasten to satisfy these at the expense, if necessary, of their teaching. Thus, the nature of the resident's job limits the effort he might put into directing students, influencing their activity, and thereby decreasing the amount of student autonomy.

Nevertheless the residents do teach, and unquestionably sometimes the students, and the faculty itself, consider that some residents are teaching well. There are several reasons why residents spend more energy, thought, and time on teaching than the hospital can actually demand of them.

One is that the residents have a sense of responsibility to the profession and to the community. They are loath to turn loose upon an unsuspecting world a poorly trained graduate. They take some responsibility for seeing that every student is given an opportunity to learn — not so much for his own sake but for the good of his future patients.

Another reason for attempting to teach well, or beyond the call of duty, is because one likes to teach. Unquestionably some of the residents do enjoy teaching and "getting something across." Some of the distaste that residents feel for less-interested students comes from a sense of disappointment and boredom — and not simply from the extra work which accrues when students cannot help to run the service more smoothly. A "good" group helps to stimulate a man who likes to teach. The residents, like other physicians, believe in the efficacy of teaching "on the floor," of teaching with the patient right there in front of the student. They find it comparatively easy to comment on cases as they go about practicing medicine, or to answer questions in the halls shortly after some interesting medical event has occurred. This kind of teaching can be fitted in and around other kinds of duties and does not necessarily require a great amount of preparation.

The resident may also have a more self-serving interest in making certain that students are taught and their work carefully supervised. If the students, during their time with the faculty, reveal ignorance of some technical point or of some set of facts about a particular patient, the faculty member involved may blame the resident for the students' failure. If the resident had done a better job, the argument goes, the students would know these things. Sometimes the resident will take the trouble to coach the students in something that either he or they expect a faculty member to quiz them on when they go on rounds. This coaching can be for the good of the students, but it can also be to prevent potential embarrassment to the resident.

Finally, by supervising the students' work closely, the resident can cut down his own workload. If students can do minor procedures, such as drawing blood, quickly and without difficulty, he is relieved of one of the many tasks that compete for his time. If, by supervising the students adequately, he can get needed help in carrying out his many responsibilities, he is inclined to do so.

Thus, even though the resident's ranking of the importance of his various tasks puts teaching in last place, he will make some effort to supervise students. This might decrease the autonomy of students if it were not that the residents tend to use the same perspectives as students. Since this is the case, even when residents do intervene in student activities they are not likely to want the students to do anything that does not seem reasonable from the perspectives of student culture.

One reason for thinking that residents share student perspectives is the similarity in background and training of residents and students. Although it is not true of all of them, the residents tended to plan to go into private practice, to have come from Kansas and nearby states in the region, to have had their undergraduate medical training at the University of Kansas, and to plan to practice in the small and medium-sized cities of the region. (This is particularly true of the residents in the "big" courses — medicine, surgery, pediatrics, and obstetrics — with whom students spent most time.) In all these ways they resemble the students they teach and, insofar as the students' perspectives depend on these facts of background, training, and ambitions, the residents' perspectives might be expected to be similar.

The residents' teaching activities do, in fact, appear to express perspectives similar to those of the student culture. Our field notes are replete with descriptions of residents teaching the students those things which are closest to the students' hearts; namely, procedures, "pearls," tips, and other bits of medical wisdom which the resident suspects will be useful for the practicing physician. Some of the residents' teaching of "pearls," tips, and procedures is at the urging of the students, but much of it is spontaneous. These matters are either important enough for the resident to teach or he is close enough to his own student days to appreciate their reception by the students. Occasionally, too, a resident is drawn into the undergraduates' discussions of their career plans and will give advice or relate relevant anecdotes about himself or his acquaintances. Sometimes both residents and students discuss the faculty, in terms that are more or less similar.

It seems safe to conclude, therefore, that when residents are drawn roughly from the same population as their students and have approximately the same kinds of training and experience — only more of it — they will rather naturally tend to teach along lines students desire and appreciate. When a resident does otherwise, we can assume that this is because he is genuinely a different kind of physician because of his background and interests or because he holds a different perspective upon a specific issue than the students, either because of his additional training or because of his different institutional position. We have already suggested, however, that relatively few residents have had a training markedly different from that of the undergraduates.

Thus, residents have some incentives for devoting attention to the activities of students but also have other compelling interests which turn their attention elsewhere. Even when they are interested, their perspectives tend to be similar to students', so that their intervention does not interfere with student autonomy. Nevertheless, residents are not undergraduate medical students. Their positions in the structure of the school and hospital are different. Their interests and perspectives differ in some ways from those of the students, even if this disparity is not as great as that between the perspectives of students and faculty.

When residents and students meet on ward or clinic, something in the nature of a contest ensues, as each tries to manage his own life in the hospital to what he considers his own advantage. The students attempt to maximize the amount of experience and responsibility they get, attempt to make a good impression on the faculty, and try to limit the amount of work they do to what they consider a reasonable and justifiable amount. The resident tries to run his service so that good medical care is given to patients and so that his superiors will be pleased with his performance; at the same time he tries to further his own medical education. Insofar as the students' behavior can affect the resident's attempts to achieve these ends, he will attempt to influence what they do. Insofar as his attempts at influence affect the students' efforts to achieve their own ends, they will resist. These attempts at influence and resistance constitute the contest played out between residents and students.

While our data do not provide any systematic information on the outcome of this contest in any large number of cases, we can inspect the strategies available to students and residents and from these arrive at the conclusion that it is very likely that the students usually prevail. This inspection of strategies thus leads us to the conclusion that, even when his own conceptions incline him to make the effort, the resident has very little ability to interfere with student autonomy.

When students and residents first meet each other, when either first comes to the service, they seek to size up each other. Of course their respective reputations may precede their confrontation. "Good" and "poor" groups of students are sometimes known before they reach a service; and "good" and "poor" residents are sometimes known through rumor and gossip before the group actually sets eyes upon them. The resident may deliberately try to influence what the students think of him by presenting a front of toughness or friendliness; or he may unwittingly show himself in such a way as to influence the students' thinking.

Whether the resident presents himself deliberately or not, the students make relatively quick judgments about such things as whether he knows his stuff or whether he doesn't; whether he is interested in teaching them or not; whether he is bent upon using them for his own purposes or is fair; whether he might be interested in teaching but is too pressed to teach well; whether he sympathizes with them and tells them what to look for on rounds or in the faculty, or whether he does not do these things. Conversely, the residents are making counterjudgments of the group: whether it is good, poor, or middling; whether the students ask good or poor questions, or no questions at all; whether they are lazy, or slow and not very bright, or alert, intelligent, and hard-working.

Following this initial sizing-up, residents and students begin to operate in ways calculated to gain what they want out of the situation. The resident who wishes to have the students play an active part and assist him in his ward work has various devices available. He can punish sloppy work or students who are laggard by such devices as making them rewrite reports of physical exams. He can reprimand

and publicly embarrass students. He can "ride" a student he thinks especially poor. But he can also employ more positive means, encouraging his students by nice treatment, pleasantries, praise and personal example; and also by implicit bargaining, such as showing the students certain procedures or allowing them to do certain procedures as well as by dropping "pearls" and bits of medical wisdom. The resident can also take pains to let his boys know they are being protected and cared for, as when he primes them for rounds or goes out of his way to have them see "interesting cases" they might otherwise not have an opportunity to observe. In general, the residents put themselves out more when they think the group of students they are dealing with is a "good" one, i.e., a group that is intelligent and competent. When they think the group not so "good," they tend to withdraw and restrict their activity with students to what is necessary and required. They justify their withdrawal in part by saying that such a group would not learn much anyway and in part by saying that, because the students are not good and cannot be trusted with much, they themselves have more work and less time for teaching.

The students have at their disposal, in turn, similar moves in this game. They will try to work quickly and well, provided that the work is interesting and teaches them something or at least that the resident takes time to teach them worthwhile things. They can engage also in various maneuvers to get from the resident the information that he would not otherwise give; we have described many of these in earlier chapters.

Students also have techniques for avoiding work which they consider is not rewarding or is not yielding dividends of instruction. Thus they may fail to show up on the floor when the resident is there; they may cut their time on the service to a minimum; they may disappear into back rooms where they cannot be found; they may slow down and cut corners. This does not mean that they do not learn on such a service or that they are wasting their time; rather, they are simply staying out of sight of a man who will not, or cannot, co-operate with them.

When they do this, the resident has relatively few countergambits available. He cannot so easily or effectively complain to his chief as he can about an unsatisfactory intern — he can simply gripe that this group is lazy or stupid. (Hence we once or twice heard residents saying that they actually cannot discipline the students effectively — or at least as effectively as they might wish.) When the students employ the tactic of withdrawal, the resident may also do so; he refuses to bother much with them except to give scheduled conferences and hardly bothers to toss off bits of information as he goes about his administrative business. On some services the students feel that they have explored thoroughly the possibilities of the service in a few days or weeks. Then they tend to withdraw from work and, if possible, from the sight of the resident. (We should say that this bargaining, the game of move and countermove, is carried on without public recognition of its existence; that is, both residents and students know what they are doing and intend to influence each other's behavior, but the matter is not discussed publicly between them.)

Residents, thus, have neither the desire nor the means to supervise students intensively enough to prevent the development and acting out of the perspectives constituting student culture. Though their position in the hospital, as subordinates of the faculty and superiors of the students, gives them the power to intervene effectively in student activities, residents do not pose any threat to the students' autonomy vis-à-vis the faculty. The residents do nothing to prevent the students from acting on assumptions we have seen to differ radically from those used by the faculty.

Autonomy and Student Culture

Students must have some autonomy — some freedom to determine what they will do and how they will do it — before such a phenomenon as student culture is possible. In this chapter, we have demonstrated, first of all, that they do have this necessary minimum of autonomy, showing that student perspectives are based on assumptions quite different from those the faculty makes with regard to issues central to the problems of medical education. The fact that students act on such different assumptions is presumptive evidence that they have a considerable degree of autonomy. We have also, in this chapter, shown that the students' immediate superiors, the residents, have neither the inclination nor the power to supervise students closely in order to prevent the growth of student culture. The residents do not provide a brake on student autonomy.

Some readers may feel that the evidence of student autonomy provided in this section of our book discloses the existence of a "bad" situation, that students ought not to be so free to choose their own level and direction of effort. Some readers may even blame the hard-working faculty of the school for this state of affairs. To so read our analysis would be a major error. What we have described is a common sociological phenomenon, present in many organizations and probably present in most schools, including medical schools.

Gouldner has pointed out that ". . . a basic source of organizational tension may derive . . . from the tendency of the parts to resist encroachment on their functional autonomy. . . ."[2] In other words, we may expect that in all organizations the units of which it is made up will strive for and, except in extreme cases, attain some measure of autonomy. A study of public school teachers provides an empirical base for this conclusion. This study concluded that the teachers were able to maintain a certain amount of autonomy over their work because they could fend off the encroachments of principals and parents either by the threat of countermeasures or by the development of a secretive relationship to outsiders.[3]

Medical students, then, have autonomy in the same way most organizational participants have it. This is not a pathological development, to be deplored, but rather a natural feature of organizational life.

One of the important sociological generalizations to be drawn from our work arises from consideration of the fact of student autonomy. The generalization is that subordinate groups in complex organizations tend to have considerably more power to determine the conditions of their existence and actions than the authority system of the organization formally allows and that they use this autonomy to develop systems of belief and action that may run counter to those their superiors desire. The tendency of subordinate groups to develop autonomous cultures within larger organizations has several bases. First, subordinates share a common position in the organization and thus have common problems arising out of the peculiarities of that position. They are likely to attempt collective solutions of their problems. Neither the solutions nor the problems that prompt them are likely to be given official recognition in the higher reaches of the organization, so that both solutions and problems will continue to reflect the unique biases of the subordinates' position. Second, since

[2] Alvin W. Gouldner, "Organizational Analysis," in *Sociology Today,* ed. by Robert K. Merton, Leonard Broom, and Leonard S. Cottrell, Jr. (New York: Basic Books, 1959), p. 421.

[3] See Howard S. Becker, "The Teacher in the Authority System of the Public School," *Journal of Educational Sociology,* XXVII (November, 1953), 128–41.

all organizations rely to some extent on the willing participation of their members in their activities, subordinates have considerable power to develop their activities autonomously by virtue of the possibility of withholding their willingness to engage in some of the organization's activities. They may simply refuse to do some things their superiors desire them to do, in which case increased supervision must be used to force compliance. Or they may bargain, by refusing to do some things as their superiors desire unless they are given autonomy with respect to other activities.

Part Four:

PERSPECTIVES ON THE FUTURE

Chapter 18

Student Perspectives on
Styles of Practice

The Dilemma of Independence and Responsibility

Mᴇᴅɪᴄᴀʟ school, obviously, is not an end in itself. Students go to medical school in order to get education and training
which will enable them, when they graduate, to do things for which
that education and training are necessary. Though the immediate
conditions of their daily lives cause them to focus their attention
largely on the present and on the difficulties of getting through
school, students do look forward to the future, to the time when they
will have graduated and will have to choose what they will do as
physicians. While they are in school they develop tentative perspectives on the situations they expect to find themselves in in the future,
perspectives which define what these situations will be like, the terms
of the choices they will be called on to make, and the most suitable
actions for them to take when the time comes.

Specifically, the student looking toward the future considers these
questions. What kind of career am I going to have? Should I go into
teaching, research, or the private practice of medicine? If I decide to
practice medicine, where should I practice? Whom should I practice
with, or should I practice on my own? Should I go into general practice or get into a specialty? Where shall I intern? Students discuss
these problems frequently and arrive at certain collective solutions.

We may think of these collective solutions as perspectives belonging to the same class of phenomena as those perspectives that make

367

up student culture. But certain important differences should be kept in mind. The perspectives of the student culture were specific and referred to situations students were involved in at the time. They define immediate situations and actions appropriate to them. We included in our analysis of these perspectives the actions students took in accord with them. Furthermore, we found these perspectives characteristic of almost the entire student body, the exceptions being easily identified isolates and deviants. Students' goals were essentially similar, and the situations in which they acted to implement their goals were the same for all.

In contrast, the perspectives students develop on problems they will face in the future have necessarily a speculative and hypothetical character. They consist of definitions of what things may or will be like and how a student might behave when he gets to the point in time when things are like that. They are essentially playful, because they call for no action in the present, with the single exception of perspectives on internships which do, in the final year, call for an act of real choice. Students employing these perspectives are playing at making the decisions they will one day make seriously.

Perspectives on the future further differ from those which are part of student culture in that there are serious disagreements among students with regard to the matters they define. We have no monolithic student agreements on the specific details of proper student action, characteristic of the freshman year, or even the vaguer but still quite homogeneous consensus of the clinical years. Instead, students disagree on goals and on proper hypothetical actions. There is no agreement, for instance, as to whether one should be a general practitioner or a specialist and, if the latter, what kind of specialist. Similarly, there is no agreement as to whether one should be more interested in helping sick people, advancing medical knowledge, making a great deal of money, or any of the other possible goals of a medical career.

Because of these differences, the objects of our analysis in this section are different. We no longer seek to describe homogeneity. We cannot follow the pattern of reasoning used so far, in which we show that students sharing certain common assumptions and facing common situations develop a collective perspective defining problems and their proper solutions. Instead, we look for consistency of a different order and find it in sets of stereotypes students hold about future possibilities.

Student perspectives on the future take account of the range of possibilities offered by the medical world they hope to move into and attribute certain characteristics to each of those possibilities. They describe a range of motives students might have in choosing one or another of those possibilities. Finally, they define the relations between motives and possibilities, by saying that if you want X you must choose Y. They lay out, in short, alternative career routes and steps and say what kind of goal is appropriate for each. Our analysis, then, is concerned with these stereotypical pictures of the future.

We have further analytic concerns. In some cases it is possible for us to say what kinds of students seem to prefer (in the hypothetical form their preferences for the future take) what kinds of career paths and thus to relate specific student preferences to specific student characteristics. We do not, in doing this, intend to make any predictions about what these students will do. We know that their ultimate decisions will be made later, after they have left school, and that in the interim between graduation and the time of decision many further influences will intervene to affect their decisions so that very little prediction is possible. Only a longitudinal study which followed students up to the point of career decision could say with any assurance what students would do. We can only identify tentatively the first groping steps toward those decisions which students do make while in school. We do not know the degree to which these groping steps commit students more or less irrevocably to future career paths.

Finally, we pay close attention to the differences in content between the perspectives students make use of in dealing with the day-to-day problems of school and those they use in thinking about the future, unhampered by the constraints of their daily situation. On the one hand, we are interested in showing how the perspectives of student culture, as students developed them to meet the problems of school life, are used in thinking about the future. On the other hand, we are interested in demonstrating that certain themes continue to appear in students' thinking about the future, even though they find no place in the perspectives students use in dealing with problems of school life.

Chapter 18 deals with student perspectives on style of practice: general or specialized, and with whom to practice. Chapter 19 takes up the internship and details student views on the criteria by which internships should be judged and the ways internships differ with respect to these criteria. Chapter 20 moves farther into the future and considers students' perspectives on the various specialties. In

Chapter 21 we present a more generalized picture of the medical student's development as he moves through medical school. In addition, we suggest a theory of the connections between the immediate and long-range perspectives of institutional participants. In so doing, we discuss the perennial question of medical students' cynicism.

Throughout, our concern is to show how the students' participation in the life of the medical school furnishes them with a way of viewing their future and to explain the nature of those views and their relation to the facts of medical school life.

We begin our analysis of students' perspectives on the future by considering the way they assess various styles of practice. "Style of practice" is not a very concrete matter, and we have made our analysis more specific by dealing with two questions about which students think a great deal: Shall I have a general practice or a specialty practice? Shall I practice by myself or in association with one or more doctors? If I choose to associate myself with others, what form should that association take?

These questions form a staple subject of debate in the columns of both medical and lay journals. Some physicians question whether one man can amass all the knowledge now available and necessary for the adequate handling of the variety of patients who come to a general practitioner's office. Others question whether or not the growing specialization of modern medical practice does not somehow lose sight of the "whole patient." Many feel that solo practice is a thing of the past, but there is intense concern in the profession about the various forms of group practice being experimented with and the possible limitations that such practices might impose on the freedom with which patients select their physicians.

We do not propose to speak to these questions here. Instead, we analyze the way students regarded these questions. In some instances, students' views mesh with those now occupying the attention of the profession; in others, they are quite different.

General Practice vs. Specialty Practice

One major decision facing students as they go through school is whether to take specialty training and embark on a specialist's career or enter general practice immediately after finishing an internship.

The University of Kansas Medical School is known to be interested, among other things, in training general practitioners for the sparsely populated western half of the state in order to raise the level of medical facilities available there. Students who apply to the University of Kansas take cognizance of this and, almost to a man, announce on their application blanks that they are interested in becoming general practitioners in a small town in western Kansas. This happens with such regularity as to be a standing joke among the faculty and students.

Whatever intentions they may announce on an application form, students' plans are in fact more various. We met many students in the course of our field work who intended to become specialists and many more who had reached no decision or who vacillated from one specialty to another. Of the sixty-two students in our random sample of interviewees, twenty-five expressed a firm intention of becoming general practitioners. Three expressed no opinion, and the other thirty-four were either considering both general and specialty practice, had definitely chosen to specialize but were not sure in what field, or had definitely chosen a particular specialty.

Would-be specialists and general practitioners are not quite randomly distributed through the four years, although there are no statistically significant differences. Table XXXII shows that students in the first and last years are most likely to choose a specialty. Since many of these choices are indefinite and, further, since this is a subject about which students are likely to change their minds, we do not concentrate on the differences among those making different

TABLE XXXII

GENERAL OR SPECIALTY PRACTICE BY YEAR IN SCHOOL *

YEAR	GENERAL PRACTICE	SPECIALTY	No Opinion	TOTAL
First	6	11	2	19
Second	7	6	1	14
Third	7	8	–	15
Fourth	5	9	–	14
Total	25	34	3	62

* The "general practice" category includes only those who expressed a firm preference for that style of practice and no other. The "specialty" category includes all those who were considering both general and specialty practice as well as those who preferred a specialty practice, whether or not they had decided on a particular specialty.

choices. Instead, we turn our attention to the perspective which comes to dominate the thinking of most students as they approach graduation, a perspective that outlines the criteria to be used in judging general and specialty practices.

Students use four main criteria in assessing the relative value of general as opposed to specialty practice. The first of these takes account of the fact that specialization will require a great deal of training after the internship, at least three and as many as five years of residency. The student asks himself: can I afford or do I want to spend that much time in training before I begin my own practice? As might be expected, in most of the cases where students use this criterion they answer in the negative. Some simply say they cannot afford it financially; perhaps they have run up a sizable debt going through medical school and wish to begin paying it back as soon as possible. Others say they could afford a residency only if their wives continued to work and that it seems intolerable to postpone having children any longer. Still others feel that, having started school when they were a little older (because of service in the armed forces or other occupational involvements), they are too old to spend any more time in training. And some say that they will have been going to school for twenty years by the time they graduate from medical school and simply cannot stand the thought of being a schoolboy (as they conceive the resident to be) any longer.

The second criterion students use in thinking about general as opposed to specialty practice addresses itself to the question of the relative broadness of each of the styles of practice. The student says to himself: "As a general practitioner I will be called on to treat every disease that anyone ever gets while as a specialist I will deal only with a small fraction of all diseases. I can know just about everything there is to know about the specialty I take up but no one can ever know enough to be prepared for everything a G.P. might be faced with. On the other hand, a specialty practice will be narrow and limited while a general practice will be infinitely varied and interesting." A senior looking forward to what lay beyond graduation expressed the criterion this way:

I asked Jack Crown, "What kind of medicine do you intend to practice when you get out?" He said, "Well, I intend to go into general practice in some small town." I said, having spoken to him about this and gotten the same answer a year ago, "You haven't changed your mind very much about that, have you?" He said, "No, I haven't. I guess that's probably what

I'll still end up doing, although I have been thinking a little bit about going into a specialty maybe." This surprised me. [We talked for awhile about possible specialties.] Then Crown said, "Actually, the reason I am thinking about a specialty is that the idea of going into general practice kind of scares me." I said, "It does?" He said, "Yes. When you think about all those people just walking in off the street and they might have anything under the sun, from a brain tumor to diabetes to cancer — and you might not recognize it. It's kind of frightening and I just don't think I know enough to handle it. I really don't. So that worries me. I sometimes think it would be a lot better to learn one field pretty well and be able to deal with that, rather than trying to do it all. I think you have to know an awful lot to be a good general practitioner, but it would be easier to be a good specialist, I think."

Two other seniors, Heston and Pound, agreed. Pound said, "Boy, I sure agree with you there, Jack. General practice would scare me too. I would never go into general practice, not me. I don't think anybody knows enough to do that, to tell you the truth." Heston said, "Well, the idea of it doesn't make me very happy either, but I don't know whether I could last through a long residency or not."

(Senior Surgical Specialties. September, 1956.)

In another mood, students will speak about the tremendous challenge of general practice, about the great variety of patients and diseases one will see and the continuing interest one will be able to maintain in it.

The third criterion students use to judge styles of practice consists of an estimate of the amount of work the particular kind of practice will mean for them. General practice is typically seen as involving a tremendous amount of hard work: you have no control over the number of patients you see; you put in long hours. They sometimes mention that the physical strain of a crowded schedule may prevent you from doing the best possible job of diagnosis and treatment on each patient. In contrast, a specialist can limit his practice more easily and effectively, seeing patients by appointment only and then no more than he can comfortably handle; and most specialties require few night or emergency calls, some none at all.

The fourth criterion by which students choose between general and specialty practice is the opportunity each affords for getting to know one's patients well. Students fear that a specialist's view might be so limited that he would not be interested in the patient as a human being; he would be simply a technician, however skilled and talented. At worst, they think of the surgeons they have heard of who meet their patients for the first time in the operating room. They think of general practitioners, in contrast, as physicians who have a large amount of intimate contact with the families they serve. As one interviewee, a freshman who was planning to be a general practitioner, put it: "One of the reasons I went into medicine is that I like to be around people, and by specializing, it seems to me, you lose a lot of the personal contact. You don't have the time to get to know the person."[1]

A few other criteria were mentioned. A girl said that she thought it would be very difficult for a woman to carry on a general practice successfully. One student mentioned that he felt there was a great need for general practitioners. Two students thought there would be more money in a specialized practice, and another said that a specialist would necessarily have to live in a larger city. These occurred so infrequently that we do not deal with them separately in the remainder of our analysis but lump them together as "miscellaneous."

Having identified these criteria in a preliminary analysis of our data, we searched our field notes and interviews systematically for all uses of criteria by students to assess the relative worth of the two kinds of practice. The relative frequencies of each criterion in both kinds of data are shown in Table XXXIII. The four main criteria just described account for all of those observed in use during the field work and 72 per cent of those used in the interviews; combining the two kinds of data, they account for 88.5 per cent of all criteria

TABLE XXXIII
CRITERIA USED BY STUDENTS TO JUDGE GENERAL AND SPECIALTY PRACTICE

CRITERION	FIELD OBSERVATIONS		INTERVIEWS *		TOTAL	
	NUMBER	PER CENT	NUMBER	PER CENT	NUMBER	PER CENT
Length of training.....	34	49	8	16	42	35.0
Broadness & manageability	30	43	21	42	51	42.5
Hard work...........	6	8	7	14	13	11.0
Patient contact	–	–	9	18	9	7.5
Miscellaneous	–	–	5	10	5	4.0
Total	70	100	50	100	120	100.0

* The question we asked students was, "What kind of practice do you intend to go into? General practice or a specialty? If a specialty, which one? Why are you making this choice?"

[1] All quotations carrying no date, course, or service name are taken from our interviews with a random sample of students.

used, thus supporting the conclusion that they are the main criteria students use in assessing the two kinds of practice.

From this tabulation it appears that the questions uppermost in students' minds when they think about the kind of practice they would like to have are those revolving around the twin problems of the length of training one will need and the broadness and manageability of the two types of practice. Students do not, however, apply these criteria randomly; rather, they have consistent stereotypes of general and specialty practice. We get a more differentiated view of student perspectives in this area by considering these stereotypes. Figures 7 and 8 represent graphically all student uses of criteria to evaluate the two kinds of practice. Each figure shows, for field observations and interview data separately, a bar for each criterion; height indicates the number of times students used the criterion. The height of the bar above the mid-line indicates the number of students who said the style of practice possessed the characteristic specified in the criterion, the height below the line the number saying that the trait was absent. Each segment of the bar is further divided into those who evaluated the presence or absence of the trait, positively, negatively, or neutrally. (The miscellaneous category is not included in this tabulation.)

Comparing the two figures, we see that students clearly see specialty training as lengthy and that this weighs against specialization for them. On the other hand, they think of general practice as quite broad but specialty practice as narrow and limited. They like the narrowness of specialty practice, when they mention it, but are divided as to whether or not the broadness of general practice is a good thing. This division apparently has some relation to the techniques by which the data were obtained, for students observed in the field dwell on the difficulties of carrying on a general practice in view of the wide variety of complaints one will have to deal with, while the students we interviewed think the broadness of general practice would be a good thing, making for a more varied and interesting work life.[2]

Students agree completely that general practitioners work harder than specialists and agree further that hard work is not a good thing; this counts against general practice and for specialization in their

[2] This discrepancy between student views as observed in the field and expressed in interviews is probably a consequence of students' tendency to make use of their idealistic long-range perspective in interviews.

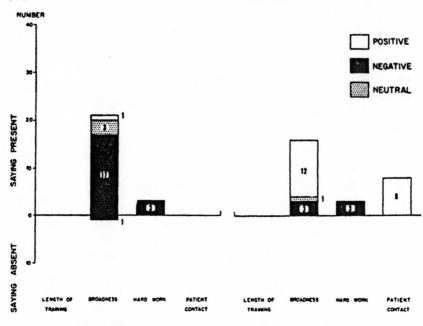

FIELD OBSERVATION   INTERVIEWS
Fig. 7 — Student Stereotype of General Practice.

eyes. Finally, they like general practice because it will provide them
with closer contact with patients (although one student liked specialty practice because it would protect him from this).

We noted earlier that though seniors and freshmen both seem to
prefer specialty practices, their reasons are different. We first decided
this when, in our field work, we observed several seniors who had
always intended to enter general practice experiencing a crisis of
conscience as they came to believe that, by the end of school, they
simply were not going to learn everything needed to practice general medicine effectively and efficiently. The conversation quoted
earlier involves one of these seniors. We now think that the perspective we have described influences many students to make such a
change, but unfortunately we do not have sufficient systematic data
to support this belief.

In spite of our lack of systematic data, we suggest that the following is a typical pattern of shifts in student thinking about the question of general versus specialty practice. As they enter medical
school, students have no very firm ideas about what kind of practice
they desire; some will say that general practice is what they want;
many, however, are likely to be unsure enough to also consider those

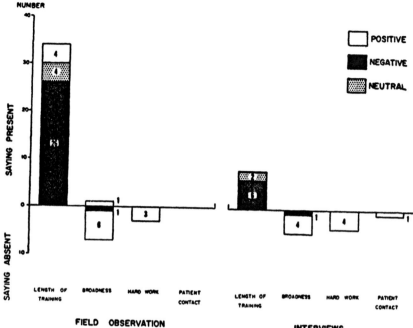

Fig. 8 — Student Stereotype of Specialty Practice.

specialties about which they have some knowledge though, as they are quick to say themselves, their knowledge is limited. As they go through school and gain greater acquaintance with various kinds of specialized practice, many pick out some constellation of specialties in which they are interested and begin to orient themselves toward it. Others get a more realistic idea of what the financial burden of residency training will be for them and decide that they cannot afford it. Finally, as graduation approaches, some of those who have decided on general practice become uneasy at the thought of exposing themselves to the hazards of handling every conceivable kind of medical problem and contemplate a switch into a specialty practice. Those who have more or less decided on specialty practice already no longer concern themselves with the alternative of general practice.

We cannot predict which students will go into general and which into specialized practices. They must finish school and an internship before they decide; many must spend two years in the armed service in addition; finally, many may go into general practice, change their minds after trying it for a few years, and take residency training. Since so many experiences that will have a profound effect

on their choice of style of practice lie in the future, we cannot say
with any assurance what any particular student will do. We can only
say that the choices are likely to be made with the criteria we have
described in mind.

Arrangements for Practice

Students, as they look ahead to practicing medicine, consider
whom they should practice with. There is a great variety of possibilities today but, with very few exceptions, students see only a few
of them. They then choose between the possibilities they are aware
of by referring to a set of criteria which specify what things are important in the arrangements one makes for practice.

The major choice is that between solo practice and some form of
group practice, the latter either a simple partnership or some kind
of clinic in which receipts and expenses are handled corporately and
each participant gets a specified percentage of the profit. Fifty-one
(82%) of our sixty-two interviewees expressed a preference for one
of these arrangements.

There are, of course, many other kinds of business arrangements
a young physician might make. Most prominent among these, and
becoming increasingly important, is medical practice as a salaried
employee of some organization: the government (and, particularly,
the armed forces), a health plan, an industry, a union, a hospital,
and so on. Only one of our sixty-two interviewees contemplated any
such arrangement; he intended to become a pathologist and thought
it likely that he might end up as a salaried employee of a hospital.
(The other ten interviewees did not express any preference.) In
short, Kansas students expect to become private practitioners in the
sense of living from fees rather than from a salary.

In choosing between solo and some form of group practice, students somewhat surprisingly favor group practice overwhelmingly.
Only three of the fifty-one interviewees who expressed a preference
preferred solo practice. To those who think of the plains states as a
last stronghold of rugged individualism, it will come as a surprise that
Kansas students are so much in accord with current trends.

Since most students favor group practice, we also asked them what
kind of doctors they would prefer to practice with. They typically
expressed their preferences in terms of age. But note that twenty-four
of the sixty-two had no preference at all in this respect. Sixteen interviewees (26% of all interviewees) prefer to practice with older men,

men who have been in practice for many years. Twenty-two interviewees (35% of the total) prefer to practice with men about their own age, either students in their own class or someone who has finished his training recently.

Bearing in mind that these choices, like those between specialized and general practice, lie far in the future and thus are necessarily tentative, we should be less interested in the percentages of students making one or another choice than in the bases for these choices; for the bases on which choices are made, being present in student culture, are likely to be more stable than the choices themselves, though no doubt subject to change too. We classified all student comments on this question in the interviews according to the criterion or criteria used. Student comments contain four criteria; these are the perspectives from which students think about the question of arrangements for practice.

The first criterion takes open account of the fact that medical practice, carried on as private enterprise, is a business. Students ask themselves how well will this particular kind of arrangement (solo or partnership with an older man or one of one's own age) handle the difficulties of starting a practice. Among these are the costs of setting up an office and the problem of building a clientele. Some mentioned this criterion as a reason for preferring group practice: "I can see a lot of advantages to a partnership with an older doctor who is already established. You don't get stuck immediately for the cost of outfitting an office, and you will have a practice in a hurry that way. That would sound like a pretty nice deal in a way." Others suggested that it would be better to go in with someone of your own age because you would get a more equitable share of the profits if you dealt with a younger man. On the other hand, some felt that an older man would have a big clientele so that even though one got a smaller share of the pie the fact that it was a bigger pie would more than make up for this.

In evaluating kinds of arrangements for practice, students use a second criterion which grows out of their desire to practice medicine as effectively as possible and recognizes that four years of medical school and an internship may not be sufficient experience for this. In particular, students realize that they may never have had the experience of actually exercising medical responsibility without supervision. So students ask: Will this set of arrangements for practice help me to practice medicine effectively and will it cushion the move from practicing under supervision to practicing without supervision?

Some students think a partnership with an older man will be better: "Because even though you've gone through your internship and all, you're not going to 'know the ropes,' so to speak. And you could learn a great deal from an older man." On the other hand, some felt that an older man would not be receptive to modern ideas the student had acquired in school: "The older doctor might feel the younger one is trying to tell him all the new concepts and would not be willing to listen to all his ideas. He'd feel too sensitive about the whole thing." Other students expressed this criterion in a different way when they justified their preference for group practice of some kind on the ground that this would make it possible to share medical responsibility and provide better service for the patient: "I think it would be nice to be in a clinic where you can call on someone if you do get into trouble."

The third criterion draws on student stereotypes about the rigors of practice. Worried that their practices might load them with more work than they could handle, students ask: Will this set of arrangements provide defenses against the threat of overwork? This criterion boils down to a concern about who will take care of the patients if one wishes to take time off: "I'd like to work with someone else. I'm not a lone wolf, by any means. It is nice. It is real convenient to refer, and it takes a lot of work off you for night and weekend calls."

The final criterion students make use of recognizes that working with someone else will impose constraints; one will not always be able to do things just as he wants. Students ask themselves: Will this set of arrangements give me sufficient independence? The few students who preferred solo practice had this criterion very much in mind, explaining that they did not want to be under anyone's thumb. The criterion was often used in explaining a preference for a partner one's age rather than older: (*Why someone your own age?*) "He's not going to have a lot of set ideas about the way things have to be. You can develop together a way of doing things. Whereas if you go into practice with someone older, you have to go along with the way he wants things done." Students also sometimes fear that an older partner will give them all the "scut" work and keep the bigger, more interesting cases for themselves; this may be combined with a fear that he will also take the lion's share of the fees: "I think if you go in with an old established physician you do most of the work. I don't know, I may be all wet on this, but I think you probably do most of the work and he takes most of the gravy." Occasionally, students feel that a lack of independence would harm the patient, especially if their older partner were not well versed in the latest treatments and refused to let the younger man do something that would help the patient.

Table XXXIV shows that all four criteria are used in approximately equal proportions by our interviewees. While our data are too scanty for a systematic analysis, we think that the criteria are probably ap-

TABLE XXXIV

CRITERIA USED BY STUDENTS IN EVALUATING ARRANGEMENTS FOR PRACTICE

CRITERIA	NUMBER	PER CENT
Difficulty of starting a medical practice	17	28
Practicing medicine effectively	19	31
Dealing with the workload	13	21
Independence	12	20
Total	61	100

plied in stereotyped ways to different sets of arrangements. Cautioning that this must be treated as speculation, we suggest that students think of solo practice as overly demanding physically and as likely to put you into situations where your lack of experience will get you into difficulties in treating patients. It will also be difficult, as a solo practitioner, to get started; on the other hand, you will be completely independent. Group practice, of any variety, is seen stereotypically as the exact opposite: a minimum of trouble in starting practice, plenty of medical assistance, optimum arrangements for time off, but grave dangers of a lack of independence. Some students think that this disadvantage of group practice can be overcome by choosing partners of one's own age; others are more concerned that one's partner should be older and experienced enough to be a real help with medical difficulties.

Conclusion

As students move through medical school, they acquire many perspectives specific to their situation as students: the perspectives of responsibility and experience, the academic perspective, the student co-operation perspective. Some are so closely related to the peculiar position and disabilities of students that we cannot expect them to survive graduation. But others have their basic roots in the culture of the medical profession and, this being the case, will have resonance far beyond student days.

The perspective built up around the twin values of responsibility and experience is a particularly good example. It emphasizes the physician's responsibility for the welfare of his patients and the physician's dependence on the kind of knowledge that is gained through firsthand experience with the treatment of disease. These values permeate the thought and activity of practicing physicians, as students themselves observe during their training, and students make use of them in envisioning their prospective careers as practitioners. The criteria students use to assess the relative merits of specialty and general practice and to judge the worth of various kinds of arrangements for practice reflect their concern with problems of responsibility and experience.

Two criteria stand out in the students' assessments of kinds of practice: the length of training required and the broadness of the demands on one's medical knowledge. In addition to the realities these criteria refer to, both criteria have immediate reference, as we shall see, to the responsibility and experience perspective; their importance to the student can be interpreted in part in terms of their relation to that perspective. Similarly, student concerns over arrangements for practice focus in large part on two criteria that are likewise related to the responsibility and experience perspective: practicing medicine effectively and achieving independence. Let us explore the relations of these criteria to this perspective a little further.

As the student looks ahead to his future practice, he sees himself treating patients who may be seriously ill, patients who may, if his skill and knowledge are insufficient or his efforts unavailing, die or suffer serious disability. He will be most fully a physician when he finds himself in this situation and will not be a real physician until he does find himself so situated. For this reason, as our analysis of the responsibility perspective showed, as long as the student remains the second-in-command, a man who cannot make the ultimate decision, he will not have achieved professional adulthood. Students chafe under this subordination even in school. To take a residency means to them just that many more years of not being "real doctors," men who can exercise medical responsibility independently. Similarly, becoming the partner of an older physician means that one will be subordinated (at least potentially) because of the operation of the value of experience. One might always have to defer in his exercise of responsibility to the undoubtedly longer experience and presumed wisdom of his senior partner.

On the other hand, as we saw in our earlier analysis, the price of exercising responsibility is the danger of "getting into trouble," making a serious mistake which will injure or kill a patient. The surest way to avoid such trouble is to have had sufficient experience in clinical medicine to know the things that no book or journal article can teach, the intangibles which prevent the fatal mistake. Students do not think they have had sufficient experience by the time they graduate; the limitations placed on their opportunities to exercise responsibility, if nothing else, make this the case. General practice will present them with the widest range of cases, the greatest possibility of getting into trouble. Conversely, specialty practice will bring them only selected cases, cases whose treatment they have had considerable experience with during a residency. In the same way, practicing in partnership with an older, more experienced physician will provide a safeguard against fatal errors due to inexperience.

In short, in appraising possible styles of practice, the student is faced with the dilemma of immediately becoming a full-fledged physician, making his own decisions and taking the responsibility for the errors he may make, or instead making a choice of further training or a situation of practice which will save him from the full load of medical responsibility but keep him in a subordinate position, something less than a full member of the profession. This dilemma comes into existence when the student, looking toward the future, uses the relevant perspectives he has acquired in the course of his medical school training.

Chapter 19

Student Perspectives on
Internships

In order to practice medicine a physician must be licensed by the state in which he wishes to practice. Most states require that a physician, to be fully licensed, must have served one year of internship in an approved hospital. Almost all students, with the exception of those few who do not intend ever to practice medicine, therefore expect to intern immediately after graduating from medical school.

We can distinguish between internships on the basis of the organization of the intern's work and on the basis of the kind of hospital in which the internship is served. First, an internship may be specialized, mixed, or rotating. A specialized internship concentrates the year's work in one specialty and is, in effect, the first year of specialized training in that field, leading directly to further training as a resident in the same field. Mixed and rotating internships consist of various combinations of work in several specialties, differing essentially in the number of specialties entering into the combination.

Second, internships differ in the kind of hospital in which they are served. Students distinguish several categories of hospitals for internship purposes. There is the large public charity hospital, epitomized for them by Kansas City General; they refer to all hospitals of this type as general hospitals. There is the private hospital, which they are familiar with both in Kansas City and their home towns. There is the teaching hospital, of which, of course, the University of

Kansas Medical Center is the chief example. Finally, there are the many hospitals run by the federal government.

Kansas students typically concern themselves only with the problem of what type of hospital to select for, in contrast to some other medical schools, hardly any students contemplated choosing a specialized internship.[1] We discovered only three instances during our observations and interviewing: one student who wished to become a surgeon and was taking a surgical internship and two others who had decided to go into pathology rather than practice medicine and had elected pathology internships.

Choice of an internship for the Kansas student thus becomes simply a question of deciding where to intern. This means primarily in what kind of hospital and only secondarily in which hospital within this type. It must be stressed that, as we shall see, this school differs from many schools in that students attach little importance to the "connections" one can make in a given hospital or to the further career steps that are either made possible or forever closed off because of where one interns. They do not conceive of an internship in a particular hospital as a necessary prelude to a "good" residency or hospital connection. In this they differ from some students in other schools who may feel that if they do not get an internship at, let us say, Massachusetts General, their careers have been seriously damaged.

Kansas students' choices of an internship, then, consist primarily of choosing between the four varieties of an internship they distinguish — general, private, teaching, or government hospital. Of these four, the most popular is the general hospital, the least popular the government hospital. Table XXXV shows the distribution of internship preferences in our interview sample. (The reader should keep in mind that this sample included freshmen whose choices were based more on fantasy than on realistic appraisal.)

[1] This fact makes it difficult to compare our findings with those of the studies carried out by the Bureau of Applied Social Research of Columbia University at Cornell Medical College and at other private medical schools. Students at the schools in which the research was done frequently chose specialized internships, and the research so far reported deals with the determinants of this choice as opposed to the choice of a rotating internship. See, for instance, Patricia L. Kendall and Hanan C. Selvin, "Tendencies Toward Specialization in Medical Training," in Robert K. Merton, George Reader, and Patricia L. Kendall, *The Student-Physician* (Cambridge, Mass.: Harvard University Press, 1957), pp. 153–74, and William A. Glaser, "Internship Appointments of Medical Students," *Administrative Science Quarterly*, IV (December, 1959), 337–56.

TABLE XXXV
DISTRIBUTION OF INTERNSHIP PREFERENCES

KIND OF HOSPITAL	FREQUENCY	PER CENT
General 21		34.0
Private 12		19.3
Teaching 11		17.7
Government 9		14.5
Don't know 9		14.5

In making these choices students make use of certain collective understandings about the nature of an internship and the advantages one might gain from one. Further, these collective understandings define the particular advantages and disadvantages associated with each kind of internship. These understandings do not, however, specify which kind of internship one should desire or choose, for students recognize that individual students may have different views of what will be important for them to get out of their internship.

In what follows we describe these collective understandings and the kinds of choices students make. It should be understood that these understandings do not have the solid homogeneity of the perspectives we earlier described as part of student culture. Insofar as these perspectives on internships deal with the unknown, students have a certain amount of latitude in which to make differing interpretations of what is important in an internship and what the characteristics of each kind of internship are. This is also true because there are no immediate situational constraints to color their thinking.

Criteria for Judging Internships

The students make their choices of internships by referring to various criteria. Though students disagree, as we shall see, on the relative importance of the criteria, the criteria are intelligible to all students, even though they may not consider some of them of great importance.

The job of the intern, though it has some basic similarities from one hospital to another, can vary widely, and it is these variations that students are concerned with. The criteria refer to aspects of an internship which vary among internships and thus make it possible to judge an internship as more or less good on each of these counts.

Before turning to a consideration of the variations students consider important, let us describe briefly the core characteristics of an internship. An intern is licensed to practice medicine under the supervision of the hospital staff. Unlike the student, the intern has the legal power to make medical decisions, assume responsibility for the welfare of patients, and perform necessary medical procedures. He typically has some immediate responsibility for the hour-by-hour medical supervision of a hospital ward, being the medical person most immediately available to handle both routine and emergency situations. The intern, of course, is supposed to be getting training for his future professional practice while he does this work.

In the course of his workday, the intern works-up patients who enter the hospital for treatment, examines and treats patients in the hospital clinics, and performs routine diagnostic and therapeutic procedures. He attends hospital conferences and makes rounds with the staff physicians. He assists the staff physicians in such medical and surgical procedures as they perform.

The intern typically serves for one year, at the end of which he is legally ready to practice medicine entirely on his own. The hospital provides token pay for his services during the year. At the end of the year, he may go immediately into practice or may decide to take a residency in some specialty.

The first criterion students use in assessing the value of an internship is already familiar to us as an integral part of student culture. They ask: To what degree will I be allowed to exercise *medical responsibility*? Although interns are legally empowered to exercise responsibility, students believe that the amount of responsibility one can exercise varies from hospital to hospital, and many students feel that the degree to which one is allowed to act as a doctor is important in judging an internship.

Students frequently expressed this criterion directly, in statements like this:

"The important thing is to get into the right kind of hospital where they let you do things, where they really give you a chance to take over patients and get some experience with all of these different kinds of procedures and with the diagnosis and treatment of various diseases. Some hospitals won't let you do that and your whole internship is just a waste. You don't learn anything more than you did in medical school and they treat you like a student. Of course, in other hospitals they let you do just about anything a doctor would do. You have to know that, before you decide on where you want to intern."

(Junior Medicine. September, 1955.)

The same criterion is reflected in student concern over whether they will get to do surgery. Even though the participants in the following conversation disclaim any desire to do major surgery, the reader will note that they do desire to try their hands at less extensive procedures:

Mores said, "I think I will get a pretty good experience where I want to intern. It's a hospital up in Michigan and they get a lot of auto accidents and so on from around Detroit. So I will probably get a lot of minor and emergency surgery. I think a doctor should know how to do that stuff." Garrity said, "Yeah, but I wouldn't like too much of it. Tonsils, appendix, hernias — things like that. But I wouldn't want to do too many gall bladders, and I certainly don't want to do any stomachs or colons or anything like that." Prentiss said, "Neither do I. Of course, you've got to know how to do some of it, just in case."

(Senior Medicine. February, 1956.)

Similarly, students make use of the responsibility criterion when they worry about the fact that "in some places the intern is the lowest thing in the world":

"[In some hospitals] there are so damn many people between you and the patient. You know, they have so many residents around, and if any interesting case or problem case comes in, why the resident is going to work on that one himself, so that you don't get such a good look at those things."

(Senior Medicine. February, 1956.)

Students make use of a second criterion familiar from our discussion of student culture when they assess internships, the criterion of *clinical experience*. To what degree, they ask, will this internship give me a chance to get knowledge of important common diseases that one can get only through firsthand observation? For an intern this is largely a question of the character of the hospital's clientele. Are the patients who come to the hospital, as one student put it, "a cross section of the kind of patients that you will be dealing with [in practice]?" Students most frequently express this criterion negatively, fearing that a given hospital's selection of cases will be too narrow or too unlike those commonly seen by private practitioners:

"One thing is that they practice a very specialized kind of medicine. I'm sure you've heard it said many times that they only get the rare and bizarre cases here, and there is a good deal of truth in that."

(Senior Medicine. February, 1956.)

A third criterion students use to assess internships takes into account the fact that the internship can include a substantial amount of *teaching* and raises the question of whether the teaching program for interns in a particular hospital is full enough or well enough taught. This concern may be expressed in queries about whether there are enough conferences or classes scheduled for interns but also comes out in worry over the character of the staff physician-intern relationship and whether this allows for sufficient intimate contact for real learning to take place:

"You can really learn a lot over there when you make rounds. It's just you and the doctor. You can ask all the questions you want to and so on. You can really pick up an awful lot of wisdom that way. It's not like those rounds we had here last week — that was really ridiculous. I'll bet there were twenty people. If you asked more than one question you felt you were taking up too much time and making a pig of yourself. That's no way to learn anything. But at another place you could really learn things."

(Senior Medicine. March, 1956.)

The students also worry about teaching when they discuss the quality of the staff under whom they might serve at various hospitals:

One senior said, "You know, I think this place right here would be a pretty darn good internship. After all, you have the best lectures you are going to get anywhere right here. A lot of very good men, and a lot of good guest speakers coming in all the time. This would be a perfect place, I think." Kern said, "Yes, it would be good from that point of view, but I don't know how much teaching you would get as an intern. Besides I just couldn't stand it around here another year, I've been here so many already."

(Senior Surgical Specialties. October, 1956.)

The last comment introduces a final aspect of the teaching criterion — the question of whether it is not important to move to some hospital other than the university medical center, in order to be exposed to different teachers:

"I've thought very seriously about applying here to K.U. I really did, but I think you can get into kind of a rut, you know. You spend four years in one institution and I think that's really enough. I think it's more important to go someplace else and get involved with some other men. Of course, you want it to be someplace where they have equally good men and where they have a pretty good teaching program. . . . You get the change in viewpoint."

(Senior Medicine. February, 1956.)

Students use as a fourth criterion for assessing internships the amount of *pay* the intern receives. This amount can vary widely, from what is really a token payment of twenty or thirty dollars a month to as much as five or six hundred dollars a month. For some students, this is an important consideration:

Discussing an internship that paid very well, one student said, "I sure could use it, too. I've got a thirteen-thousand-dollar debt to pay off, and the sooner I start paying it off, the better."

(Junior Medicine. September, 1955.)

Some students make use of a fifth criterion in judging an internship: the opportunity to *travel and live in an interesting place*. This kind of hedonistic, nonmedical criterion figures heavily in some men's thinking:

"I'll tell you. My ideas are a little funny on this subject, I think. But I feel very strongly that I would like to travel and see the world and have a lot of adventure and glamour and romance before I get too old to enjoy it. You know, when you get to be sixty years' old you might have the time for those things and the money but you're not young enough to enjoy it any more. I think there are a lot of good things in this world and that they are meant for young people to do. People who are young and agile and flexible and can really enjoy them. What I intend to do is take an internship in some place like Honolulu where I can really enjoy life."

(Senior Medicine. March, 1956.)

A sixth criterion has to do with *hospital facilities and working conditions*. Here students make a judgment on the basis of the size of the hospital, the number of patients, the number of interns, and other characteristics which affect the intern's workload and opportunities for patient contact. Their main concern here is that, while there should be enough patients in the hospital to provide sufficient opportunities for learning and the exercise of responsibility, there should not be so many patients in relation to the number of interns that the intern has to work very hard just in order to finish his routine, uninteresting work.

The seniors had just received their internship appointments and were discussing the case of one man who had been the only one to apply for a particular hospital in town. Wallis said, "You can just imagine being the only intern in that whole hospital. Boy, he'll be worked to death. He'll probably have only every other night off and on the nights when he is off they probably won't let him go until nine o'clock. He's really going to work his tail off . . . It wouldn't be worth it, having all that stuff piled on you."

(Senior Medicine. March, 1956.)

A seventh criterion we found students making use of in assessing internships was the degree to which an internship would provide one with *professional contacts* useful in one's later career. For instance, a student might regard an internship as valuable because it paved the way to a residency he wanted:

"You just can't take any old internship just because it pays well if you want to get a good residency. Maybe you can get a bad residency someplace, but you can't get those real good ones unless you have interned at a good place."

(Senior Surgical Specialties. October, 1956.)

Similarly, a student might feel that interning at a particular hospital would help him get established in practice:

Burton was discussing interning at one of the private hospitals in town. "Another thing is that if a person wanted to practice in Kansas City, he would be able to get on the staff there without any trouble, I think. Most of the private hospitals will make a place on their staff for their interns. It's a kind of courtesy, and that's pretty important if you want to practice in town. It's a big help if you have a good hospital connection like that."

(Senior Medicine. March, 1956.)

Finally, some students take into account in considering internships various factors which are not generalized enough to be thought of as criteria of selection, but instead are specialized facts about their own career preferences or the characteristics of some particular hospital. Thus, a student interested in a surgery residency said that he was interested in a specialized surgical internship. Two students, in considering internships in the armed services, weighed the effect of taking such an internship on their obligation to spend two years in the armed forces. Several students discussed a rumor that Catholic hospitals enforced certain religious principles which might interfere with an intern's medical activities. One student was interested in research and desired an internship which would give him time for this. In the following analyses, we have lumped all these various comments on internships into a "miscellaneous" category, as being too scattered and infrequent to require separate consideration.

Our field data reveal eighty-five instances in which students make some judgment on internships. Table XXXVI shows that the seven criteria described above account for all but six of these judgments and that the criteria of amount of responsibility given the intern, the amount of pay, and the adequacy of the teaching are most frequently used, totaling 68 per cent of the judgments made.

TABLE XXXVI

FREQUENCY OF USE OF VARIOUS CRITERIA FOR ASSESSING
INTERNSHIPS

(Field Observation)

CRITERION	NUMBER	PER CENT
Responsibility	27	32
Clinical experience	6	7
Teaching	15	18
Pay	16	19
Travel	7	7
Facilities and working conditions	5	6
Professional contacts	3	4
Miscellaneous	6	7
Total	85	100

We can further support the conclusion that these criteria constituted the bases of student selection of internships by turning to the results of our interviews with a random sample of the student body. We asked them to list the advantages and disadvantages of each of the four kinds of internships — general, private, teaching, and government — as they saw them. Table XXXVII shows their answers classified into the same categories as those used for the field data in Table XXXVI and further demonstrates that the criteria described above are the ones students most frequently use in dealing with the problem of choosing an internship. (The main difference between the two tables — the marked increase in the number of references to clinical experience in the interviews — does not disturb this conclusion.)

In short, these criteria set the terms in which students view internships. Two of the criteria are projections into the future of perspectives included in student culture: responsibility and experience. Since these are perspectives which were customary among the student body, we may assume that all students were familiar with their application to the problem of choosing an internship. Similarly, the criterion of teaching should be familiar to anyone who has been a student, and the criterion of pay is a common enough one in our society. This is not, of course, to say that all students made use of these cri-

TABLE XXXVII

FREQUENCY OF USE OF VARIOUS CRITERIA FOR ASSESSING
INTERNSHIPS
(Interviews)

CRITERION	NUMBER	PER CENT
Responsibility	91	27
Clinical experience	63	19
Teaching	95	28
Pay	45	13
Travel	2	—
Facilities and working conditions	23	7
Professional contacts	2	—
Miscellaneous	15	5
Total	336	99

teria in judging internships, but that all students were aware of them as possible criteria to use in making such judgments. Since the four categories contain most of the judgments students expressed, we can conclude that students generally make such decisions with reference to this array of criteria.

Stereotypes of Kinds of Hospitals

In understanding how students make use of the criteria just described in choosing internships, we must first of all understand that they tend to see these criteria as varying not so much among individual hospitals as among the major types of hospitals already listed. That is, they tend to discuss the amount of responsibility given an intern in private hospitals generally rather than in Private Hospital X which they are particularly interested in. In other words, students have stereotypes of the way each kind of hospital measures up on the criteria we have outlined. We will now describe these stereotypes, taking up each major variety of hospital in turn. In making these descriptions we use data already discussed: the statements students were observed to make during our field observations and the judgments they were asked to make during interviews. Most of the statements recorded in the field were made in the context of a discussion of some particular type of hospital. Only sixteen of the eighty-five judgments we recorded did not have such a referent, being statements of criteria to be used in judging specific internships. These are not included in our analyses. All of the judgments expressed in the interviews were tied to a consideration of a specific type of hospital, having been made in answer to questions about these types. In summarizing the data on each kind of hospital, we divide the judgments according to whether the kind of hospital was ranked as scoring positively or negatively on each criterion.

The reader will note as we proceed that the stereotypes of kinds of hospitals do not always give each hospital a score on every criterion. Rather, students tend to see in each type one or two outstanding characteristics, either positive or negative, and ignore the other criteria. This may mean that they think the type adequate in all other respects, or it may mean that one large advantage or disadvantage will override, for them, other considerations. We do not know which of these suppositions is true, but we think that this may vary for different stereotypes and different students.

The student stereotype of the general hospital is outlined in Table XXXVIII. Clearly, the outstanding fact about the general hospital, for students, is that it is a place where they can do the kinds of things they will do in practice. They will have full responsibility for patients, do surgery, and in general bear the burdens of a full-fledged physician. This is the only stereotypical feature of the general hospital which appears in our field notes. In the interviews, where students were asked to list advantages and disadvantages for each type of hospital, students also noted frequently that the teaching would not be very good but that they would have a good selection of patients on whom to exercise responsibility.

Students have a much cloudier picture of what an internship in a private hospital will be like, as Table XXXIX shows. Their major con-

TABLE XXXVIII

STEREOTYPE OF THE GENERAL HOSPITAL

	FIELD OBSERVATIONS		INTERVIEWS	
CRITERION	+	−	+	−
Responsibility	11	1	31	—
Clinical experience	—	—	16	4
Teaching	—	1	4	28
Pay	—	2	—	5
Travel	—	—	—	—
Facilities and working conditions	1	1	—	11
Professional contacts	—	—	—	—
Miscellaneous	1	—	—	—

cern is the amount of responsibility they will have, but they are not agreed as to whether the private hospital will be satisfactory in this respect or not. Some of this confusion is caused by the fact that some students compared the general hospital to the private hospital, concluding that they would not have as much responsibility in the latter; others compared it to the teaching hospital, where they saw the presence of many residents as necessarily diminishing the area in which they would have a free hand. Beyond this, they see the private hospital as likely to provide them with access to patients of the kind they will see in practice and as having adequate teaching programs.

Students see the excellence of the teaching as the major characteristic of the teaching hospital, as we might expect (see Table XL). Although they approve of this, they think it likely that the teaching hospital will be unsatisfactory in the selection of patients it offers, having too few patients with common diseases and far too many pa-

TABLE XXXIX
STEREOTYPE OF THE PRIVATE HOSPITAL

CRITERION	FIELD OBSERVATIONS +	−	INTERVIEWS +	−
Responsibility	5	6	3	26
Clinical experience	1	−	12	8
Teaching	4	2	12	12
Pay	2	−	10	−
Travel	−	−	−	−
Facilities and working conditions	1	−	2	4
Professional contacts	2	−	2	−
Miscellaneous	−	−	−	−

TABLE XL
STEREOTYPE OF THE TEACHING HOSPITAL

CRITERION	FIELD OBSERVATIONS +	−	INTERVIEWS +	−
Responsibility	−	3	2	19
Clinical experience	1	3	3	10
Teaching	6	1	30	−
Pay	−	2	−	4
Travel	−	−	−	−
Facilities and working conditions	−	−	1	3
Professional contacts	−	−	−	−
Miscellaneous	−	−	1	−

tients with unusual and rare conditions, and in the amount of responsibility the intern has.

The government hospital stereotype differs markedly from the others. It ignores, relatively, the characteristics so prominent in the other stereotypes and concentrates on two quite different advantages: the high pay (service hospitals typically pay the intern an officer's salary and allowances) and the opportunity to live in such desirable cities as Honolulu or San Francisco. Students think of the major disadvantage of such hospitals as the restricted range of patients they are likely to have — mostly young adult males (see Table XLI).

TABLE XLI

STEREOTYPE OF THE GOVERNMENT HOSPITAL

CRITERION	FIELD OBSERVATIONS		INTERVIEWS	
	+	−	+	−
Responsibility	−	−	10	−
Clinical experience	1	−	3	17
Teaching	−	−	8	1
Pay	7	−	26	−
Travel	3	−	2	−
Facilities and working conditions	−	−	1	1
Professional contacts	−	−	−	−
Miscellaneous	1	−	4	10

This set of stereotypes organizes the world of prospective internships for the student. It contains, in effect, a prediction of what one will be getting into if he chooses a hospital of a given type. It also hints to the student at a particular set of motivations he might reasonably use in making his own choice; that is, it defines the good and sufficient reasons current among students for choosing one variety of internship or another. It tells him what kinds of advantages he may reasonably expect from an internship and what kind of hospital to choose in order to get those advantages. Given the consistency of these stereotypes, it is likely that they are held in common by the bulk of the student body and thus have the legitimacy of those things that "everyone knows."

Internship Choices and
Career Plans

Students thus tend to agree on the constellation of advantages and disadvantages to be found at each kind of hospital. They believe that the general hospital will give them much responsibility but poor teaching; that the private hospital will give them less responsibility but better teaching and clinical experience; that the university hospital will furnish excellent teaching but little else; that the government hospital will offer good pay and a chance to see the world. But, as we have seen, students do not agree on which internships to choose. This diversity of choice is a consequence of differing career plans, filtered through the mesh of student definitions we have just described. Students with differing career plans are likely to wish to maximize different criteria, and this leads them, as they follow the guidelines of student thought, to choose different internships.

Student disagreement on the importance of various facets of an internship stems from divergence in students' images of their professional future. What you want out of your internship is a function of what you think you will be doing once you have finished the internship. The most important influence on internship choice is the choice the student tentatively makes between general and specialized practice. The student who looks forward to starting general practice a year after he leaves school looks on the internship as the last chance he will have to perform medical procedures in order to learn; after the internship, he will be doing the same procedures in earnest, not just getting himself ready for "the real thing."

Hagen told me that he was going into general practice. I asked, "Where are you going to intern?" He said, "I hope to intern at General, here in town." I said, "Why that one?" He said, " . . . I used to work over there and I saw what the interns got to do and they got quite a bit to do compared with some of these other hospitals, especially with a private hospital like X. At X every patient has his own doctor so the intern just doesn't get to do much, but over at General, well it's a different story — the intern is the patient's doctor over there. Usually he's just about the only M.D. the patient sees and they are his patients and he does pretty much what he wants with them. I think that would be a much better experience for me. More useful." I said, "You mean for going out into general practice?" He said, "Yes."

(Senior Medicine. February, 1956.)

"I'll probably go right out into general practice after I finish my internship and I figure that General Hospital would be a pretty good place to pick up the kind of experience I need for that."

(Senior Medicine. March, 1956.)

The vision of immediately going into practice causes the student to feel an immense pressure to get what experience he can while he can still get it under some supervision. Student stereotypes make it clear that if this is what you want the general hospital is the place to take your internship.

On the other hand, the student who looks forward to a specialized practice has no such immediate and intense pressure for practical training bearing on him. He knows that after he finishes his internship he will take several more years of training in some specialty, so that unsupervised medical practice still lies a long way in the future. He will have many more opportunities, during his residency, to get training in exercising responsibility; he does not think it so crucial to have this during his internship. Nor will the rotating internship, with its emphasis on getting a little bit in each of many specialties, seem to him to be preparation for the kind of career he is going to have, for in his practice he will concentrate on only one of those specialties.

"If you're planning to take a residency I don't think it makes an awful lot of difference what kind of internship you have. You'll get your real training in your residency."

(Senior Medicine. February, 1956.)

The would-be specialist thus has considerably more leeway in making his choice. Since the internship is not really so important, he is free to consider all the possibilities and does not feel bound by the necessity of getting experience in the exercise of responsibility. He applies other criteria more readily, and is more likely to be concerned with the quality of teaching, travel, pay, and so on. His choice of criteria to use in choosing an internship, and hence of internships themselves, is not so constrained by an imminent plunge into medical practice as that of the would-be general practitioner. We would therefore expect the choices of prospective specialists to be more widely scattered.

We can test these notions, derived from a few clear-cut field experiences like those cited above, more systematically by turning to our interviews with a random sample of students. We asked them what kind of hospital they intended to intern in and why they made that choice. Table XLII shows that would-be general practitioners are much more likely than would-be specialists to give the opportunity to exercise responsibility as their reason for choosing a particular internship, while the reasons given by would-be specialists are scattered over several categories. Similarly, Table XLIII shows that would-be general practitioners are much more likely to choose a general hospital internship while the choices of would-be specialists are

TABLE XLII

CAREER PLANS AND MAJOR CRITERION USED IN CHOOSING AN INTERNSHIP
(Interviews)

CRITERION	GENERAL PRACTICE	SPECIALTY	DON'T KNOW	TOTAL
Responsibility	10	5	1	16
Clinical experience	8	7	1	16
Teaching	2	10	1	13
Pay	1	4	–	5
Travel	–	1	–	1
Facilities and working conditions	–	1	–	1
Connections	1	1	–	2
Miscellaneous (and combination of two or more of the above)	3	5	–	8
Total	25	34	3	62

TABLE XLIII

INTERNSHIP CHOICE AND CAREER PLANS

KIND OF HOSPITAL	GENERAL PRACTICE	SPECIALTY	DON'T KNOW	TOTAL
General	13	8	–	21
Private	5	7	–	12
Teaching	2	9	–	11
Government	1	6	2	9
Don't know	4	4	1	9
Total	25	34	3	62

divided, roughly equally, among the four possible choices. In short, a man who intends to become a general practitioner will probably put most weight on the criterion of responsibility. He then makes the choice of internship student stereotypes dictate as most logical for someone who wishes to maximize responsibility and chooses a general hospital.

Conclusion

The material we have presented indicates that students have definite ideas about what things it is possible to get out of an internship and equally definite ideas about what kinds of hospitals are most likely to give you one or another of these things. These ideas were very likely customary perspectives, in the sense in which we have used that term earlier. That is, they were, first of all, frequently used; we have seen that all student criteria used to assess internships could be subsumed under these few categories. Second, they were widespread;

we have seen that their use by a random sample of interviewees paralleled that observed in the field. Also, it is likely that they were collective or shared, in the sense that the criteria were mutually intelligible to all students, either because, like the responsibility and experience criteria, they are part of student culture, or because they are common lay terms like teaching, pay, or travel. Finally, many of the incidents observed in the field consisted of discussions among students in which these criteria were used to communicate ideas about internships.

Further, our material demonstrates that students' choices of internships are constrained by these perspectives. Those students who, because they intend to enter general practice, look forward to practicing medicine immediately after completing their internships tend to emphasize the need for opportunities to exercise responsibility during the internship. In accord with student stereotypes they choose the general hospital internship as most likely to give them what they want. Conversely, would-be specialists make use of a diversity of criteria in choosing an internship and correspondingly choose a wider variety of internships.

Choice of internship, then, poses essentially the same dilemma for the student as choice of a style of practice, though in a slightly different way. Should one prepare himself immediately for the independence of medical practice, with its attendant dangers and responsibilities? Or should one take advantage of the opportunity to be a student for another year, adding to one's knowledge and accumulating clinical experience under the supervision of others who will bear the major responsibilities for the welfare of patients? The internship can be a kind of moratorium, in which the student takes on the legal responsibilities of a practicing physician without actually being called on to exercise them. Our data show that students have a realistic eye on the immediate future: those who will not be required to begin practice immediately use the internship as a moratorium, but those who believe they will be practicing medicine on their own in a year do not.

The terms of this dilemma clearly have their origins in student culture, and particularly in the responsibility and clinical experience perspectives. The student has learned while he was a student that both responsibility and clinical experience are important and necessary things to have, and it is this knowledge that gives shape to his consideration of the internship.

Chapter 20

Student Views of Specialties

W<small>HEN</small> he finishes his internship, the young doctor faces the question whether he will go into general practice or specialize in some narrower area of medicine. If he chooses to specialize, he must take a residency in some field, getting further specialized training with intensive supervision. In an earlier era many doctors became specialists by becoming particularly interested in some branch of medicine, devoting more and more of their time to it, and finally voluntarily restricting their practice. Today, one becomes a specialist by taking a residency, engaging in a specialized practice for a few years, and then taking the examinations set by the board which governs the specialty. A man who practices a specialty now must restrict his practice to work in that specialty and not do medical work of other kinds.

All this means that the decision to become a specialist is more fateful than it used to be. One cannot gradually slide into a specialty after a period of experimentation in practice, but must make his decision early and stick by it. Students recognize this latter fact, although they do not always understand its historical and political context. Recognizing that the choice must be made early and that it is a fateful one, students who contemplate going into a specialty (and many of those who do not) look carefully at the specialties they have experience with in school, wondering what they would be like over a professional lifetime. They discuss specialties among themselves at great length, make tentative choices, change them, and in general have the question of which area of medicine they will enter well in mind while they are in school.

In this chapter we discuss students' ideas in this area, outlining the perspectives from which they view the various specialties. As in our discussion of internships, we consider first the various criteria students use in assessing the specialties they consider and then look at how students rate particular specialties on these criteria.

But we do not go on, as we did in the earlier chapter, to make an analysis of those who choose one specialty as against another, and this omission requires explanation. The explanation is simple. We believe that students' choices of specialties are at this time for the most part make-believe, an experimental trying-on of roles about which they know very little. Their choices do not usually (except for the few who take specialized internships) commit them in any way, and they lose nothing by changing their minds, even by changing them several times. They do not even lose face, because no one really expects them to stick by these choices. Since this is the case, students' choices of specialties are neither firm nor stable. On the one hand, most students who express a preference for a specialty do so in a tentative and uncertain way; they say "I've been thinking that I might go into pediatrics," instead of "I am going to be a pediatrician." Furthermore, they are apt to express a preference for several specialties simultaneously: "Well, it's between medicine, pediatrics, or ENT." Alternatively, when students do express a firm choice they are apt to change it at any moment to another one that sounds equally firm. In one case a student expressed firm preferences for five specialties in as many weeks.

Though we believe that the choices students make are typically playful, containing very little serious intention and not leading to definite commitments, we cannot prove this. Nor can anyone prove the opposite, that these choices were firm and stable and led to predictable actions, from the data we have. We could only ascertain the consequences of these choices made in school from a longitudinal study which followed students for a sufficient time to find out what specialties they actually entered.

We must make one qualification, however, though we have little support for it, in view of the above considerations. Certain men impressed us as much more likely than their fellows to stick with the choices they expressed, though we do not know whether they did or not. In the last section of this chapter, we discuss some of our reasons for accepting this impression as valid.

Criteria Used in Assessing Specialties

In analyzing the various criteria students used to assess different specialties we had available two bodies of data. First, we had all the informal conversations we had heard or participated in during the course of the field work. In these conversations, students often talked about the kind of practice they hoped eventually to have and particularly about the specialties they might enter. They argued with each other the merits and bad points of many specialties. Second, we had the answers our random sample of student interviewees gave to this question: "What would be the usual reason for a man going into each of these specialties? What would be a good reason not to go into each of them?" We presented the student with a list of seven specialties and asked him to discuss the reasons for and against going into each one of them. The seven specialties we asked them about were: internal medicine, general surgery, pediatrics, obstetrics and gynecology, dermatology, neurology, and neurosurgery.

We found a total of one hundred and forty uses of various criteria to assess specialties in our field notes and fifteen hundred and two separate comments in our interviews. We have categorized these under twelve rubrics, for although there was much variety in the way these ideas were expressed these twelve basic themes contain all the ideas students consider when making their judgments. We now discuss each of the criteria, putting each one in the form of a positive statement which might or might not be true of a given specialty.

1. *This specialty allows one to make an adequate amount of money.* Students frequently take into account the financial aspects of a specialty practice, noting such things as the amount of income one can expect, the degree to which the specialty is crowded so that competition with others would lower one's chances of making an adequate income, and the difficulties of establishing a practice in that specialty which might lower one's income in the early years of practice.

2. *This specialty allows one to have convenient working hours and not work too hard.* Students feel that some specialties allow one to keep limited hours so that the times when one is not in the office or hospital may be spent on recreation or with one's family. In contrast, other specialties subject one to the possibility of being called out in the middle of the night to attend to medical emergencies and thus make it difficult to carry on a normal life. Similarly, some special-

ties — surgery, for example — require long hours of tiring physical labor, while others are free from this.

3. *This specialty has great prestige with the public, with one's medical colleagues, or both.* This criterion is self-explanatory.

4. *This specialty allows one to have a close relationship with patients of a kind one likes, a relationship that has no depressing or unpleasant aspects.* Some specialties, students recognize, allow one little or no contact with patients; the clearest example is the pathologist, who may never see a live patient. On the other hand, when there is a closer relation with patients, the patients may be of a kind one does not like. For instance, many students feel that pediatrics would be difficult because of the necessity of dealing with children or their parents. Others feel that specialties where many patients die would be unpleasant.

5. *This specialty allows one to exercise medical responsibility.* The concept of medical responsibility, let us recall, implies the drama of the physician coming to the aid of a patient who, in the archetypical case, would lose his life without the doctor's intervention. Students feel that many specialties do not provide the conditions under which they could feel that they were exercising responsibility of this kind. That is, the patients a man in a given specialty sees may typically have nothing really serious the matter with them, so that his intervention in the case can never be dramatically lifesaving. Or, alternatively, the kind of patients one sees may have diseases about which the doctor can do nothing, in the present state of medical science, so that the possibility of intervening successfully is foreclosed. Finally, students sometimes feel that the amount of responsibility for patients' lives and well-being associated with a specialty is too great, at least for them, to shoulder.

6. *This specialty has great intellectual breadth.* Students discussing various specialties frequently made use of words like "variety," "challenging," "interesting," and so on. They distinguished between those specialties which covered a wide area and those which were narrow, those which would challenge a man to use all his knowledge and capacities and those which would not, those which would continue to provide interest and intellectual stimulation and those which would soon become dull, boring, and routine. They may complain that a specialty is too narrow and would not require them to make use of all the training they have received in school.

Students also apply this criterion in the opposite direction, seeing some specialties as requiring too much knowledge because of the variety of patients they attract. Although they view the use of knowledge as a good thing generally, they conceive of certain specialties as requiring an amount of knowledge beyond their own capacities.

7. *This specialty presents medical problems which are, in the present state of knowledge, manageable.* In many specialties, as students conceive these, the work has been limited to a relatively few pathological states for which methods of diagnosis and treatment are precise and definitive. This does not mean that the physician's treatment is always successful, but rather that he always knows exactly what is going on and what he must do. There is little or no guesswork. In other specialties, diagnostic methods are not so sure, the range of cases one must cover is so wide that one cannot possibly be precise in applying them, and the choice of treatments cannot be scientifically determined.

8. *For this specialty one must have special skills or personality traits.* When they use this criterion, students point to some skill they consider to be necessary for the specialty, like the innate manual dexterity they consider important for a surgeon, and say that if one has that skill the specialty might be good for him, but not otherwise. Or they point to some trait of character or personality, such as the fondness for children they think necessary for pediatrics. The kind of skill or personal characteristic thought necessary varies widely between students and according to the specialty they are thinking about; when we speak of students using this criterion, we mean simply that they feel that possession of some skill or trait is a necessary prerequisite without which one would not want to enter that specialty.

9. *This specialty requires a long residency.* The number of years of residency training required before one enters a specialty varied, at the time we did our field work, from two years for pediatrics to five or more years for some kinds of surgery. Students see each additional year of residency as just that much more time standing between them and the freedom of independent practice and a much larger income. Accordingly, they may judge specialties in terms of the sheer length of the additional training required. Occasionally, they may turn this criterion around and see the long residency as good, because the work of the specialty requires long intensive training.

10. *This specialty may arouse nonspecific feelings, either positive or negative, in one.* Students frequently say of a specialty, without further specification, that it would be "enjoyable," or "appealing," or "unpleasant," and so on. While these vague terms of approbation or disapproval carry no specific content, they seem to reflect very real student evaluations whose bases the students themselves cannot explain.

11. *This specialty requires that a person practicing it live in a large city.* Students occasionally make the point that some specialties are so narrowly defined that one would have to live in a large city in order to have a sufficient pool of potential patients. Insofar as one has definite ideas about where he wants to practice this can be a disadvantage.

12. *One may have a good experience while working in this specialty in school.* Some students, through various circumstances, particularly enjoy their work on some particular service they are assigned to as students and give this as a reason for preferring a particular specialty.

Students do not make equal use of all of these criteria. They do not, that is, ask of each specialty whether it scores high or low on each of these criteria. Left to their own devices, and not required to place a check mark somewhere along a scale for each criterion, students make much more use of some than others and apply some much more frequently to one specialty than another. Hence, our first interest is to see which criteria students most make use of. Table XLIV shows the relative frequency of use of each of the twelve criteria, in both our field work and interview data.

The results of this tabulation may be surprising. First, students give relatively little attention to such criteria as money, hours, and prestige, the criteria which we may with most justice think of as non-medical and reflecting the cynical outlook of a person whose concern is for his own success and well-being. Second, students pay most attention to the criterion of intellectual breadth, to the notion that their future work either must make use of all they know or must not be so broad as to preclude their knowing enough to do a good job. The other criteria which rank high show a similar concern with the medical characteristics of the work, particularly concern for the possibility the specialty allows for helping patients who need a doctor's care and concern for being able to handle this responsibility ade-

TABLE XLIV

RELATIVE FREQUENCY OF USE OF CRITERIA TO ASSESS SPECIALTIES

CRITERION	FIELD WORK		INTERVIEWS	
	NUMBER	PER CENT	NUMBER	PER CENT
Money	20	14	61	4
Hours	24	17	137	9
Prestige	2	2	46	3
Patient relationship	19	13	129	9
Responsibility	6	4	243	17
Intellectual breadth	47	34	398	27
Manageability	5	4	152	10
Special personal traits	7	5	197	13
Long residency	4	3	35	2
Nonspecific feelings	2	2	91	6
Live in city	—	—	8	—
Liked specialty in school	4	2	5	—
Total	140	100	1,502	100

quately. In short, students' concerns as reflected in these criteria are the concerns contained in their idealistic long-range perspective.

But students' use of these criteria also reflects the impact of their experience in medical school. While in school, they acquire some familiarity with a medical culture, in addition to specific technical knowledge and skills. What is most important about our finding that they fail, in assessing specialties, to use such criteria as money, hours, and prestige is not that these are the criteria a "cynical" physician might use, but that these are criteria a layman would be likely to use.

When laymen think about occupations with whose inner workings they are not familiar, they must rely on such ideas as have common currency. When they assess occupational success, for example, they use those criteria they are familiar with, criteria that can be applied to any kind of work irrespective of its unique content, criteria like money, hours, and prestige. But when a member of a particular occupation thinks about his own aspirations, he is likely to use instead of these common cultural standards an esoteric set of standards common only among his colleagues. For all occupational cultures contain, among other things, a set of standards for judging one's work which can only be understood by those who know from their own experience what the problems of that kind of work are.[1] The member tends to set his own standards and assess himself in relation to those

[1] See Everett C. Hughes, *Men and Their Work* (Glencoe, Ill.: Free Press, 1958), pp. 88–101.

standards which lie in the occupational culture. When thinking about possible careers in an occupation which offers some diversity from which to choose, he will assess those possibilities in terms furnished by the occupational culture. He may also use criteria understood and used by those outside his line of work, but he will always be mindful of the criteria his colleagues use.

Thus, practicing physicians probably think about money, hours, and prestige when they think about their specialties, but they also use criteria unique to medicine, criteria quite similar to those used by the medical students we observed and interviewed. The students themselves, as we have seen, mainly use their own version, derived from their school experience, of these esoteric criteria in assessing the various possibilities of specialty practice.

Stereotypes of Specialties

Students exhibit considerable consensus on the characteristics of various specialties. But these perspectives define situations which lie far in the future for all students; situations they know relatively little about. Consequently, we might expect the students to exhibit some disagreement on the characteristics of specialties. Furthermore, specific student goals for the future vary greatly and with them the evaluation of certain features of specialties as good or bad. So, while there is consensus in student perspectives on specialties, there is disagreement too. We take account both of variations in perception of specialty characteristics and variations in evaluation of those characteristics in the following analysis.

We have made use only of our interview materials, because the data from our field notes contain so few comments about any particular specialty as to make an analysis of student stereotypes unprofitable. (For what it is worth, however, the field workers agree that none of the features of these stereotypes strike them as out of line with what students said and did while being observed.) Our findings are presented in a series of diagrams, each containing a bar for each of the ten most commonly used criteria. (The criteria of having to live in a city and having enjoyed the specialty in school are left out because they occurred so seldom.) The height of each bar indicates the number of times students used the criterion. The height of the bar above the mid-line indicates the number of students who said the specialty possessed the characteristic specified in the criterion, the height below the line the number saying that trait was absent. Each segment of the bar is further divided into those who evaluated the presence or absence of the trait positively, negatively, or neutrally.

Internal medicine (Fig. 9) has, as the core characteristic of its stereotype among students, a positively evaluated intellectual breadth. Students see it as the broadest of the medical specialties, requiring great knowledge and a willingness to continue learning. Students also apply frequently the criterion of manageability, but differ on whether internal medicine possesses this characteristic or not. Those who think it is easily manageable evaluate this positively, but the largest single group of comments disapproves of the absence of this trait. The only other large group of comments concerns patient relationships, and those comments are divided between those who feel they would have a chance to know their patients well and those who feel that their patients would probably be old people with chronic disease and thus unpleasant to deal with.

Students have quite a different picture of *general surgery* (Fig. 10). First of all, they think of it as something for which you must have certain personal traits: a certain kind of personality, a pleasure in

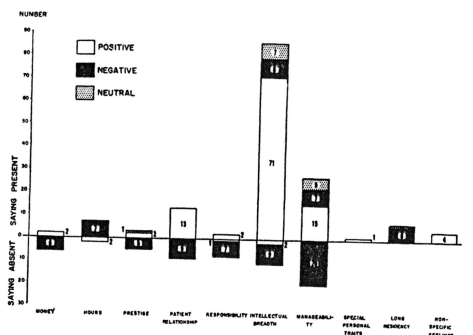

Fig. 9 — STUDENT STEREOTYPE OF INTERNAL MEDICINE.

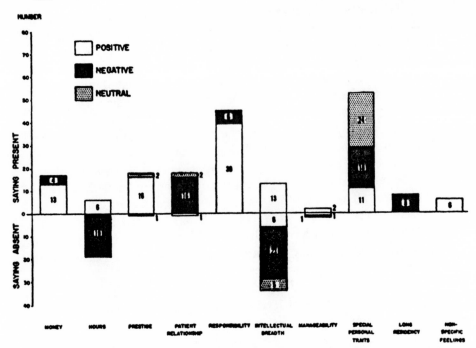

Fig. 10 — STUDENT STEREOTYPE OF GENERAL SURGERY.

working with your hands, the strength for long hours of physical work, and so on. Second, they see surgery as a specialty which is narrow, technical, and lacking in variety and intellectual breadth, though a sizable minority think it is just the other way around. Third, they see surgery, with no dissent, as a specialty which affords ample opportunity for the exercise of medical responsibility, though some think there is too much of this. Finally, they agree that it provides good income and much prestige, but that the hours are bad, with too many emergencies and night calls.

The student stereotype of *pediatrics* (Fig. 11) also emphasizes the necessity for certain personal traits, in this case without any exception the necessity for being the kind of person who likes and gets along with children. It also contains a strong suggestion that the patient relationship will be unsatisfactory because of the difficulty of communicating with children and dealing with their parents. The stereotype contains other negative features: bad hours and a lack of breadth, because the pediatrician is confined to working with children. On the other hand, the stereotype contains some good fea-

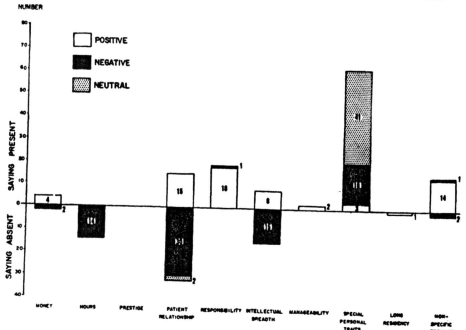

NUMBER

POSITIVE

NEGATIVE

NEUTRAL

SAYING PRESENT

SAYING ABSENT

MONEY   HOURS   PRESTIGE   PATIENT   RESPONSIBILITY   INTELLECTUAL   MANAGEABILITY   SPECIAL   LONG   NON-
                          RELATIONSHIP   BREADTH   PERSONAL RESIDENCY SPECIFIC
                                                                                     TRAITS   FEELINGS

Fig. 11 — STUDENT STEREOTYPE OF PEDIATRICS.

tures: the residency is short, and one can really help his patients, thus exercising medical responsibility.

In talking about *obstetrics and gynecology* (Fig. 12), students exhibit complete consensus on the fact that the hours are bad and the work hard. They have in mind, of course, the numerous night calls and lengthy deliveries which can take up so much of an obstetrician's time. In addition, they think OB likely to be boring, because of the lack of variety in the problems dealt with. On the positive side, they think one gets close to his patients, that patients are grateful and co-operative, that there is plenty of drama and responsibility, and that there are a variety of nonspecific gratifications: it is "appealing," "rewarding," "gratifying," and the like.

Three negative features dominate the stereotype of *dermatology* (Fig. 13). First of all, it is seen as tremendously limited, routine, and dull, using very little of the material they have learned in school. Second, there is little opportunity to exercise medical responsibility because the diseases one treats are thought of as essentially not serious. As many students put it to us, with a similarity of phrasing that argues convincingly that this is indeed a collectively held stereotype,

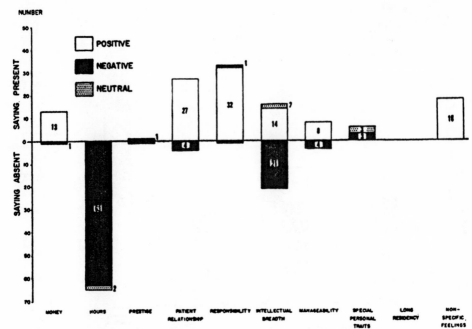

Fig. 12 — STEREOTYPE OF OBSTETRICS AND GYNECOLOGY.

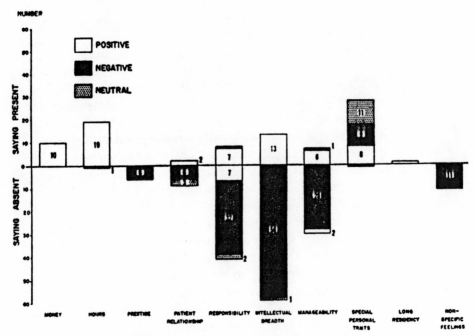

Fig. 13 — STUDENT STEREOTYPE OF DERMATOLOGY.

"You can't kill them and you can't cure them." That is, since the patient is in no danger, no lifesaving miracles can be performed. The third negative feature is the fact that very little is known about how to diagnose and treat skin diseases. On the positive side, students see only the convenient working hours (which are a function of the lack of serious disease, because of which there are no emergencies or night calls) and the good income.

Neurology (Fig. 14) possesses a stereotype that is also dominated by three characteristics. First, students think it an intellectually challenging area of medicine: a neurologist must really "know his stuff," the field is fascinating, interesting, and exacting, a field that will call on all one's mental abilities. Second, it is manageable: if one really knows the material, he will be able to make precise diagnoses. Third, however, neurology suffers from a lack of opportunity to exercise medical responsibility. Students think this because they think it impossible to intervene successfully in most neurological diseases; there are too many cases where cure is impossible and the doctor makes a brilliant diagnosis, only to have his patient die anyway.

Finally, *neurosurgery* (Fig. 15) is seen by some as possessing a

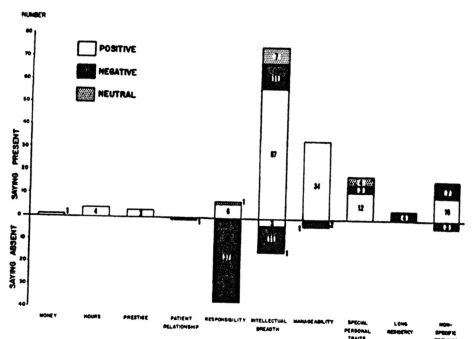

Fig. 14 — STUDENT STEREOTYPE OF NEUROLOGY.

great deal of medical responsibility because brain surgery is so difficult and the chances great of making a fatal mistake. On the other
hand, some students think there is little responsibility involved because so many patients are in such hopeless condition that the surgeon can do nothing to help them. Somewhat surprisingly, in view of
the narrow range of the specialty, students think it interesting and
challenging, remarking on the detective-like character of the diagnostic processes used. The other major feature of the student stereotype is its emphasis on the necessity for certain personal qualities if
one wants to be a neurosurgeon: an interest in science, high mental
capacity, and so on.

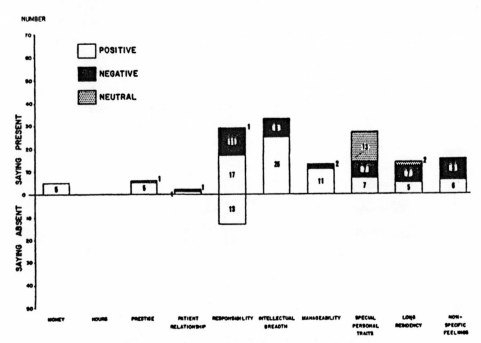

Fig. 15 — STUDENT STEREOTYPE OF NEUROSURGERY.

Students' stereotypes of specialties differ in important ways from
the realities of various kinds of specialty practice as practicing specialists see them. The differences arise because the students' school
experience, taking place as it does in a heavily specialized training
and research center, gives them an unrepresentative sampling of the
kinds of cases various specialties actually get and because their posi-

tion as students makes them see those cases from a quite different perspective than that of the practitioner.

The medical center, like all medical training centers, receives a biased selection of patients. Doctors in the area send there for treatment their most difficult cases, those requiring the care of men intensively specialized. The medical school faculty member sees a higher proportion of difficult cases and probably a higher proportion of hopeless cases than the average member of his specialty; similarly, he sees a lower proportion of the routine, easily diagnosed, and easily handled cases than the average member of his specialty. But students are likely to be unaware of this and to judge the specialty on the basis of what they see while they are on a particular specialty service.

Thus we have seen that students think that neurologists have little opportunity to exercise medical responsibility because so many of their cases are hopeless ones in which the physician may be able to make a penetrating diagnosis but be unable to do anything for his patient. Cases like this bulk large in the practices of the neurologists on the faculty because these are the kind of cases other doctors are most likely to send in. But the neurologists at the medical school tell us that in fact half of the patients of the average neurologist are epileptics, who can be helped markedly; students, however, do not see this side of neurology.

Even when the faculty sees the same kinds of cases as does the average member of their specialty, students are likely to get a distorted view of what the practice of that specialty is really like. This is so because students' duties and responsibilities make them see cases differently from their superiors on the faculty. For instance, students are likely to overestimate the number of hours an obstetrician puts in on a case. They appear to think that an obstetrician in ordinary practice spends as much time with a woman in labor as students do while they are serving on the obstetrical service. But they forget that the necessity of spending the time they do with women in labor is dictated by the educational philosophy of the faculty rather than by medical necessity and that, this being the case, the practicing obstetrician does not spend any more time with a patient than medical necessity requires.

In short, our analysis of student stereotypes of medical specialties lends weight to the general proposition that students view not only their school activities but also those activities and choices which still lie ahead of them in their professional careers from perspectives appropriate to their position as students in the organization of the medical school.

The Possibility of Stable
Specialty Choices

We noted earlier that we had the impression that, though most student choices of specialties were essentially playful, a few students had made firmer choices that probably would not change. Clearly, we have no way of knowing whether this impression was correct or not. But, for what they are worth, we present our speculations on the point.

One group of students who seem to have made a stable choice still baffles us, in the sense that we cannot understand why their choices should be any firmer than those of their more changeable fellows. We distinguish these men by the fact that they announced a specialty choice when we first met them during the field work and did not vary from that choice over a period of many months. We became convinced that their choices would not change when they applied for specialized internships which would commit them to practice of a particular specialty. One would-be surgeon, for instance, took a surgical internship after insisting to us for several months that his sole desire was to be a surgeon; we believed him.

While we do not know what accounts for such steadfastness, it is our impression that the man who makes an early choice and sticks by it in this fashion is most likely to be found in one of two specialties: psychiatry or surgery.[2] It may be that this kind of commitment can only be made to a specialty whose character is well-known to laymen. That is, choices of this kind are probably made before one enters medical school; in fact, one goes to medical school not to become a physician but to become a surgeon or psychiatrist. This fanatic interest in one specialty makes the student "different" from his fellows, and this difference isolates him somewhat from the currents of fashion that sweep through the groups of working associates he belongs to. Thus, he is able to maintain the special interest.

[2] Another study shows that, of all specialties, surgery and psychiatry are most likely to be chosen prior to entering medical school. See "Patterns of Influence: Medical School Faculty Members and the Values and Specialty Interests of Medical Students," by Robert E. Coker, Norman Miller, Kurt W. Back, Lloyd H. Strickland, and Thomas G. Donnelly (unpublished paper presented at the meetings of the Association of American Medical Colleges, Chicago, November, 1959).

A second group of students who seem to have made a stable choice of a specialty give us a somewhat firmer basis for speculation. Although we observed only three cases of this type in any detail, we suspect that the pattern occurs more commonly. We describe the pattern in its ideal form. The process begins with a student of upper middle-class background who, although he has decided that he will not be a general practitioner, has no particular preference among the specialties. As he becomes aware of the character of the various medical specialties, some one among them catches his interest. Since he has decided that he will specialize, he does not feel the urgency of preparing himself equally for all the contingencies of medical practice felt by the man who looks forward to a career as a general practitioner. He allows himself to be captured by this interest and exhibits it to fellow students and the faculty. The faculty are always on the lookout, we may assume, for students who exhibit such specialized intellectual curiosity, particularly if the special interest meshes with some interest of the faculty member.

In any case, it seems likely that a student who exhibits this kind of interest will understandably be given special treatment by the faculty. In second-year pathology, for instance, a man who proclaims a special interest in neurology may be given a brain to autopsy as a reward. In other specialties as well, the student who is interested will get more specialized faculty attention and instruction. In the clinical years, when students place so much stress on being allowed to "do things," i.e., to perform medical procedures, the student who exhibits a specialized interest may well be given greater privileges in this important area.

A vicious circle, whose consequence is an ever-increasing commitment[3] by the student to the specialty, goes into operation. As a result of his special interest he gets more instruction and becomes more proficient in the particular specialty. Further, he is rewarded with special opportunities to "do things" not available to other students: he may be allowed, for example, to attempt complicated deliveries other students are not allowed to try in obstetrics. These developments increase his interest in the specialty and make him more at-

[3] A model of processes of commitment to occupational identities is presented in Howard S. Becker, "The Implications of Research on Occupational Careers for a Model of Household Decision Making," in *Consumer Behavior, IV. Household Decision Making*, Nelson Foote (ed.), (New York: New York University Press, 1961), pp. 239–54, and "An Analytical Model for Studies of the Recruitment of Scientific Manpower," in *Scientific Manpower 1958* (National Science Foundation, 1959), 75–79.

tractive than ever to the faculty, who then give him even more instruction and privileges.

At the same time, the student becomes known to other students as a man particularly interested in this specialty, and they begin to treat him as an expert on the subject. Discussions of neurological problems are referred to the student "neurologist" for settlement, and so on.

In all of these ways, the student finds it easier, more interesting, and more rewarding to continue his interest in the particular specialty. He thus becomes quite specialized in his own knowledge and skills, and it seems natural and sensible to him, when the time comes, to apply for a residency in the specialty of his interest, a residency the faculty will work hard to make sure is a "good" one.

Let us remind the reader that much of this is hypothetical. We have observed students in some stages of this process, but have made no intensive study of it. The above speculations might best be regarded as tentative hypotheses to be checked out and refined in future research.

Chapter 21   The Development of the Medical Student

W$_E$ began our study with a concern about what happens to medical students as they move through medical school. This concern receded as we became more and more preoccupied with what went on in the school itself and, particularly, with the problem of the level and direction of academic effort of medical students. Nevertheless, there are some things we can say about how medical students change and develop as they go through school.

There are two views commonly held concerning what happens to students as a result of their schooling. One is that they are socialized into a professional role. Mary Jean Huntington [1] has shown that medical students are more likely, with each succeeding year in school, to say that they thought of themselves as a doctor rather than as a student on the occasion of their last contact with a patient. She interprets this to mean that medical students gradually develop a professional self-image in the course of their medical training. Similarly, Renée Fox [2] has analyzed the development of the medical student as a process of learning and assimilating the traits the student will need in order properly to play the role of physician once he has left school. For instance, she argues that students get a thorough training in dealing with the many areas of uncertainty they will have to face as physicians and that medical schools, whether purposely or not, are

[1] "The Development of a Professional Self-Image," in *The Student-Physician*, Robert K. Merton, George Reader, and Patricia L. Kendall (eds.), (Cambridge, Mass.: Harvard University Press, 1957), pp. 179–87.
[2] "Training for Uncertainty," *ibid.*, pp. 207–41.

organized to make sure that students get that training. Training for uncertainty is only one of the kinds of training students get in preparation for their future professional role, in Fox's view. Other areas of such training are detached concern, time allocation, and so on.

We have not found this framework useful in analyzing our data on the Kansas medical student. We have already seen in earlier chapters that the Kansas students do not take on a professional role while they are students, largely because the system they operate in does not allow them to do so. They are not doctors, and the recurring experiences of being denied responsibility make it perfectly clear to them that they are not. Though they may occasionally, in fantasy, play at being doctors, they never mistake their fantasies for the fact, for they know that until they have graduated and are licensed they will not be allowed to act as doctors.

We have explained earlier why we felt it not fruitful to think of the student's training as providing him with the attitudes and values necessary for professional practice. We do not feel that we know what attitudes and values will help the student adjust most easily and adequately to the professional role he is going to play, for we do not know what that role consists of. Furthermore, the argument that certain things are learned latently which will have an effect on the student's behavior in the distant future strikes us as quite speculative.

A second, and extremely common, view of the development of the medical student is one that stems from lay concern with medical practice but has been investigated by social scientists. This is the view that one of the important effects of medical school is to make the student considerably more cynical than he was when he entered.[3] Laymen and medical educators alike are inclined to accept this as obvious; indeed, attitude studies seem to support this view.[4] Our data suggest that this oversimplifies a complex process. The term *cynicism* and its antonym *idealism* are used loosely. They require more specific definition.

People ordinarily think of cynicism and idealism as general traits of persons. The cynic so conceived is a man who has no belief in the ultimate worth of what he is doing and no interest in doing good

[3] This problem has been analyzed more intensively in Howard S. Becker and Blanche Geer, "The Fate of Idealism in Medical School," *American Sociological Review*, XXIII (February, 1958), 50–56.
[4] See, for instance, Leonard D. Eron, "Effect of Medical Education on Medical Students," *Journal of Medical Education*, X (October, 1955), 559–66.

to others; the idealist, a man who thinks his work worthwhile and who want to help others. According to this view, these attitudes inform every area of a man's thought and activity. It is more likely that these are not general traits but ways of looking at people and situations. Consequently, they vary according to the person or situation one is looking at. A student may be cynical about some things but quite idealistic about others. Those studies in which students' "cynical" attitudes are measured by asking them to agree or disagree with general statements about human nature (such as: "Most people are out for what they can get") obscure this point by not taking account of the specific referents of the attitude. A person's attitude may be cynical or not, depending upon the audience to whom he is interpreting his actions. He may speak cynically to an audience of his peers but idealistically to an audience of laymen, or he may do the reverse. We should recognize that cynicism and idealism are not general attributes of the actor, but judgments made by either the actor or someone else about his activity and feelings in certain circumstances. No act or attitude is in itself cynical or idealistic. It depends upon the situation and how one looks on it. Many things may appear cynical to laymen which would appear neutral or even idealistic to medical students or practicing physicians.

Two sets of ideas characteristic of medical students seem particularly cynical to other people. As a result of their experience in school students acquire a point of view and terminology of a technical kind, which allow them to talk and think about patients and diseases in a way quite different from the layman. They look upon death and disabling disease, not with the horror and sense of tragedy the layman finds appropriate, but as problems in medical responsibility. The technical attitude which prevents the student from becoming emotionally involved in the tragedy of patients' diseases seems to the layman cruel, heartless, and cynical.

In a more sophisticated way, some observers (in this case not only laymen, but also members of the medical faculty) think students cynical because they set for themselves some standard of a reasonable and proper level of effort. When, for instance, members of the faculty complain about the "eight to five" student, they are complaining that students do not make as complete an effort as might be made. Similarly, our finding that freshmen decide it is necessary to select some of the material they are presented with for intensive study while ignoring other material will seem to some people an unjustifiably cynical approach to the study of medicine.

Where the immediate situation of the student dictates the development of a perspective of the kind we analyzed in our consideration of student culture, the layman is likely to see the development of ingrained, long-lasting cynicism. While this would be a misreading of our analysis, the problem warrants our making a more differentiated analysis, using a dimension of which cynicism and idealism are endpoints, of what happens to students as they move through medical school. We shall point out both the ways in which students become "cynical" in the layman's view and the ways in which, looked at from other vantage points, students may be said to be continuingly idealistic.

We believe that medical students enter medical school openly idealistic about the practice of medicine and the medical profession. They do not lose this idealistic long-range perspective but realistically develop a "cynical" concern with the day-to-day details of getting through medical school. As they approach the end of school they again openly exhibit an idealistic concern with problems of practice. In other words, the students simultaneously maintain an idealistic view of the broader problems of medical practice, a view which has its roots in lay culture, and a narrower view which sees the only important problems as those posed by the daily exigencies of school itself. This relation between what we might refer to as extra and intramural interests occupies our attention for the rest of this chapter. The process we describe may be easily generalized to other kinds of institutions and thus have a sociological significance beyond the case under consideration.

We have already seen that medical students enter school with broad and idealistic concerns. They are not interested in medicine as a way of getting rich; this may be because they feel so sure of doing well financially in medicine. In any case, income is not a major concern of students when they enter school. They come in with a complement of ideas about healing the sick and rendering service to mankind. They resent any hints that they may have crasser motives. They are determined to learn all the facts that the medical school will give them, in order that they may do the best possible job of caring for the patients they will later have. They work long hours and are willing to work even longer ones.

These idealistic notions have little relevance to the students' activities in medical school. The work they do in the first year appears to them far removed from anything having to do with sick patients and, besides, there is so much of it that they cannot possibly learn everything as they had expected to do. No matter how hard they work, they are told by the faculty, and believe, they will not be able to learn it all. This being the case, they must decide which of the many facts they are brought into contact with they will try to remember and make use of. For awhile, some students try to make this choice by thinking ahead to their prospective medical practices and seeing what will be most needed there. But they really know nothing of what will be needed in medical practice so that this is not a workable criterion.

What is much more pressing is their discovery that they must first of all pass the examinations set for them by the faculty; if they do not they will not practice medicine at all. Though the examinations sometimes appear unrelated to the problems of medical practice and arbitrary, they are still facts of life with which the students must deal. So the students, some quickly and others more reluctantly, take the view that the way to get through the first year of school is to find out what the faculty wants them to know and learn it. This concerns them deeply, for it seems to them a violation of the idealistic notions with which they entered their training. But they find it absolutely necessary to concentrate on learning in order to get through school and to give up their idealistic concern with learning in order to alleviate suffering. In the course of the upsets caused by the examinations of the first year, the students engage in increased communication across lines that formerly divided them, so that by the end of the year the entire class is united on the basic proposition that the important thing is to get through school.

It is this immediate concern with getting through school that appears cynical to many outside observers. Students do not worry much about the fact of death; they are not very much bothered by the fact that the cadavers they now dissect were once living human beings. A cadaver is primarily a device for acquiring certain facts they may be asked for on an examination. They have little time for concern with what kind of a person the cadaver once was. Successful students put such questions aside.

With the advent of the clinical years, students' concerns become more closely entangled with the fate of living patients. But here again, the pressures of school are so great that they take first place in the students' minds. Students become engrossed with the problem of "working" faculty and house staff for as many nuggets of clinical experience and as many opportunities to exercise medical responsibility as possible. They worry about always presenting a good front to their superiors and never making a bad impression. They organize to share their collective work more equitably and to prevent situations in which one student will make the others look bad by working too hard. Students do these things because they are so earnest about using their time in school to acquire the knowledge and experience they think they will need in practice, and because they want so much to graduate and be licensed to practice. They see many of the requirements faculty make as interfering with their pursuit of knowledge by encumbering them with "busy work"; students' dislike of doing admission laboratory work on patients, for instance, falls in this category.

Again, these concerns make students appear cynical to an outside observer. As we have seen, students are not concerned with their patients in terms that are found in lay or medical culture. Instead, they tend to view patients in terms that are adapted from student culture, terms that reflect their concern with doing well as students. For instance, a patient who dies reminds them less of medicine's tragic inability to control disease than of the autopsy they will have to attend. From the students' point of view, the autopsy is a procedure which will take a great deal of their time and from which they will get information they might acquire more quickly from the pathologist's report. At the same time, they will also have to prepare an autopsy report which may, if it is not done properly, make a bad impression on the faculty. The requirements of their immediate situation force these practical considerations on them. This attention to short-run considerations in situations containing tragic elements is the kind of student behavior that dismays laymen, although to the students it seems reasonable and necessary.

The medical student in his fourth year thus appears to the outsider as a pretty tough and cynical customer. But toward the end of that year, as he approaches graduation, he reveals that medical school has had some other effects on him. His concern with getting through school becomes inappropriate for he is now almost through school.

(Though he may still fear that he will not graduate, he really knows that this is irrational and that the chance of his not graduating is very slim.) He begins to look ahead, beyond medical school, to internship and practice. He knows that in these situations one does not worry about impressing a faculty member, but about taking care of one's patients as best one can while living the life of a physician in a community. He thinks about the many problems he will face and the many pressures he will be subjected to and wonders how he will behave when he meets the realities of medical practice. The question of how he will be able to do his best for those he serves occupies his mind and he finds no ready answers. In short, he loses his concern with the immediate situational problems of medical school and once again openly exhibits those broad concerns with service to humanity that characterized him as an entering freshman.

The medical student is now idealistic with a difference. His idealism is more informed and knowledgeable, for he has learned a lot about what to expect and fear in medical practice. He has picked up some ideas about how one can overcome some of the problems to be faced. His idealism is more specific and more professional than it was when he entered. The layman, not seeing things the way the student does, or indeed the way the doctor does, may miss the idealistic content of much of these student concerns. From the medical point of view, however, this idealism is evident.

We believe that this new idealism is simply a more informed version of the idealism with which the students entered. That idealism, however, is inappropriate to the facts of life in school, so the student becomes concerned with those things which are important while he is in school. He does not evaluate school matters in broad idealistic terms because those terms are not relevant. But when he is asked to think about the future, about things beyond school, his idealism reveals itself and when he approaches the end of school it bursts into full bloom.

Our evidence for the existence of this late-blooming idealism is necessarily indirect. We asked students no questions having immediate reference to this problem. But the character of students' perspectives on their medical futures, coupled with scanty but telling incidents from our field work and answers to certain subsidiary questions in the interview provide a solid base for the proposition that students leave school in as idealistic a mood as they entered.

One excellent indication of the continuing, though underground, existence of student idealism is found in the criteria they use to evaluate specialties. We saw in the last chapter that the most frequently used criterion is that of intellectual breadth. This came as a surprise to us, for it is not something that is often mentioned in student discussions of school and schoolwork. But when they are able to think beyond school to the future this criterion comes up more frequently than any other. It is a criterion which assigns maximum importance to knowing all there is to know, in order that one may treat his patients more effectively. The use of this idealistic criterion with reference to the future recalls strongly the freshman insistence on learning everything the school has to teach. On the other hand, such crass criteria as income and the number of hours one puts in in a specialty play a relatively unimportant part in student evaluations.

Another evidence of student idealism we have already seen is the manner in which certain students, toward the end of their undergraduate medical education, begin to think about specializing. They do this, not because they seek greener pastures in a specialty practice, but because they feel that this is the only way in which they will be able to do justice to their patients. They think of a general practice as requiring so much knowledge and so much skill that one man cannot possibly handle it adequately; therefore, they reason, the only honorable thing for them to do is to become more skilled in some one branch of medicine so that they may thereby hope to give their patients the best possible medical care. It should be remembered that in doing this students think of a general practice as one that will be quite rewarding financially, perhaps not quite so much as a specialty practice, but enough so that the extra years of training are not warranted in view of the financial sacrifice involved in taking a residency.

Underlying idealism among students can be found in the standards they say they intend to apply when they set up their own practice. For example, many students volunteered the information that they hoped never to treat a patient without first establishing a diagnosis. This is an ideal the faculty preached to them, but one which is sometimes honored more in the breach than in practice by practicing physicians. Many diagnoses are difficult to make and the average practitioner often cannot afford the time (or perhaps his patient cannot afford the expense of the necessary tests) to live up to this high standard. Yet students matter-of-factly state that they intend to operate their practices in this way, with all that this implies about reduced income (because one necessarily sees fewer patients) and increased difficulty and strain. The following conversation illustrates the kind of observation which led us to see the students' insistence on establishing a diagnosis as an idealistic attitude:

Perkins told a story about an OB man at a local hospital. He said this doctor had operated on a young girl for a fibroid tumor but had discovered, on opening her up, a five-month-old fetus. He said, "I guess she lied to him and said she wasn't pregnant and he didn't think of it because she wasn't married. But he didn't know a thing about it. He didn't even try to make a diagnosis. The thing was that he could have done a Friedman test on her and found out if she was pregnant first, but he didn't do it. After all, when you have a mass in the abdomen of a twenty-seven-year-old woman the first thing you have to rule out is pregnancy. Then you start thinking about fibroids and carcinomas and things like that. But the first thing is pregnancy. I even saw the chart. The extern who worked her up was just a junior medical student. He put right down on the chart, 'Rule out pregnancy,' and they never did a thing about it."

One of the other students suggested this might have been an honest mistake. Perkins said, "Maybe he was honest but that isn't the right way to practice medicine. After all, the big thing in medicine is to make the right diagnosis. Any clunk can carry out the treatment once you know what the trouble is."

(Senior Surgical Specialties. October, 1956.)

Closely related to this is another evidence of student idealism. We asked them how many patients they expected to see in a day when they had established their practices. This question was suggested to us by student comments on their preceptorships. Many students expressed great concern over the number of patients the G.P.s they worked with saw in a day and could not see how one could give adequate medical service when seeing that many patients. If each patient gets a complete diagnostic work-up and treatment is not attempted without a firm diagnosis, it follows that the doctor must spend more time with each patient and simply cannot see seventy or eighty or one hundred patients in a day. He must reduce his patient load considerably. Students typically expressed concern about this problem and thought much about what could be done about it. For example:

"That's another thing that worries me about general practice — this business of seeing seventy or eighty patients a day. I know a lot of those fellows do it and I don't know how they do it. That means you would spend no more than seven or eight minutes with each patient. Why, you'd hardly get to say hello and goodbye in that time. I just can't imagine how anyone carries on a practice like that. Of course, I suppose a lot of the patients you'd see that way wouldn't really have anything wrong with them and wouldn't need anything but to have their prescription refilled or dressing changed or something like that. But even so, it must be awfully hard — I don't see how they do it. I don't think I could, but I don't see how I could turn them away either, so that's one of the things that makes me kind of shy of general practice."

(Senior Surgical Specialties. September, 1956.)

Many students, when asked how many patients they expected to see in a day, arrived at their answer by figuring out how long it would take to give each patient a complete work-up and how many hours they could work efficiently in a day. Typically they hoped to be able to limit themselves to a relatively small number of patients: 60 per cent of our interviewees said they expected to see no more than twenty-five a day; another 20 per cent could not give any figure; only 20 per cent expected to see more than twenty-five per day. The heavy preponderance of students who wanted to keep small the number of patients they saw indicates that the idealistic problem of providing the best possible care for patients was a major concern.

This conclusion is strengthened by the explanations students gave when we asked them to explain the basis on which they had made their estimate of the number of patients they would see. Twenty-eight of the sixty-two students interviewed gave no reason, but twenty-one said they had chosen the number they did because one could not treat any more patients than that and still do a good job. The other explanations consisted of caveats pointing out that any number mentioned would be arbitrary, since the number of patients one saw would depend on such variables as the kind of specialty one was in, the cases one saw, and the success of one's practice. One student suggested that the number might not be up to the physician who, if he were the only doctor in a given area, would have to see everyone who came to him, no matter how many there were.

Among the possibilities that students see for dealing with this problem of the number of patients is some form of group practice. Students believe that if one associates himself with several other physicians he will be able more easily to control his own workload and thus do a better job. While it is true that some of the concern for group practice stems from a desire to avoid the rigors of solo practice, it is still true that many students see it as a way of providing better medical care.

Students' views of their future careers frequently refer, as we have seen, to the dilemma of independence versus responsibility. Should one immediately become a full-fledged independent practitioner or is it better to arrange one's practice so that one has older (and, perhaps, more experienced) colleagues who can share the heavy burden of medical responsibility? To see such a dilemma at all implies a real concern for the welfare of one's patients which must be interpreted as idealistic.

When we asked students, "What is your idea of a successful physician?" the answers again revealed the presence of long-range idealistic views. We supposed that this question would be likely to provoke materialistic answers: references to large incomes, large houses, and large cars. We erred in making this assumption, for 87 per cent of our sixty-two interviewees gave answers that could only be categorized as idealistic. They typically spoke of the successful doctor as one who really helped his patients, as a man who had worked hard and acquired all the skill and knowledge necessary to give such help. Many students, of course, also mentioned a large income or a large practice, but only 13 per cent failed to give any kind of an idealistic answer. We further find support for our contention that students never lose their idealism but simply find it irrelevant to their daily concerns in school in the fact that, looking to the future as they do in answering this question, the percentage of students giving idealistic answers does not change much from year to year. Only among the sophomores does it fall to 64 per cent; 93 per cent of the seniors, 95 per cent of the freshmen, and 93 per cent of the juniors give idealistic answers (see Table XLV).

TABLE XLV

STUDENT ANSWERS TO "WHAT IS YOUR IDEA OF A SUCCESSFUL PHYSICIAN?"

ANSWERS	FRESHMEN	SOPH-OMORES	JUNIORS	SENIORS	TOTAL
Medical idealism	18	9	14	13	54
Respected by patients and community	3	3	1	6	13
Comfortable living................	2	3	5	4	14
Personal satisfaction..............	2	2	3	4	11
Participation in the community.....	0	3	1	0	4
Large practice....................	2	2	3	3	10
Esteem of colleagues.............	1	0	1	0	2
Get along with patients...........	2	1	0	0	3

Finally, we may interpret as expressions of student idealism answers to the following question, asked in our student interviews: "Would you like to practice in a hospital or community where everything you do is reviewed by a committee of other physicians?" Of the sixty-two students questioned, thirty-five (or 56.5%) answered "Yes." Only twenty-two (or 35.5%) did not like the idea; five students (or 8%) said it made no difference, or that it might be a good idea, or that they did not know. In other words, better than half of the students gave unqualified support to this idealistic idea. Furthermore, although the reasons given for the "No" answers can be interpreted as rationalizations, and the true motive behind the answer ascribed to fear of being found out in inadequate practice or some similarly low motive, these reasons express idealism too, though in a different way. The most frequent reason given against the notion of having physicians' work reviewed was that it would frighten the doctor so that he would not take some of the chances it is necessary for a physician to take if he is to practice adequately and give his patients the best possible care.

All of these signs indicate that students maintain their idealism throughout school, even though they do not apply it to the immediate situations of school life. When they leave medical school it again comes to the fore, but it now has a more specific character, consisting of concrete ideas about how certain problems of medical practice are to be faced. Those who fear that medical students leave school too cynical should take heart from the students' interest and concern over such problems as treatment on the basis of a firm diagnosis, the number of patients one should see, and so on.

This analysis of medical students' idealism and cynicism may have a certain general relevance. Sociologists often speak of the way generalized values influence behavior through a variety of situations. There is no doubt a great deal to this contention, but our findings from the medical school indicate that this is not all of the story. To put these in more general form, we may first of all note that the proposition that values influence behavior is insufficient; it is equally true that situations influence values. When the medical students find the idealistic values they bring from their lay backgrounds irrelevant and not applicable in the medical school situation, they use others which have more immediate bearing while maintaining their idealistic values for situations in which they will be more appropriate.

In short, people find it possible to maintain two sets of values, between which there are possible contradictions and incompatibilities, at the same time. Immediate situational pressures constrain behavior in the present and play an important part in shaping the values participants make use of. But this influence need not have any effect beyond the situation in which it operates. Values operate and influence behavior in situations in which they seem to the actors to be relevant. Where that relevance is not clear, the values are not used and others, more appropriate to the problems to be faced, are brought into play. But this does not mean that the original values are gone forever. Instead, these values may simply lie dormant, ready to be made use of as soon as an appropriate situation presents itself.

Recognizing this relation of values to situations allows us to be more specific about the relations between immediate and long-range perspectives. Long-range perspectives are diffuse and generalized and do not state specific imperatives to be followed under specific conditions. Rather, they suggest a mood in which one will approach specific situations and generalized values one will try to maximize. But the immediate situations in which action must be taken constrain behavior in specific ways and actors must come to terms with these immediate situational imperatives. The patterns of thought and action they develop in meeting these imperatives are their immediate perspectives. Long-range perspectives influence actors' behavior in immediate situations insofar as they are seen by the actors as relevant and possible to use. Where the long-range perspective appears to be irrelevant to the situation at hand or impossible to make use of under the circumstances, it will have no influence on immediate perspectives. Nevertheless, actors may continue to hold their long-range perspective, using it to think about future situations whose situational constraints they are not aware of.

The experience of medical students suggests a process which may operate in many arenas of life. It is frequently the case that people are taken out of the main stream of ordinary life to participate in a somewhat enclosed and isolated institution for a more or less specified period of time. Such participation in isolated institutions is frequently, though not always, brought about for the purpose of effecting some change in the attitude, values, and behavior of those who participate. In addition to schools of all kinds, prisons and mental hospitals immediately come to mind as examples of such institutional participation.

Medical students come to medical school in order to be changed. They willingly submit to a long ordeal in order to come out of it something different from what they went in. Even in this case, however, where the desire of participants to be changed is so high, we find that the effects of institutional participation are quite complicated. Going to medical school does have an effect on students, but this effect is not a simple one. Students do not simply become what the medical school wants them to become. Indeed, their own broad and idealistic notions about what they ought to become are pushed aside as they turn their concern to the immediate business of getting through school. To be sure, they attempt throughout to make use of the school to further these idealistic ends, but this is neither a fruitful nor a rewarding procedure. So they become "institutionalized." That is, they become engrossed in matters which are of interest only within the school and have no relevance outside it. When their participation in the school ends, they give up these concerns, realizing that they are no longer of any value.

Nevertheless, participation in the school has had some effect, for the long-range perspective that students brought with them has remained and been transformed by the school experience, being made more professional and specific. There is enough congruence between their long-range perspectives and the immediate perspectives they develop in response to the problems school sets for them to allow this kind of transformation to take place. Pedagogically speaking, the worst situation would be that in which there was such disparity between the students' long-range perspective and the immediate perspectives enforced by the situation that no such transformation could take place. In the medical school we studied the situation probably approaches the optimum, for the immediate perspectives students acquire in school have an effect of the kind the faculty desires on their long-range perspectives.

Nevertheless, it is quite possible that this effect does not last once the young physician enters practice, or that it persists only if the immediate situation of practice is one to which the values contained in the long-range perspective seem appropriate. Just as students make use of values which appear appropriate to their situation in school, the practicing physician will use those values which seem appropriate to the situation he is practicing in. A recent study of general practitioners in North Carolina [5] shows that many of them do not persist in the habit of making extensive and thorough examinations of patients they presumably acquired in school. Furthermore, after the physician has been out of his school a decade, variations in the thoroughness of the examination are not related to such variables as the school he attended or his rank in the graduating class. This suggests the validity of our view that values learned in school persist only when the immediate situation makes their use appropriate.

A recent study of a prison suggests that a similar relation between immediate and long-range perspectives can be found in such institutions as well.[6] Prisoners come in desiring to be rehabilitated and exhibiting substantial attachment to law-abiding values. But once in prison they become concerned with achieving prestige and power within the prison walls and one of the ways of doing this is to drop one's concern with rehabilitation and "going straight." This adjustment to prison folkways is temporary, however, and the nearer convicts come to completing their sentence the more likely they are to drop their interest in prison affairs and once more concern themselves with the possibility of a life within the law.

It is quite possible that such processes occur in many other settings. We think it likely, for instance, that the experience of attending an undergraduate college has precisely this character for many students.

[5] Osler Peterson, "An Analytical Study of North Carolina General Practice, 1953–54," *Journal of Medical Education*, XXXI (December, 1956, Part 2).

[6] Stanton Wheeler, "Aspects of Socialization In a Correctional Community," unpublished article.

CODA

W_E have followed our students from their first day in medical school to the time when, as graduating seniors, they must and do envision their futures in professional practice. Now, in conclusion, we draw together the several themes that have informed our analysis.

Student Culture

We have shown that the students collectively set the level and direction of their efforts to learn. There is nothing unusual about such a finding. What is significant — as we insist throughout — is that these levels and directions are not the result of some conscious cabal, but that they are the working-out in practice of the perspectives from which the students view their day-to-day problems in relation to their long-term goals. The perspectives, themselves collectively developed, are organizations of ideas and actions. The actions derive their rationale from the ideas; the ideas are sustained by success in action. The whole becomes a complex of mutual expectations.

To these perspectives, we give the name *student culture*. In so doing we follow the essence of anthropological practice; for culture is commonly defined as a body of ideas and practices considered to support each other and expected of each other by members of some group of people. Such a group forms a *community of fate*, for however individualistic their motives, they share goals, a body of crucial experiences, and exposure to the same perils. We do not follow that

435

accidental part of anthropological usage, which attributes the persistence of culture solely to the initiation of each generation by its predecessor, to tradition. In fact, our evidence suggests that if the perspectives — the student culture — we describe go on from generation to generation of students, it is because each class enters medical school with the same ideas and objectives and finds itself faced with the same combination of short-run and long-term problems.

A perspective, to be more precise, contains several elements: a definition of the situation in which the actors are involved, a statement of the goals they are trying to achieve, a set of ideas specifying what kinds of activities are expedient and proper, and a set of activities or practices congruent with them. The freshmen defined their situation as one in which there was more work than they could possibly do. They developed the idea that they must necessarily learn what the faculty wanted them to learn, although it sometimes seemed to them that these were not the things they themselves would have thought necessary for a medical practitioner. They developed ways of acting, studying, and working which made it possible for them to achieve this goal in the situation they had defined. Similarly, the students in the clinical years saw their situation as one in which the goal of learning what was necessary for the practice of medicine might be interfered with by the structure of the hospital and by the necessity of making a good impression on the faculty. As they came in contact with clinical medicine, they developed new goals that were more specific than those they had had before. They learned to want clinical experience and to want the opportunity of exercising medical responsibility but were often frustrated in their attempts to realize these desires by the necessary constraints imposed by the organization of the hospital. They developed ideas about how they must deal with the faculty, with patients, and with each other, and modes of activity in which these ideas are put into practice. They developed ways of co-operating among themselves to handle the work they must do, to deal with the problem of making a good impression on the faculty and of getting as much clinical experience and medical responsibility as possible. These perspectives, taken together, constitute student culture in the medical school.

Student culture consists of collective responses to problems posed for students by the environment. Theoretically, we expect students to develop such a culture when they face certain common problems in isolation from others and in close contact with one another. Under these circumstances various solutions for the problems of the environment will be tried out and those that work best will be made use of by all the students, insofar as it is possible for them to communicate their thoughts and discoveries to one another. The culture they thus evolve will have a peculiarly student flavor insofar as they are isolated enough by the circumstances of their work to prevent them from being influenced by others, such as older students, their families, and so on.

So far as the actions of students are determined by student culture, they are collective rather than individual actions. This means that they cannot be understood as the products of individual motivation for, while individual motivation plays a part in the development of the actions, the final activity is one that is carried out jointly with the other members of the student body.

Student Autonomy

The fact that the ideas and activities that make up student culture are collective has one important consequence. Because others share this point of view and engage in the same kinds of activities, giving themselves the same reasons for doing so, the ideas and activities acquire a certain legitimacy in the eyes of the students. They are seen as the "right" things to do and think in the circumstances; there is a rationale for doing as one does. The ideas one uses to order one's work seem justified by their success in practice. This public and legitimate character gives student culture a certain strength in the face of possible opposition and thus makes it possible for students to deviate from what others, particularly the faculty, might want them to do. Acting collectively with regard to the problems they share as students, students find the social support and reinforcement necessary to behaving, in some measure, autonomously.

We have already seen that students make use of this possibility for autonomous behavior in dealing with problems of the level and direction of academic effort. There are disparities of several kinds between what their superiors in the school organization, the faculty, would like to see them do and what students actually do. Students and faculty disagree in part about how hard students should work, about how much effort they should put in on their academic studies. It is more important that students and faculty disagree over the direction in which effort should be put forth. First of all, students are likely to respond to the necessity of convincing the faculty that they are doing a good job as students by directing their efforts toward that end; other things being equal, they will do the thing which makes a good impression on the faculty. Second, students will strive to learn those things and engage in those activities which they think will stand them in best stead when they get into medical practice; hence the importance of such themes as clinical experience and medical responsibility in student culture. Neither of these directions of student effort seems quite appropriate to the faculty, who would prefer students to do the best they can without reference to the effect their activities have on the faculty's picture of them and who think that the "practical" direction of student concerns is misplaced.

It may seem paradoxical that the students, subordinated as they are to the faculty of the school, have so much autonomy with respect to their academic effort. After all, the administration and faculty of a medical school have relatively more power over the students than in almost any other educational institution one can think of. Their power grows in large part out of the fact that medical students are strongly committed to a career in medicine. The student typically cannot think of any other career for himself and furthermore would regard it as a tremendous disgrace, costly in terms of self-esteem, to fail in medical school. Students want very much to be doctors. They regard their teachers as men who really know what is best for them. For all these reasons, the medical student is perhaps more likely than any other kind of student to do what his faculty wants him to do and be what his faculty wants him to be.

Nevertheless, students do have considerable autonomy, and this should not be surprising, for it attests to the truth of some general sociological propositions for which support can be found in many other organizations. Superiors in an organization control the behavior of their subordinates in part because the subordinates consent to having their behavior controlled. The effectiveness of passive resistance by some nationalistic and racial movements makes the point; power cannot be exercised by leaders in the way they are accustomed to exercise it if subordinates will not co-operate in allowing it to be exercised that way. Similarly, students of prisons have often noted that in a certain sense it is the prisoners who really run the prison; the warden and his guards can run it in the way they would like only if the prisoners co-operate with them and assist in running it that way.

This is not to say, of course, that being a medical student is anything like being a member of an oppressed minority or a prisoner in jail. But the comparison is instructive because it leads us to see that, whatever power lies in the hands of organizational superiors, that power is effective only to the degree that subordinates co-operate with their superiors. The amount of autonomy subordinates have will vary from situation to situation and organization to organization. Similarly, the areas in which autonomy is exercised by subordinates will vary. Medical students have very little autonomy in many areas of their activity; but with respect to the setting of levels and directions of academic efforts they have a great deal.

Medical·education is now in a state of ferment. Medical educators are trying in many ways to improve the quality of the education they give their students. Our analysis suggests that reforms in medical education will be most effective when they take into account the collective character of student behavior and recognize the fact that students, as a subordinate echelon in the medical school, have a certain degree of autonomy with respect to these issues.

Pragmatic Idealism

What use do students make of their autonomy? What is the content of the perspectives that make up the culture they fashion for themselves? Do they become tough and cynical, as popular folklore would have us believe, or do they retain the idealistic outlook typical of students before they enter medical school?

We have already indicated our main conclusions with respect to this problem: students retain an idealistic view of medicine even though they reorient it in the direction of greater realism and adaptation to the immediate situation and to the medical practice they envision for themselves. The perspectives they develop while they are in school and those with which they leave school for internship and medical practice may be characterized as being pragmatically idealistic. That is, students continue to be idealistic but not in the vague and nonspecific way that characterized them as freshmen. Rather, they have come face to face with the realities of medical school and have gained, in addition, a much clearer picture of the realities of medical practice, though they by no means know all there is to know about this as yet. They transform their naïve idealism into a specific set of perspectives designed to deal with the specific problems they encounter and expect to encounter.

Freshmen medical students find their idealistic long-range perspective an insufficient guide to medical school. The first year offers them little opportunity to participate in the medical drama of fighting disease and saving lives. Instead, they must learn a great many scientific facts and theories, whose relevance to medical practice is not always clear to them. When they discover that this is the situation, they put their long-range perspective aside and develop more pragmatic and specific perspectives which enable them to deal with the problems posed by the first year of medical school. Their idealism is irrelevant to the problems they must now deal with but, though they put it aside, they do not lose it. Indeed, they put it aside because they think that it is necessary to finish school before they can put their idealistic notions into practice, and they realize that they will not finish school without some more specific guide as to what to do while they are there. When students reach the clinical years, they find themselves in a situation in which once more it might be possible for them to activate their idealistic goals. They now deal with patients whose diseases can be cured or not by the intervention of medically trained people. But students find that, though medical activity is going on all around them, they are prevented from playing any but the most subordinate roles in this activity because they are novices. So they devote their attention and their energy to getting as much as they can of the training and experience necessary for one who is to be allowed to play a full part in this activity. Once again their idealistic long-range perspective must be pragmatically subordinated to a perspective tied to the immediate situation; in this case, a perspective that helps them solve the problems of getting the training and experience they want and at the same time satisfying the faculty that they are doing a good job in dealing with the problem of what, out of all the material they are presented with, to study and when.

But this experience in the clinical years does not extinguish student idealism any more than did the experience of the freshman year. It remains present throughout, though there is seldom an occasion when it can be brought into practice. But something important happens to student idealism in the clinical years: it is transformed and made more specific and meaningful for the situation of medical practice. Students learn ways of specifying an idealistic act and the kind of detail necessary to make idealism relevant to real-life situations. They develop such specifically idealistic notions as never treating a patient without establishing a diagnosis. They recognize that one of the barriers to good medical practice may be a workload so heavy that one cannot do a good job for all one's patients, and they begin to search for ways of organizing a practice that will allow them to overcome this difficulty. Some students who had intended to take no training beyond the internship now decide that without further training they will be unable to do the best job they are capable of and revise their career plans accordingly.

One implication of our analysis of medical students' idealism is especially relevant for educators. The emotional and attitudinal responses that students make while they are in school may be specific to the school situation. Students do not necessarily carry over such attitudes beyond school. Though they may decide that it is necessary for them, while in school, to do certain things that appear not to be idealistic, they may well see these compromises as necessary only while they are in school and as having no relevance once they have graduated.

Another implication is perhaps of more interest to social scientists. The complexities of the development of student cynicism and idealism suggest that a simple analysis in terms of such traits is not sufficient for an understanding of what happens to medical students. One cannot simply say that students are idealistic or cynical. Rather, one must specify the particular things about which they are idealistic or cynical, the range of application in time and space of their idealistic or cynical attitudes, and the audiences to whom their responses appear to be idealistic or cynical. This last point is of extreme importance, for what may seem to be cynicism when viewed from the outside may in fact be idealistic when viewed from the perspective of the actor.

Situation and Conduct

The proposition that immediate situations exert a compelling influence on individual conduct has pervaded our entire book. Like most sweeping generalizations, this is a half-truth, but the element of truth in this proposition is often ignored and we want to re-emphasize its importance.

When we say that immediate situations exert a compelling influence on individual conduct, we intend to distinguish that influence from the influence of social factors which lie outside the immediate situation. Such factors include membership in other groups whose standards or social controls might affect the person's performance in the immediate situation, and the fact that the individual may hold generalized values which might constrain his behavior in the situation. While both of these phenomena do exert considerable influence over human conduct, we contend that much of human conduct is oriented to the immediate pressures and social controls originating in the situation in which the person is presently acting, and that he will organize his behavior so as to take account of and in some way adjust to them. He adapts his behavior to the situation as he sees it, ignoring possible lines of action which appear preordained to fail or unworkable, discarding those which may cause conflict — in short, choosing the action which seems reasonable and expedient.

One of the most important reasons for the influence of immediate situational constraints lies in the fact that they are so much more specific than statements of belief and value usually are. For instance, if an entering medical student says to himself, "I'm going to medical school in order to learn how to save lives," this tells him nothing about what he should do when he is faced with the problem of what portions of his course in anatomy are most important for him to remember and incorporate into his fund of information. Long-range perspectives, by their very nature, do not deal with such details. Therefore, the person has a great amount of leeway in coming to some decision as to how his long-range perspective can best be implemented in any particular situation. It is in this area of ambiguity and leeway that situational pressures and constraints operate.

The implication of this for those who desire to change people's behavior is that changes can be brought about by altering the circumstances and situations people have to contend with. In the medical school, it is likely that the most effective way of altering students' behavior with respect to levels and directions of academic effort would be so to alter the situation which students face that they would have different problems to deal with. If this were done, students would probably adapt to the changed situation and develop quite different kinds of perspectives. But the changes made in the situation would have to be such as, given the students' long-range perspectives and the collective character of their activity, would provoke the desired kinds of responses.

In one sense, this gives cheer to those who would improve human conduct and institutions. For it is surely far easier to change the situational constraints imposed on people than it is to change their values or group memberships. Yet we should not be overly sanguine. The institutional practices that create situations and their constraints are deeply rooted in organizational structure and culture. An attempt to change them attacks the vested interests and privileges of some groups in the organization and forces the innovator to run the risk of stirring up organizational trouble and "politics." Further, any change in institutional practice has many and varied ramifications, so that its consequences could not be restricted to the specific areas the innovator wants to affect.

To attempt to change human conduct by manipulating institutional practices thus requires of the innovator the courage and strength to resist conservative pressure, the wisdom to foresee the consequences of his actions, and the resiliency to meet the new problems generated by the ramified effects of his actions.

APPENDIX

AT the end of the second year of field work we interviewed a random sample of the student body, using the interview guide reproduced below. We typically asked all the questions in the order given and using approximately the same wording. We sometimes skipped questions that had already been answered in response to a prior question and often changed the wording of particular questions.

The interview guide was constructed on the basis of our participant observation material. Many of the questions are simple rephrasings of statements we heard students make during discussions with us or fellow students. We intended to use the interview data to provide more systematic material on conclusions derived from our field work. We have used it in this fashion in our analyses of student backgrounds (in chaps. 4 and 9) and in our description of student views of their professional futures (part iv). We have not used the interview data in our analysis of student perspectives to any great extent because there was a marked difference between what we observed students doing while they were in school and the way they talked about school in retrospect. We hope to present a systematic analysis of this difference at another time. Briefly, it seems that students adopted a more judicious and "mature" attitude toward their school experience during the interview than they did while acting in school situations. For instance, when asked whether students get enough chance to perform various procedures, most students said they did, even though this is a chronic source of dissatisfaction for them in the hospital.[1]

[1] For a preliminary discussion see Howard S. Becker and Blanche Geer, "Participant Observation and Interviewing: A Comparison," *Human Organization*, XVI (Fall, 1957), 28–32. For similar findings in the study of a labor union see Lois R. Dean, "Interaction, Reported and Observed: The Case of One Local Union," *Human Organization*, XVII (Fall, 1958), 36–44.

445

INTERVIEW GUIDE

1. How did you happen to choose medicine?
2. Did you ever seriously consider any other kind of work? What kind?
3. What did your mother and father think about you going into medicine?
4. What do they think about your future plans in medicine?
5. Do you have any friends, relatives, or whatever who practice medicine? What influence have they had on you?
6. Have you learned anything about what medicine is really like from talking with, hearing the talk of, or watching such people?
7. How are you financing your way through school (per cent from each source)?
8. How hard has it been?
9. How hard will it be in the future?
10. Are you married or planning to be? Date of marriage?
11. Any children?
12. Does your wife work? If so, what does she do? How much education has she had?
13. Will her training enable her to help you after you start practicing?
14. What kind of future plans would she like you to make?
15. Where were you born? When?
16. Where were you raised? How big a place is it?
17. Where else have you lived?
18. What does (or did) your father do for a living?
19. How well does he make out financially?
20. How much education did your father have?
21. How much education did your mother have?
22. What do your brothers and sisters do for a living?
23. How much education have they had?
24. What have you done since you left high school?
25. Have you ever worked in a hospital or lab or anything else medical? If yes, do you think this made any difference?
26. Where did you go to high school?
27. What kind of school was it?
28. Was there much competition for grades?
29. Where did you go to college?
30. What did you major in?
31. Much competition there?
32. Did you take any postgraduate work in another field? What field? Why? Why didn't you continue?
33. Did you ever take courses in comparative anatomy, embryology, physiology, or histology?

34. What difference did you notice between college and medical school?
35. Was this good or bad? Why?
36. How many other medical schools had you applied to? Which ones?
37. If you had applied to others, which ones would they have been?
38. Why didn't you apply to others?
39. What fraternity, if any, did you belong to in college?
40. Did you join a medical school fraternity? Which one? When?
41. Why did (or didn't) you join one?
42. What did the fraternity do to help or hinder your work in the first year?
43. What is your idea of a successful physician?
44. What kind of practice do you intend to go into? G.P. or specialty? What specialty?
45. Why? .
46 a. Do a lot of people ask you about that?
46 b. What would be the usual reason for a man going into each of these specialties? What would be a good reason not to go into each of them?

| Medicine | Pediatrics | Dermatology | Neurosurgery |
| General Surgery | OB-GYN | Neurology | |

47. What kind of a place do you intend to practice in? (Location? Size?)
48. Why?
49 a. Would you like to practice in a hospital or community where everything you do is reviewed by a committee of other physicians?
49 b. Would you rather be the only doctor in town or practice in a place where there are other physicians? Why?
50. What kind of arrangements do you intend to make for practice? (Group or solo? With older men or age mates?) Why?
51. What kind of patients do you want to have when you get into practice?
52. (Ask about other dimensions than the one they use.)
53. When you get out into practice, what kinds of medical problems do you think you will have to deal with most frequently?
54. What makes you think that?
55. How many patients do you expect to see a day?
56 a. Imagine that you are about thirty-five years' old. What will your medical day be like?
56 b. Is there any man on the staff here who is just the kind of doctor you'd like to be?
56 c. Is there any man on the staff here who practices the kind of medicine you'd like to practice?
57. What kinds of things should a G.P. do? What kinds of things shouldn't he do? (This refers to medical things.)

58. Specifically, should a G.P.:
    a. Do tonsillectomies, herniorrhaphies, appendectomies?
    b. Send any difficult case to a specialist or treat it himself?
59. Do you think your training will be good enough for you to be able to handle everything you should or will as a G.P.?
60. Do you think you will be ready to go out and practice medicine on your own after you finish school and do a year of internship?
61. What kind of a car should a doctor drive?
62. Do you think being a medical student sort of separates you from other people?
63. Do you think being a doctor will?
64. What are the most important courses you're taking this year? What makes them important?
65. Which courses are least important? Why?
66. In each of the other years you have been in school, which courses were most important? Which least? Why?
67. Have your ideas changed about the relative importance of courses you had in earlier years? Why?
68. What thing(s) about your work this year has given you the most trouble?
69. What was your biggest single problem during your first months in medical school?
70. How did it work out?
71. Why is that kind of thing a problem for beginners?
72. Was there any other time during school when you had problems of this kind?
73. Can you think of any particular things about medical school that have been traumatic? What? Why?
74. What do you do if a lecturer doesn't show up and you have an hour or two to kill?
75. When that happens, why don't you read? Work-up patients? Etc.?
76. What do you think the faculty thinks about this?
77. Do you have a system for studying?
78. Which is most important:

| Own reading | Lectures | Old exams |
| Own lab work | Former students' advice | |

79. We all know that textbooks (Morris, Anderson, Cecil) have more information than anyone can remember. How do you decide which things are most important to read up on?
80. Do you do much studying with other students in your own year? Other years?
81. Do you get much help in deciding what and how to study from other students?

82. Do you get much help from other students in deciding how much work to do and what things to concentrate on?
83. Who do you live with here?
84. Do you think, on the whole, that the grades the faculty gives are fair?
85. How do you know?
86. What basis do you think the faculty grades on?
87. If you are judged against your own capacity, how do you think the faculty knows what that is?
88. Would you prefer a system where you are given all your grades or one where you are not? Why?
89. Can you trust the faculty to let you know when you are in trouble in time, if you don't get grades?
90. What about counseling? Would you use a counselor?
91. How would you feel (what would you do) if you flunked out of medical school?
92. How would your family, your wife, feel?
93. How would you feel if you had to give the differential at C.P.C. and you gave a good discussion (the staff member in charge says so) but missed the diagnosis? [2]
94. Do you think that students get enough chance to carry out procedures such as lumbar punctures, passing gastric tubes, etc.?
95. Why does the faculty do this (either way)?
96. How important is it to get this kind of experience?
97. What procedures have you gotten to do so far?
98. Very often it's hard to get someone to check your work in the clinic. Why does this happen?
99. What kind of patients do you like to get assigned to you to work-up on the wards or in the clinic? Why?
100. What kinds of patients are there?
101. Have you taken any electives? What were they?
102. How did you get interested in that? If none taken, why?
103. Is it a field you'd like to go into?
104. Have you done any work in research while you've been in medical school?
105. Why (why not) did you go in for this?
106. How much free time should a medical student have?
107. What should he use it for?
108. If you were in a position to reorganize the curriculum, what changes, if any, would you make?

[2] Questions 93–99 were asked only of third and fourth-year students.

109. In connection with medical school, what do the following words mean to you?[3]

Responsibility	Details
Facts	Crock

110. What do you think about doing the lab work?
111. What makes the faculty think you should do it?
112. What kind of hospital do you intend to intern in?
113. Why?
114. What are the advantages and disadvantages of each kind of internship?

General hospital	University hospital
Private hospital	Armed services hospital

115. What city or cities would you like to intern in? Why?
116. Is there some particular hospital you want to go to? Why?
117. If you take a residency in some specialty, where will you do it?
118. What are the reasons for and against taking a residency?
119. If you are married or plan to be, how does this affect your plans for internship and residency training?
120. Would you ever consider going into research? Why or why not?
121. Would you like to be associated with a teaching hospital? Why or why not?
122. How do you think K.U. rates as compared with other medical schools? What are the top five or ten schools, in order? How do you know?
123. Do you think it's a good or bad thing for the medical students to have so many residents and interns around? Why?
124. Consider the case of an eighty-year-old woman with a malignant tumor. She receives radiation treatments which are painful, etc., but may give her an extra six months or a year. What do you think about that?
125. Supposing an intern or resident and a staff member disagree about a plan of treatment for a patient. The staff member overrules the intern. Outside of the fact that the staff member is his boss, why should the intern do what he says?
126. Many people think that an M.D. should know something about art, politics, social problems, etc. How important do you think this is?
Very important
Of some importance
Not important
127. Do you play much bridge around school? Pool? Do you play either well? When did you learn to play bridge?

[3] This question did not elicit meaningful replies in our first interviews, and we did not continue asking it.

128. Where have you traveled, outside of the army?
129. What kind of wife do you think a doctor should have?
130. Did you read any novels about medical schools or medicine before you entered?
131. Do you remember the titles?
132. What is your parents' religion?
133. What is your religion?
134. How active are you in religious things now? When you were in college? When you were in high school?
135. Do you think there are any particular ways in which medical school is harder for a girl? Why?
136. What do you think the girls in your class will do after they graduate?
137. If you had it all to do over and knew what you know now, would you go to medical school?
138. Suppose it is ten years from now. You and most of your classmates have finished all your training and your compulsory time in the service and are now out in the kinds of practices you will probably have for the rest of your lives. What are the different kinds of things the fellows in your class will end up doing?

Index